BIRTH ASPHYXIA AND THE BRAIN

BASIC SCIENCE AND CLINICAL IMPLICATIONS

Edited by

Steven M. Donn, M.D.
Professor of Pediatrics
Director, Division of Neonatal-Perinatal Medicine
Medical Director, Holden Neonatal Intensive Care Unit
C.S. Mott Children's Hospital
University of Michigan Health System
Ann Arbor, Michigan, U.S.A.

Sunil K. Sinha, M.D., Ph.D.
Honorary Professor, School for Health
University of Durham
Consultant Paediatrician and Neonatologist
The James Cook University Hospital
Middlesbrough, U.K.

Malcolm L. Chiswick, M.D.
Professor of Child Health and Paediatrics
University of Manchester
Consultant Paediatrician
Neonatal Medical Unit
St. Mary's Hospital for Women and Children
Manchester, U.K.

Futura Publishing Company, Inc.
Armonk, New York

Library of Congress Cataloging-in-Publication Data

Birth asphyxia and the brain : basic science and clinical implications /
edited by Steven M. Donn, Sunil K. Sinha, Malcolm L. Chiswick.
   p. ; cm.
   Includes bibliographical references and index.
   ISBN 0-87993-499-9
     1. Asphyxia neonatorum—Complications. 2. Fetal Brain—Ab-
normalities. 3. Fetal brain—Diseases. I. Donn, Steven M. II. Sinha,
Sunil K., M.D., PhD. III. Chiswick, Malcolm L.
     [DNLM: 1. Asphyxia Neonatorum—complications. 2. Brain Dis-
eases—etiology. WQ 450 B619 2001]
   RG629.B73 B55 2001
   618.3′268—dc21

                            2001040958

Published by:
Futura Publishing Company, Inc.
135 Bedford Road
Armonk, NY 10504-0418
www.futuraco.com

LC#: 2001040958
ISBN#: 0-87993-499-9

Every effort has been made to ensure that the information in this book
is as up to date and accurate as possible at the time of publication.
However, due to the constant developments in medicine, the author(s),
the editors, and the publisher cannot accept any legal or other responsibility for any errors or omissions that may occur.

Printed in the United States of America.

This book is printed on acid-free paper.

*T*he fact is, that there was considerable difficulty in inducing Oliver to take upon himself the office of respiration – a troublesome practice, but one which custom has rendered necessary to our easy existence; and for some time he lay gasping on a little flock mattress, rather unequally poised between this world and the next: the balance being decidedly in favour of the latter. Now, if during this brief period, Oliver had been surrounded by careful grandmothers, anxious aunts, experienced nurses, and doctors of profound wisdom, he would most inevitably and indubitably have been killed in no time.

Oliver Twist
Charles Dickens, 1837

Contributors

Susan Anderson, M.S.N., M.B.A. Coordinator of Patient and Staff Relations, University of Michigan Health System, Ann Arbor, Michigan, U.S.A.

Stephen Ashwal, M.D., F.A.A.P. Associate Professor of Pediatrics and Neurology, Chief, Division of Child Neurology, Loma Linda University, Loma Linda, California, U.S.A.

John D.E. Barks, M.D., F.A.A.P. Associate Professor of Pediatrics, Division of Neonatal-Perinatal Medicine, Director of Neonatal Research Programs, University of Michigan Health System, Ann Arbor, Michigan, U.S.A.

Laura Bennet, Ph.D. Senior Lecturer, Research Centre for Developmental Medicine and Biology, The University of Auckland, Auckland, New Zealand

Malcolm L. Chiswick, M.D., F.R.C.P. (Lond), F.R.C.P.C.H., D.C.H. Professor of Child Health and Paediatrics, University of Manchester, Consultant Paediatrician, Neonatal Medical Unit, St. Mary's Hospital for Women and Children, Manchester, U.K.

Michael P. Collins, M.D., M.S. Assistant Professor, Department of Epidemiology, College of Human Medicine, Michigan State University, East Lansing, Michigan; Medical Director, Grand Traverse County Health Department, Traverse City, Michigan, U.S.A.

Steven M. Donn, M.D., F.A.A.P. Professor of Pediatrics, Director, Division of Neonatal-Perinatal Medicine, Medical Director, Holden Neonatal Intensive Care Unit, C.S. Mott Children's Hospital, University of Michigan Health System, Ann Arbor, Michigan, U.S.A.

A. David Edwards, M.B.B.S., M.A., F.R.C.P., F.R.C.P.C.H. Weston Professor of Neonatal Medicine, Chairman, Division of Paediatrics, Obstetrics and Gynaecology, Imperial College of Science, Technology and Medicine, Hammersmith Hospital, London, U.K.

Donna Ferriero, M.D. Professor of Neurology and Pediatrics, Chief, Division of Child Neurology, University of California-San Francisco, San Francisco, California, U.S.A.

v

Alistair J. Gunn, M.B.Ch.B., Ph.D., F.R.A.C.P. Senior Lecturer, Department of Paediatrics, Research Centre for Developmental Medicine and Biology, Faculty of Medical and Health Sciences, The University of Auckland, Auckland, New Zealand

Mark A. Hanson, M.D. Professor of Obstetrics and Gynaecology, Centre for Fetal Origins of Adult Disease, University of Southampton, Southampton, U.K.

Akira Ishida, M.D., Ph.D. Assistant Professor of Pediatrics, Akita University School of Medicine, Hondo, Akita, Japan

Michael V. Johnston, M.D., F.A.A.P. Professor of Pediatrics and Neurology, Kennedy Krieger Institute, Johns Hopkins University School of Medicine, Baltimore, Maryland, U.S.A.

Malcolm I. Levene, M.D., F.R.C.P., F.R.C.P.C.H., F.Med.Sc. Professor of Paediatrics, University Division of Pediatrics and Child Health, Obstetrics and Gynaecology, Leeds General Infirmary, Leeds, U.K.

Huseyin Mehmet, B.Sc., Ph.D. Weston Senior Lecturer in Neurobiology, Head, Weston Laboratory, Division of Paediatrics, Obstetrics and Gynaecology, Imperial College of Science, Technology and Medicine, Hammersmith Hospital, London, U.K.

Wako Nakajima, M.D., Ph.D. Assistant Professor of Pediatrics, Akita University School of Medicine, Hondo, Akita, Japan

Nigel S. Paneth, M.D., M.P.H., F.A.A.P. Professor of Pediatrics, Chair, Department of Epidemiology, Michigan State University, East Lansing, Michigan, U.S.A.

Donald M. Peebles, M.D., M.R.C.O.G. Department of Obstetrics and Gynaecology, University College London, London, U.K.

Tonse N.K. Raju, M.D., F.A.A.P. Professor of Pediatrics, Division of Neonatology, University of Illinois College of Medicine at Chicago, Chicago, Illinois, U.S.A.

Mary Rutherford, M.D. Medical Research Council Clinical Scientist, Honorary Senior Lecturer in Paediatrics, Imperial College School of Medicine, Hammersmith Campus, London, U.K.

Ola Didrik Saugstad, M.D., Ph.D., F.R.C.P.E. Professor, Department of Paediatric Research, Rikshospitalet, University of Oslo, Oslo, Norway

Faye S. Silverstein, M.D. Professor of Pediatrics and Neurology, Director, Division of Pediatric Neurology, University of Michigan Health System, Ann Arbor, Michigan, U.S.A.

Sunil K. Sinha, M.D., Ph.D., F.R.C.P., F.R.C.P.C.H. Honorary Professor, School for Health, University of Durham, Consultant Paediatrician and Neonatologist, The James Cook University Hospital, Middlesbrough, U.K.

Marianne Thoresen, M.D., Ph.D., F.R.C.P.C.H. Department of Child Health, University of Bristol, St. Michael's Hospital, Bristol, U.K.

William Trescher, M.D. Assistant Professor of Neurology, Kennedy Krieger Institute, Johns Hopkins University School of Medicine, Baltimore, Maryland, U.S.A.

Robert C. Vannucci, M.D., F.A.A.P. Professor of Pediatrics and Neurology, Department of Pediatrics, The PennState Geisinger Health System, The Milton S. Hershey Medical Center, The Pennsylvania State University College of Medicine, Hershey, Pennsylvania, U.S.A.

Susan J. Vannucci, Ph.D. Department of Pediatrics, The PennState Geisinger Health System, The Milton S. Hershey Medical Center, The Pennsylvania State University College of Medicine, Hershey, Pennsylvania, U.S.A.

Jenny A. Westgate, M.B.Ch.B., D.M., F.R.A.N.Z.O.G. Associate Professor, Department of Obstetrics and Gynaecology, Faculty of Medical and Health Sciences, The University of Auckland, Auckland, New Zealand

Paula Whittell, L.L.B. (Hons.) Solicitor, James Chapman and Company, Manchester, U.K.

John S. Wyatt, M.B.B.S., F.R.C.P., F.R.C.P.H. Professor of Neonatal Paediatrics, Royal Free and University College Medical School, University College London, London, U.K.

Foreword

At the dawn of the third millennium, hypoxic-ischemic encephalopathy (HIE) remains the most common neurologic disease of the perinatal period at all gestational ages. The pendulum has swung from the long-held belief that nearly all "cerebral palsy" resulted from birth asphyxia—to the other extreme, that HIE is responsible for only a tiny minority of cases, as many other genetic and acquired causes of this syndrome have been recognized. We are now returning to a more central position. Despite the discovery of many cerebral dysgeneses that are primordial lesions with clinical manifestations often similar to HIE, the latter is still among the most important causes of long-term neurologic handicaps dating from the perinatal period. Not only does this etiology apply to term infants, but many neurologic complications of prematurity may also be traced back to HIE as the primary etiologic factor. Even congenital infections, such as cytomegalovirus disease, cause fetal brain injury largely through vascular lesions from viral invasion of endothelial cells more than of neurons or glia.

This book is an excellent summary statement of our contemporary knowledge of both the clinical manifestations and the pathogenesis of HIE, providing a detailed analysis and exhaustive review of each aspect. The authors of the individual chapters are the most knowledgeable authorities in their fields, representing the best from both sides of the Atlantic and beyond. They have synthesized a uniformity of medical and scientific quality, clarity of style, and thoroughness of scope that is singularly uncommon in multiauthored monographs, while not neglecting historical aspects that have guided the evolution of thinking about the process. I am impressed with the relevance to clinicians that the authors of basic neuroscience have contributed in their chapters on various biochemical and physiologic aspects of HIE, including the role of neurotransmitters and chemical neurotoxins. The role of inflammation in neonatal brain injury is another modern discussion involving cytokines and the nature of the microglial response. The extrapolation of animal models to the human situation also is handled well by several authors, making such correlates meaningful to clinicians. Controversial issues of management and even the unpleasant, but regrettably important, medico-legal aspects of perinatal HIE are discussed in detail.

As we learn more about HIE in the fetus and neonate, additional neuropathologic issues need to be addressed and explained. An example is *pontosubicular degeneration,* a lesion of late gestation, maximal at 32 to 37 weeks gestation. This entity is well known to most pediatric neuropathologists and may even be the most common cerebral lesion in this age group, but neonatologists and pediatric neurologists are less familiar with it because, presently, no definitive methods exist for clinical diagnosis of this postmortem finding. The pathogenesis, apart from a statistically strong association with fetal HIE, is poorly understood, though recent evidence shows a dramatically increased rate of apoptosis associated with activation of caspase-3. Without such fundamental data on pathogenesis, rational approaches to prevention and treatment are impossible. Equally important is communication between clinicians and pathologists and between physicians of all disciplines and basic neuroscientists. Another example is *pontocerebellar hypoplasia,* a progressive, autosomal recessive, neurodegenerative disease beginning in fetal life and continuing postnatally, one that blurs the distinction between "hypoplasia" and "atrophy" by involving structures during fetal development. Not only are the cerebellum and brainstem involved, but the cerebral cortex and many other supratentorial structures are as well. The genetic basis and pathogenesis are unknown.

Apart from exemplifying the need for more specific study and understanding of both common and uncommon lesions of the perinatal brain, the two examples cited above represent the concept of the continuing importance of postmortem examination. Economic pressures to defer autopsies are now strong and clinicians receive poor information from some pathologists with little interest in neonatal neuropathology. A shifting emphasis in medical education may deprecate the value of postmortem examination in the era of imaging and molecular biology. With modern immunocytochemical and other neuropathologic techniques, a new opportunity has emerged to understand fetal and neonatal neurologic disease at a depth not previously possible, not merely for intellectual satisfaction, but also for enhanced service to the family by providing final peace of mind and, in some cases, genetic counseling.

Throughout the various chapters, the authors have preserved the important context of normal development, ranging from classical anatomic embryology to physiologic and biochemical changes that are the foundation of the term "maturation." Endocrine and neurotransmitter functions are considered in this same context. This focus on maturation makes HIE in the fetus and newborn meaningful in a manner that distinguishes it from asphyxiating brain injury in the adult.

When first invited to write this Foreword, I felt sincerely honored.

After reading the manuscript, I knew that I was even more privileged than I had initially realized for the opportunity to contribute my enthusiastic encouragement to the readers of the text. This volume is deserving not only of publication and wide recognition by physicians in all disciplines of neonatal care, but also of being the first of multiple editions to update the fountainhead of new and exciting data anticipated over the next several years.

Harvey B. Sarnat, M.D., F.R.C.P.C.
Professor of Pediatrics (Neurology)
and Pathology (Neuropathology)
University of California-Los
Angeles School of Medicine
Cedars-Sinai Hospital
Los Angeles, California, U.S.A.

Preface

The practice of medicine is an art, based on science.
Sir William Osler

Despite a myriad of advances in the fields of obstetrics and pediatrics, birth asphyxia continues to be a leading source of both neonatal mortality and long-term neurologic disability. The incidence of hypoxic-ischemic encephalopathy has been estimated at 1 per 1,000 live births, with most affected infants born at term and normally formed. This makes it especially difficult for parents to accept. Numerous epidemiologic studies have demonstrated little change in the incidence of birth asphyxia, even with the advent of electronic fetal monitoring and the liberal use of cesarean delivery. Birth asphyxia continues to be a challenge for obstetricians, who must devise reliable methods for the prediction and early diagnosis of fetal asphyxia. The only sure treatment for the affected fetus is removal from the hostile intrauterine environment. Obstetricians are burdened with the risk of litigation if they delay intervention because of public outcry about unnecessary cesarean deliveries when the infant is normal. The challenge for pediatricians and neonatologists in the coming years will be to better understand the mechanisms of brain injury, the prediction of long-term neurologic disability, and the introduction of efficacious neuroprotective strategies.

The landmark early work of investigators such as Dawes, James, Myers, Brann, and others served to establish the basic pathophysiology of the events of birth asphyxia and hypoxic-ischemic brain injury. These investigators demonstrated how changes in brain blood flow and oxygen delivery could result in neuronal injury and death. Advances in neuroimaging during the 1980s and 1990s helped to link structural injuries to functional disabilities and contributed to an understanding of etiology. The past decade has been characterized by the emergence of cellular and molecular biology, which has examined neurologic injury at a very basic level, providing new insights into both pathophysiology and potential therapeutic interventions.

In both the United States and the United Kingdom, litigation related to birth injury has increased exponentially over the past two decades. One of the key issues in such cases is the causal link between "birth asphyxia" and long-term neurologic disability or death. Much of the expert testimony – as well as a general misunderstanding of the etiology of cerebral palsy – stems from the original work of William John Little published nearly 140 years ago. It is unfortunate that not only vast sums of money, but professional reputations have rested upon his observation of a presumed causal link.

The objective of this volume is to present a state-of-the-art review of asphyxial brain injury to the fetus and newborn. We begin with a historical overview of birth-related injury, from the work of Little through that of Freud and Osler. This is followed by an epidemiologic review of the relationship of birth injury to later neuromotor disability. The next section of the book examines mechanisms of injury from a cellular and molecular perspective. This includes a review of the biochemical neurotoxic cascade; cytokine-mediated brain injury; the role of glucose and acidosis on neuronal injury; cerebral energy depletion; apoptosis and necrosis; the role of neuronal and vascular nitric oxide; and free radical-mediated processes. The next section provides an overview of clinical birth asphyxia, and includes chapters on prenatal injury, intrapartum injury, clinical management, neuroimaging, and hypothermia as a potential intervention. The final chapter discusses the medico-legal and risk management aspects of asphyxial brain injury.

One of the problems that has caused great confusion in this arena is nomenclature. Throughout this book a variety of terms will appear, and they will be used as follows. *Asphyxia* refers to a failure of the organ of respiration, leading to hypoxia, hypercapnia, *and* acidosis. *Hypoxia* refers to a reduction in oxygen; it technically refers to alveolar hypoxia, but it is often used synonymously with *hypoxemia,* the preferred term to describe a reduction of oxygen in the blood. *Ischemia* refers to a reduction in blood flow. *Prenatal* will describe the period of time prior to labor and delivery. *Intrapartum* will describe the period of time encompassing labor and delivery. *Cerebral palsy* refers to a static encephalopathy characterized by spastic and/or athetoid motor changes, which may or may not be accompanied by epilepsy and/or mental retardation.

The contributors to this text are international experts in the field. They have spent considerable portions of their careers in the laboratory or in the neonatal intensive care unit investigating the continuing problem of birth asphyxia. We are indebted to them for taking the time to share their expertise and experience. We would also like to thank Dr. Sarnat, a true giant in the field of pediatric neurology, for writing the Foreword to the text. The efforts of our secretaries, Susan Peterson, Vicky Cowley, and Marlene O'Donnell, were greatly appreciated in the preparation of this volume. Sue deserves special recognition for assembling the entire manuscript written by contributors who spanned the globe.

Most importantly, we would like to express our sincere gratitude to Marcy Kroll, our Production Editor at Futura Publishing Company, Inc. Her attention to detail and meticulousness in the editing process has resulted in cohesiveness and consistency of style, which we greatly appreciate. This was not an easy task considering the scope of the subject and the diversity of the contributors. Her effort in this project should not go unrecognized.

Finally, the stimulus for this book was our concern that, although medical researchers were advancing our understanding of hypoxic-ischemic brain injury in the newborn, there was a need to compile some of this work and make it available for both scientists and clinicians. As we reviewed the individual chapters that were submitted for this volume, it soon became clear that there were areas of knowledge that were significantly interrelated, further confirming the need for an overview of this important material. We recognize and accept some degree of inevitable overlap between chapters and even the differing perceptions of some individual contributors addressing the same topics; such reflects the current state of knowledge of birth asphyxia. A broad, interdisciplinary understanding of the basic science of asphyxial injury sustained around the time of birth is important because it stimulates investigators to reflect on newer hypotheses that can be tested, and which will hopefully generate new strategies for prevention and treatment of this tragic condition. The opinions expressed herein are those of the individual chapter authors. They should not be misconstrued as the only acceptable standards of practice, but rather personal preferences.

Steven M. Donn, M.D.
Ann Arbor, Michigan, U.S.A.

Sunil K. Sinha, M.D., Ph.D.
Middlesbrough, U.K.

Malcolm L. Chiswick, M.D.
Manchester, U.K.

Contents

PART I

History and Epidemiology

CHAPTER 1

Cerebral Palsy and Its Causes: Historical Perspectives

Tonse N.K. Raju

Thy mother felt more than a mother's pain, yet brought forth less than a mother's hope.

Shakespeare, *Henry VI,* Part III Act V, vi, 49[1]

All truths are half-truths.

Alfred North Whitehead (1880–1956)[2]

Introduction

In 1992, the American College of Obstetricians and Gynecologists (ACOG) and the American Academy of Pediatrics (AAP) recommended that the term "perinatal asphyxia" be reserved for newborn infants with persistently low Apgar scores, severe acidosis, and manifestations of early symptoms of injury to the brain and systemic organs.[3] In addition to a scientific need, there was a practical reason for this joint statement. The advent of electronic fetal monitoring and biochemical tests in the 1970s to measure fetal acid-base status had led to an enormous increase in the spurious diagnosis of "birth asphyxia." Low Apgar scores had become a proxy for asphyxia, and doctors, parents, and lawyers frequently associated *any* degree of asphyxia as a cause of brain damage. Thus, a rigorous, if restrictive, definition was offered by the ACOG and AAP. This definition was timely, since it sought to prevent the continued misuse of the term "perinatal asphyxia" and to minimize the often erroneous association of asphyxia with cerebral palsy (CP) and mental retardation.

From a historical perspective, the timing of the ACOG/AAP definition of perinatal asphyxia could not have been more opportune. It coincided with the 150th anniversary of the first clinical description of

From Donn SM, Sinha SK, Chiswick ML (eds): *Birth Asphyxia and the Brain: Basic Science and Clinical Implications.* © 2002, Futura Publishing Co., Inc., Armonk, NY.

spastic diplegia by an orthopedic surgeon from London, William John Little (1810–1894; Figure 1A). When Little wrote a series of articles titled *Deformities of the Human Frame* in *The Lancet* during 1843–1844, they barely drew much attention or triggered debate.[4] However, his 1862 paper linking "abnormal parturition, difficult labor, prematurity, and asphyxia" with intellectual impairment and neurologic deficit in later life became sensational, heralding decades of debate and confusion concerning the causes and classification of CP.[5–10]

Did Little really conclude that *all* CP resulted from asphyxia or imply that *all* asphyxia led to CP? What were the reasons for "150 years of catastrophic misunderstanding" about the causes of CP?[10] In the annals of the history of CP, what place should be accorded to Little? Untangling answers to these difficult questions may be worthwhile for the purpose of providing a historical perspective (Tables 1 and 2).

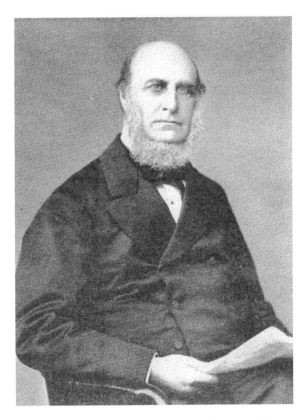

Figure 1A. William John Little (1810–1894).

INFLUENCE OF ABNORMAL PARTURITION, ETC. 293

Dr. TYLER SMITH observed that the object of the author seemed to be to show that his (Dr. Smith's) view of the cause of retroversion of the gravid uterus had been anticipated by Morgagni and others. His own paper, which had been referred to, was exclusively directed to the subject of retroversion; but it was remarkable that in the quotations given by Dr. Aveling there was not a single practical observation upon retroversion of the gravid uterus. The displacements referred to were the different forms of lateral obliquity of the pregnant organ. Only one of the authors cited spoke at all of retroflexion, and then in a purely speculative manner. His own view, as opposed to that of William Hunter, that retroversion of the gravid uterus was caused by the impregnation and development of the previously retroverted uterus, was published in 1856, and it had not yet been shown that this fact had been understood by previous writers.

ON THE INFLUENCE OF ABNORMAL PARTURITION, DIFFICULT LABOURS, PREMATURE BIRTH, AND ASPHYXIA NEONATORUM, ON THE MENTAL AND PHYSICAL CONDITION OF THE CHILD, ESPECIALLY IN RELATION TO DEFORMITIES.

By W. J. LITTLE, M.D.

SENIOR-PHYSICIAN TO THE LONDON HOSPITAL; FOUNDER OF THE ROYAL ORTHOPÆDIC HOSPITAL; VISITING-PHYSICIAN TO ASYLUM FOR IDIOTS, EARLSWOOD; ETC.

(Communicated by Dr. TYLER SMITH.)

PATHOLOGY has gradually taught that the fœtus in utero is subject to similar diseases to those which afflict the economy at later periods of existence. This is especially true if we turn to the study of the special class of abnormal conditions, which are termed deformities. We are acquainted, for example, with abundant instances of deformities arising *after* birth from disorders of the nervous system—disorders of nutrition, affecting the muscular and osseous structures, —disorders from malposition and violence. Each of these classes of deformity has its representative amongst the de-

Figure 1B. The first page of Little's famous paper published in the *Transactions of the Obstetric Society of London* in 1862.[16]

Little's Early Life

William John Little was born in London where his father owned the Red Lion Inn, the infamous locale of the notorious highwayman, Dick Turpin. Little was a sickly child; having barely survived measles,

Table 1

Milestones in the Early History of Cerebral Palsy*

Year	Name	Comments
1812–1820	Reil, and later, Cazauvielh	Reported "cerebral atrophy" in an adult who had "congenital paralysis."
1830–1831	Billard, Cruveilhier, Breschet, Lallemand, Rokitansky	Presented isolated cases of "cerebral atrophy" in children.
1820–1830	Andrey, Heine, Depeck	Described some clinical features of cerebral diplegia under the term "cerebral spastic paralysis."
1828	Joerg	Stated that " . . . too early and unripe born children may present a state of weakness and stiffness in the muscles persisting until puberty or later."
1843–1844	Little	Presented 11 lectures at the Royal Orthopaedic Hospital which were published in *The Lancet* (1843–1844).[4] In his 8th and 9th lectures, described the clinical features of spastic diplegia in children and implied, but did not elaborate, on its etiology.
1853	Little	Published a monograph based on the above lectures: *On the Nature and Treatment of Deformities of the Human Frame.* Noted an association between prematurity, prolonged labor, asphyxia, neonatal convulsions, and the use of obstetrical forceps with later spastic diplegia in children.
1861	Little	After years of study and contemplation, spoke at the Obstetric Society of London, in which he boldly proposed an association between difficult delivery, prematurity, asphyxia, and CP – later called a "learned bombshell."
1889	Osler	Published *The Cerebral Palsies of Children,* in which he used for the first time the term cerebral palsy for a specific group of nonprogressive neuromuscular disabilities in children. Also provided an excellent classification of forms of CP.
1891–1897	Freud	Published three monographs and many papers on CP. Agreed with Little about abnormal parturition and spastic diplegia, but extended the concept to include prenatal factors dating back to early pregnancy and to the period of fetal brain development. Argued that spastic diplegia was "cerebral," not "spinal." Also provided one of the most comprehensive classification systems for spastic diplegia.

*From references 17, 27–29.
CP = cerebral palsy.

Table 2

Other Milestones on Cerebral Palsy and Its Etiology

Year	Name	Comments
1885	McNutt	In two influential papers, presented autopsy findings of infants manifesting cerebral hemorrhages. Concluded that all developmental delays and mental retardation occurred from birth trauma with brain hemorrhage.
1885–1888	Gower	Described "birth palsies" and identified "first-born" children as being at risk; noted that other physicians attributed CP to teething.
1860–1880	Various authors	Reflected much uncertainty about the clinical aspects and varieties of CP; the importance of pre- and perinatal factors were debated.
1875–1885	Mitchell, Sinkler	Suggested that injury to the brain may occur from force used with forceps during labor.
1900–1924	Collier, Winthrop, Phelps, and others	Suggested "arrested brain development" as an additional cause for CP. Clarified that most infants who developed CP were intellectually normal. Improved upon the classification system.
1953	Apgar	First to standardize the "language of asphyxia." With a set of scores, she provided a means for describing an infant's condition at birth. This led to the practice of assigning an Apgar score and the erroneous designation of arbitrary scores as suggestive of global asphyxia, and consideration of any brain damage later in life to be the result of a low Apgar score at birth.
1981	Nelson, Ellenberg	Using Collaborative Perinatal Project cohort and follow-up data, showed that in the latter half of the 20th century, Apgar scores did not have a predictive value for CP; in the U.S.A., although severely asphyxiated infants were at a higher risk for poor outcomes, birth-related events accounted for only a small fraction all CP cases, and an overwhelming majority of infants with CP had normal birth histories.
1990s	Modern MRI scans	Revealed that over one-half of cases of CP may result from developmental defects of the brain, implying that "fetal distress" and poor Apgar scores may be signs, and not causes, of brain damage.
1992	ACOG/AAP	Proposed the modern definition of perinatal asphyxia.

*From references 17, 27–29.

CP = cerebral palsy; MRI = magnetic resonance imaging; ACOG = American College of Obstetricians and Gynecologists; AAP = American Academy of Pediatrics;

pertussis, and other ailments, he developed poliomyelitis at the age of 4 years. He was sent to the countryside near Dover for recuperation and schooling. Although he recovered from polio, contractures in his leg muscles led to a residual clubfoot deformity.[11–14]

It is ironic that Little, a man who devoted all of his life to treating patients with disabilities, had to endure ridicule for his own deformity. His schoolmates constantly teased him with the nickname, "canard boitu" or "lame duck."[11] After an early education in Dover, Little studied French at the celebrated Jesuit College at St. Omer. When he was 16, he decided to become a doctor and apprenticed for 2 years under a local surgeon, James Sequeira. After training for 3 more years at the London Hospital, Little obtained a licentiate from the Society of Apothecaries of London in 1831. The following year he was admitted to the Royal College of London.

Little continued his surgical training in London, Berlin, Leipzig, and Dresden. While in Berlin, he persuaded the pioneer German surgeon, Louis Stromeyer, to perform the surgical procedure "subcutaneous tenotomy," the newly introduced operation of cutting the Achilles tendon. Following this procedure, Little was completely cured of his foot deformity.

Delighted by its results, Little learned the procedure and improved it. By the age of 27, he was the foremost authority in England on the treatment of clubfoot. He established a thriving surgical practice in London and founded the Royal Orthopaedic Hospital, which received the Royal Charter in 1845. It was there that Little would see and treat patients with "deformities of the human frame."

Little's Views on Cerebral Palsy

Based on the lectures he had given at the Royal Orthopaedic Hospital during 1843–1844, Little wrote a book titled, *On the Nature and Treatment of the Deformities of the Human Frame,* in 1853.[15] This had been edited and improved from the original *Lancet* series.[4] The points of interest related to CP in this monograph are as follows:

- The nature of the illness: "A peculiar distortion which affects the new-born children which has never been elsewhere described . . . the spasmodic tetanus-like rigidity and distortion of the limbs of new-born infants."

- About its cause: "[he had] traced to asphyxia neonatorum, and mechanical injury to the foetus immediately before or during parturition . . ."

- Birth histories: " . . . The subjects were born at the seventh month, or prior to the end of the eight month of uterogestation. [Two infants were term, who . . .] owing to the difficulty and slowness of parturition, were born in a state of asphyxia, resuscitation having been obtained at the expiration of two and four hours. . . . ."

- About treatment: " . . . tenotomy has now been added to every part of the frame . . . "

In this book, Little also described spastic paralysis as characterized by higher tone in the lower than in the upper extremities. He even proposed that obstetric factors were at the root of neurologic disabilities. Interestingly, this book did not lead to much controversy, perhaps because it had been intended for orthopedic surgeons, and hence, obstetricians took little note of it.

Over the following decade, Little studied and treated many patients with orthopedic problems. Utilizing his superb observational skills, he made brilliant, but deliberately cautious deductions. He analyzed the birth histories and clinical courses of his patients. Although he had not done many autopsies, he attempted to correlate the clinical findings with the available pathologic data described by others. With this new set of concepts about the etiology of CP, Little was now ready for a receptive audience.

In 1861, he found one. He had himself invited to a meeting of the Obstetrical Society of London, and, on October 2, 1861, he delivered his lecture. The title was anything but obscure in its implications: *On the Influence of Abnormal Parturition, Difficult Labours, Premature Birth, and Asphyxia Neonatorum, on the Mental and Physical Condition of the Child, Especially in Relation to Deformities.*

Introducing the concept, Little observed that, just as the fetus may be harmed by "strange evil forces" before and after birth, it may be harmed from similar forces *during* birth. The nature and severity of such evils, he proclaimed, determined the outcome. A normal survival was possible, and death was well known. Besides, he said, there might be a third type of outcome — one of "neonatal apoplexy," congenital paralysis, and survival with long-term mental and physical deformities.

The main theme of Little's lecture was that, when assessing children with disabilities, the long-forgotten history related to their birth must be obtained. This practice had not been routine. Little then suggested that a history of prematurity, prolonged labor, difficult delivery, or the use of forceps may be found frequently in such cases. He asserted that, even when there was no obvious trauma, inadequate supply of "oxygen and materials for nutrition," or insufficient removal of "carbon and other residues" from the fetal blood through the placenta, may lead to brain "damage." He stressed that when there is a delay in initiating "pulmonary respiration" after birth, the same processes lead to brain damage.

Little's lecture and the ensuing discussion were published in the *Transactions of the Obstetric Society of London* in 1862 (Figure 1B).[16] It was a long lecture by current standards; in today's medical journals it would be approximately 33 pages in length, with the last 20 including an appendix, two figures, and full descriptions of the birth histories and clinical data from 63 cases.

Using the modern system, Accardo was able to reclassify almost all of Little's cases, which was a testimony to Little's brilliant and accurate descriptions.[11] Thirty-four of 57 patients had diplegia, 13 had hemiplegia (right, 9; left, 4), 8 had quadriplegia, and 1 in each group had double hemiplegia and choreoathetosis. Prolonged or difficult labor was seen in 33 of 57 patients (57%), and prematurity had occurred in 26 of 57 (46%).

Little's presentation was so powerful and his evidence so compelling, that the audience was stunned with disbelief. Many in the audience recounted that they had seen newborn infants with asphyxia who had recovered. Even apparently "stillborn" or "dead" infants had survived and done well. One obstetrician asserted that it was teething that caused convulsions and hemiplegia in children. Another cited the celebrated scholar, Dr. Samuel Johnson, who was "born almost dead and did not cry," and yet his name became "synonymous with intellectual grandeur." He asked Dr. Little to analyze the "nervous disorder" that Johnson suffered from — implying that it was not CP.

Little was polite in response, and agreed that many other "cerebrospinal" causes later in life also may lead to "infantile spastic and paralytic contractions." He was even conciliatory. He concluded that "for each congenital case of spasticity, there may be twenty or more from other causes incidental to later life."[16]

Little's lecture has been referred to as a historic milestone and a "learned bombshell."[9] His hosts thanked him for the "novelty" of his theory, but they were not eager to accept his seemingly far-fetched conjecture. They were certainly reluctant to embrace the notion that somehow their practice would cause such a disabling condition as CP.

Osler and Freud

It is difficult to ascertain the chronology that followed Little's historic presentation, but publications of that era indicate that interest in

CP increased enormously in the final decades of the 19th century. Two major contributions merit scrutiny.

Sir William Osler (1849–1919; Figure 2A) had always been interested in neurology, which he pursued upon moving to Philadelphia as Professor of Clinical Medicine at the University of Pennsylvania in 1884.[17,18] In 1888, Osler delivered five lectures on various aspects of neurologic diseases in children. From his experience with 151 cases of CP at the Philadelphia Infirmary for Nervous Diseases, he published *The Cerebral Palsies of Children* (Figure 2B).[19]

It is not generally appreciated that it was Osler, the great visionary and wordsmith, who first used the term *cerebral palsy* to refer to this nonprogressive neuromuscular disease in children. In his monograph, Osler reported 120 children with hemiplegia and 20 with bilateral hemiplegias. Besides his usual wit and clarity, Osler's major work also provided an excellent classification of forms of CP.

As to the etiology of CP, Osler agreed to some extent with Little, that CP "usually dates from birth." However, Osler favored the notion that trauma leading to "meningeal hemorrhage and compression of brain and spinal cord" was the major cause of CP. Osler's opinion was certainly influenced by reports from such well-known individuals as Sarah McNutt and Warton Sinkler of New York, and William Gower of England.[20–25] True to his cautious nature, Osler stressed that it was nearly impossible to be certain of the cause of CP.

The third major contribution in the 19th century to literature related to CP was that of Sigmund Freud (1856–1939; Figure 3A).[17,26–29] Before he became well known in psychiatry, Freud was deeply interested in neurology. In 1885–1886 he went to Salpêtriére in France on a fellowship and trained in clinical neurology under Jean-Martin Charcot (1825–1893). Over the next decade, Freud became a superb clinician and established a practice in Vienna. He also studied and wrote about many neurologic problems in children and adults.

Between 1891 and 1897 Freud published three monographs and several papers on spastic diplegia in children (Figure 3B).[17] Contemporary reviewers soon noted that these works were "masterly and comprehensive." Before long, Freud was considered an authority on children's paralytic conditions.

Agreeing with Little, and somewhat distancing himself from Osler, Freud asserted that asphyxia and birth trauma could lead to brain damage. However, Freud went a step further. He extended Little's explanations and noted: " . . . since the same abnormal processes of birth frequently produce no effects . . . diplegia still may be of congenital origin. [In some cases] difficult birth . . . may be merely a symp-

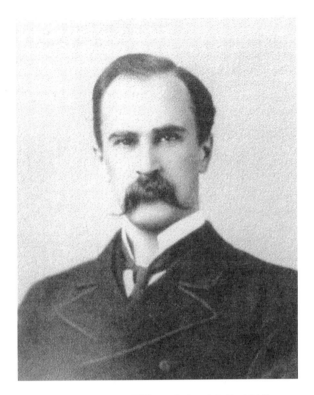

Figure 2A. Sir William Osler (1849–1919).

tom of deeper effects which influenced the development of the fetus." He proposed that "difficulties during labor and delivery, including asphyxia," might be the *result* of early developmental defects of the brain, rather than being the proximate *cause* for CP.

This was a brilliant proposition. With a single stroke of genius, Freud had dismissed the hypothesis of "spinal" pathology for CP and made it truly "cerebral" in origin. His suggestion that abnormal brain development was an important cause of CP is now becoming increasingly clear.

In spite of this, however, Freud was still aligned with Little. Freud also believed that CP *can* arise from brain damage resulting from asphyxia, difficult labor, and abnormal parturition — but he added two caveats. First, since there is not always a history of asphyxia at birth, causes beyond the intrapartum period must be investigated. Second, and most interestingly, he implied that even obvious intra-

THE

CEREBRAL PALSIES

OF

CHILDREN

A CLINICAL STUDY FROM THE INFIRMARY FOR NERVOUS DISEASES, PHILADELPHIA.

BY

SIR WILLIAM OSLER

FELLOW OF THE ROYAL COLLEGE OF PHYSICIANS, LONDON;
PROFESSOR OF CLINICAL MEDICINE IN THE UNIVERSITY OF PENNSYLVANIA; PHYSICIAN TO THE UNIVERSITY HOSPITAL, TO THE PHILADELPHIA HOSPITAL, AND TO THE INFIRMARY FOR NERVOUS DISEASES.

FIRST PUBLISHED 1889

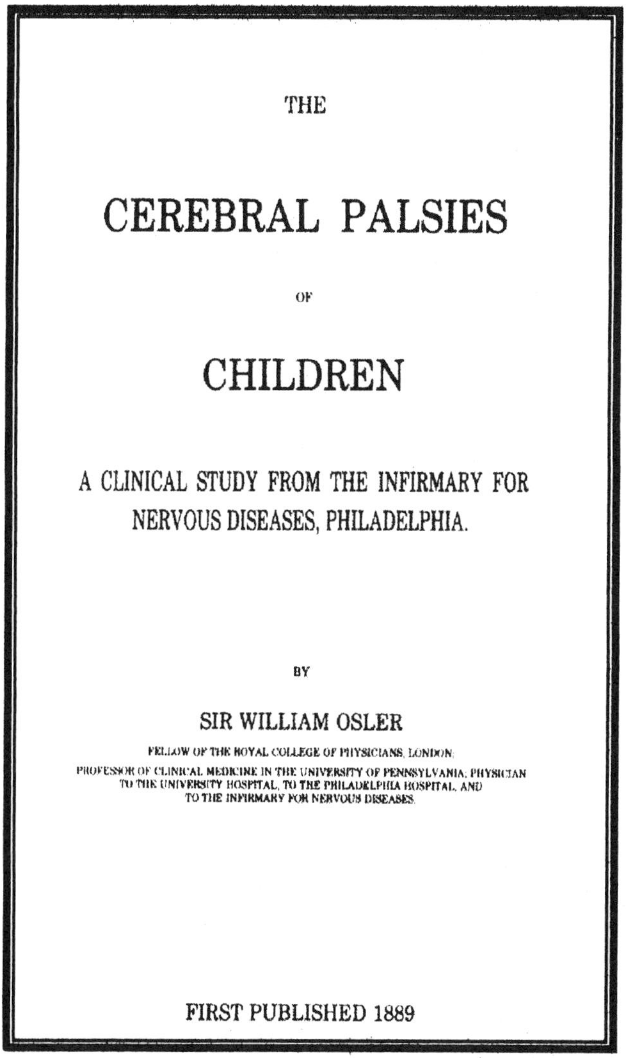

Figure 2B. Osler's monograph on cerebral palsy in children.[19]

partum asphyxia might be the *result* of developmental abnormalities of the brain. Moreover, it should be noted that Freud was one of the earliest scientists to provide a thoroughly comprehensive classification system of CP.

The Continued Misunderstanding and Confusion About Cerebral Palsy

At the dawn of the 20th century, the battle lines were drawn. There was considerable debate about the etiology and classification of CP. Even its terminology was not unanimously accepted and a plethora of terms was used to describe CP. Some of these were "Little's disease," birth palsy, spinal sclerosis, and spastic tabes in childhood.

At least two leading theories existed about the pathology of CP. The "cerebral" origin of CP regarded the pathology to be in the brain, and the "spinal" origin placed it in the medulla oblongata, brainstem, and the spinal cord. Similarly, two sets of causes were considered. One agreed with Little's proposition, that adverse perinatal events and asphyxia lead to brain damage manifested later in life; the other suggested that asphyxia was not a major cause of CP, since many asphyxiated newborns developed normally. The latter attributed other factors as causes of CP, such as familial or congenital causes, infections, and even teething.

Historians of science must set the record straight about the etiology of CP. Little was correct in most of the essentials, if not in all of the details. Even in the context of today's practice, we may see that many of Little's observations are correct. Table 3 summarizes some of Little's contributions to the subject of CP. To understand why the confusion about CP persisted for such a long time, we must also focus on the knowledge of the central nervous system and on medical practice as it existed in the second half of the 19th century.

The neuronal doctrine of cerebral function was unknown during Little's career. It was difficult for neurologists or pathologists to explain the complex clinical features of CP because of its changing symptoms and signs as the child matured.

As an orthopedic surgeon, Little did not have access to autopsy material; as such, he had to correlate the clinical findings from his patients with the autopsy reports from other patients. Since Little traced the birth histories of children who had disabilities, his research was essentially "retrospective," with the attendant investigational limitations. We do not know if Little's patients included healthy children — had he seen many healthy children who had had asphyxia at birth, perhaps he might have been more tempered about linking asphyxia with CP.

In the mid 19th century, few if any written records of prenatal and natal histories were maintained. Therefore, Little had to rely on ver-

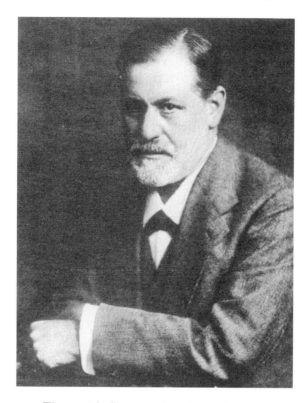

Figure 3A. Sigmund Freud (1856–1939).

bal histories from the parents of his patients, or from other caregivers of institutionalized children. Such histories may have been inadequate or incomplete. Postnatal ailments, such as jaundice, poliomyelitis, encephalitis, and meningitis occurred quite frequently, and might have further caused confusion about the causes of CP.

Today, investigators might conduct multivariate analyses and assess "relative risks" or "odds ratios" to determine a possible etiologic association. These techniques might have enabled Little to estimate the independent risks of asphyxia, prematurity, or abnormal parturition with CP. In Little's time, statistical science was virtually unknown. Beyond a descriptive presentation, few analytical methods were available. Thus, the ongong issue of "association versus causation" plagued Little.

The state-of-the art of obstetrical practice in Little's time left much to be desired. In the absence of radiographs, assessing either the pelvic

REVUE

NEUROLOGIQUE

ORGANE SPÉCIAL D'ANALYSES

DES TRAVAUX CONCERNANT LE SYSTÈME NERVEUX
ET SES MALADIES

DIRIGÉ PAR

E. BRISSAUD ET P. MARIE

PROFESSEURS AGRÉGÉS A LA FACULTÉ DE MÉDECINE DE PARIS
MÉDECINS DES HOPITAUX

Secrétaire de la Rédaction : Dr H. LAMY

PARIS

G. MASSON, ÉDITEUR

120, BOULEVARD SAINT-GERMAIN, 120

1893

Figure 3B. Freud's monograph on spastic diplegia in children. From Accardo,[26] with permission. (Continued.)

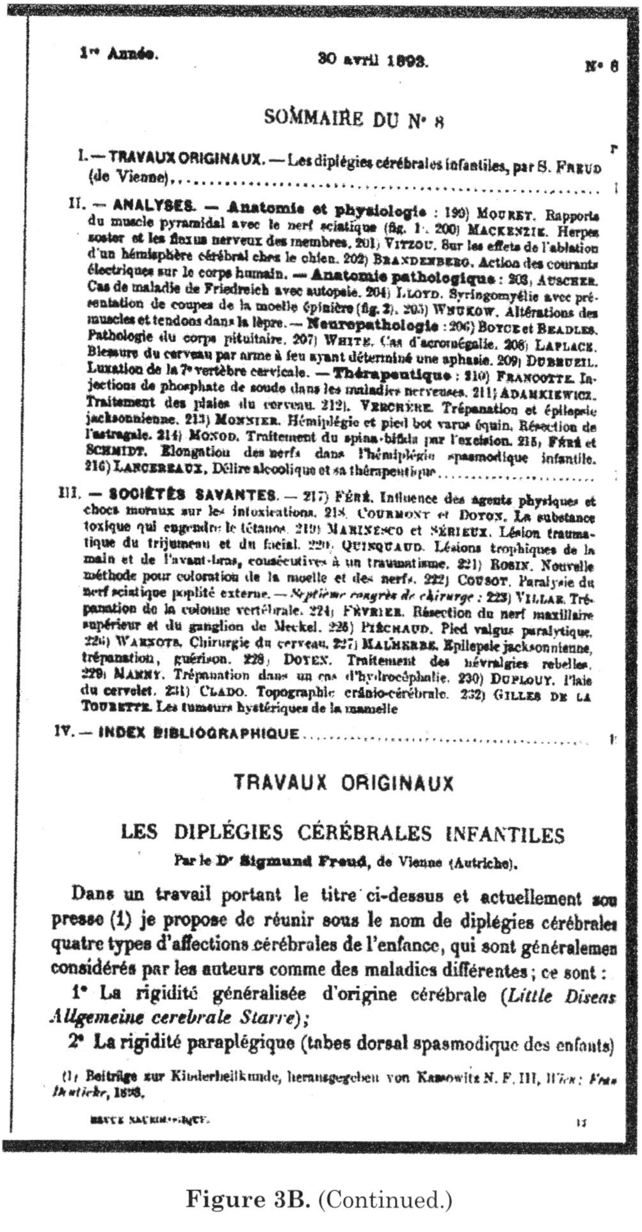

1ʳᵉ Année.　　　　30 avril 1893.　　　　N° 8

SOMMAIRE DU N° 8

TRAVAUX ORIGINAUX

LES DIPLÉGIES CÉRÉBRALES INFANTILES

Par le Dʳ **Sigmund Freud**, de Vienne (Autriche).

Dans un travail portant le titre ci-dessus et actuellement sous presse (1) je propose de réunir sous le nom de diplégies cérébrales quatre types d'affections cérébrales de l'enfance, qui sont généralemen considérés par les auteurs comme des maladies différentes ; ce sont :

1° La rigidité généralisée d'origine cérébrale (*Little Diseas Allgemeine cerebrale Starre*);

2° La rigidité paraplégique (tabes dorsal spasmodique des enfants)

(1) Beiträge zur Kinderheilkunde, herausgegeben von Kassowitz N. F. III, *Wien : Franz Deuticke*, 1893.

REVUE NEUROLOGIQUE.　　　　　　　15

Figure 3B. (Continued.)

Table 3

Contributions of Little to the Subject of Cerebral Palsy

Little Was Right

Clinical Description
- Provided an accurate description of various types of CP, particularly spastic diplegia.
- Recognized early symptoms of CP, including eating and swallowing difficulties and excessive drooling.
- Reiterated that a majority of infants with asphyxia recovered completely — an assertion that was generally ignored.
- Noted the association between microcephaly in infancy and CP.
- First to suggest that neonatal convulsions increased the risk for poor outcome.

Causes
- Provided uncontestable proof that prolonged and complicated labor, and delay in establishing "pulmonary respiration" may lead to asphyxia and to later neuromotor disability.
- Noted that a majority of infants with cerebral diplegia were premature at birth.
- Noted that brain damage may occur in the absence of external injury to the head, neck, and body.
- Argued that just as "abnormal" factors can damage the fetus, brain damage may occur in the absence of overt injury to the skull or external surface of the body.

Pathogenesis, Pathology, and Susceptibility
- Theorized that fine lesions occur in the brain substance, with one region being affected more than the other.
- Recognized that compared with adults and children, newborn infants have greater resistance to asphyxia.

Little's Minor Errors

CP and Mental Development
- Indicated that most patients with spastic paralysis were intellectually impaired.

Spinal versus Cerebral Pathology
- Because of his lack of personal experience in neuropathology, was unable to correlate clinical findings of his patients with pathology. Relied heavily upon the findings of others. Implied that the most common pathology in CP was to be found in the medulla oblongata.

Prenatal and Postnatal Causes
- Although he stated that other disorders may lead to paralytic conditions in children, he could not elaborate on any prenatal or postnatal causes (such as poliomyelitis, meningitis, or kernicterus) for spastic diplegia.

CP = cerebral palsy.

outlet or the fetal weight was at best an educated guess. Prolonged and obstructed labors were common, often leading to fetal and maternal demise. In the absence of antiseptics and antibiotics, instrument-assisted deliveries were dangerous. Obstetricians particularly feared cesarean sections, since they often led to fatal peritonitis in the mother. Thus, the use of forceps and the associated trauma were common.

Most importantly, Little attempted to convince the obstetricians that trauma during birth and asphyxia could lead to long-term neurologic deficits. However, as a guest of the Obstetric Society, he had to be cautious, for he knew that his hypotheses would implicate an entire profession. He must have anticipated a reluctant opposition; perhaps this was the reason that he gathered as much "evidence" as he could and then strongly defended his presentation.

Beyond Little's Era

After nearly150 years, it is becoming increasingly clear that CP is the "final common pathway" resulting from numerous etiologies, not the least of which may be "abnormal parturition" and perinatal asphyxia.[30–33] Furthermore, we also know that complications related to prematurity, such as intracranial hemorrhage, brain infarction, and sepsis increase the risk for CP. Advances in neuroimaging have revealed that CP may be caused by developmental defects of brain, and yet, a large proportion of CP remains idiopathic.

Thus, the contributions of Little, Osler, and Freud to the understanding of CP remain the most fundamental. As brilliant as their works are, their errors also help us understand the complex historic process of discovery. This perspective shows us the dangers of generalizing causal observations and focusing upon only narrow viewpoints. However, William Little remains a quintessential pioneer. He described CP and drew attention to a set of factors others had long forgotten — birth-related events. As such, Little opened the eyes of an entire generation of scientists. He continued to practice and publish into his 70s. Increasing deafness forced him to retire at Kent, where he died at age 84, just as he had lived — quietly, and with dignity.

Cerebral Palsy in Arts and Letters

One of the oldest pictures of a physically disabled person may be that of Raphael's *The Healing of the Lame* (Figure 4).[34] Raphael was

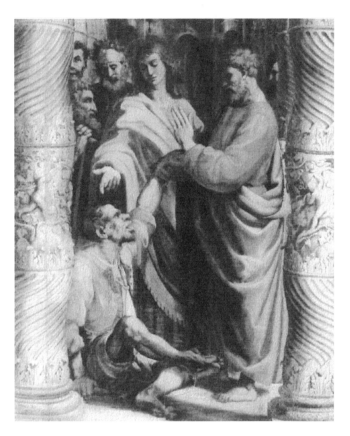

Figure 4. Detail from the picture, *The Healing of the Lame* (c1515–1516), by Raphael (Raffaello Sanzio 1483–1520).

known to use models and persons from real life for his drawings. The "lame" person in this picture appears to be exhibiting CP.

Toward the end of his discussion, Little quoted the following lines from the famous "Now is the winter of our discontent" soliloquy from Shakespeare's *Richard III*[1]:

> *Deformed, unfinish'd, sent before my times*
> *Into this breathing world scarce half made up . . .*

Sir Thomas More had stated that Richard was born prematurely with "feet forward" and neonatal teeth, which were "bad omens" explaining Richard's "deformity of frame" and "cruelty of character." Little added literary references to his otherwise heavy presentation and, at the same time, he tried to provide a historical example of CP in a man born "before his time."[16]

Ever since Little made reference to it, King Richard's deformity has been quoted by others as an example of CP. However, some historians have raised doubts about Richard's physical deformity.[35] Others have made a convincing claim that King Richard, as described by both Shakespeare and Thomas More had hemiplegia, rather than diplegia.[36]

One of most poignant musings on the burdens of difficult birth is the quotation uttered by Shakespeare's King Henry VI to the future King Richard, noted at the beginning of this chapter. If King Richard indeed had CP, this sentence — albeit rendered for a different effect in the play — implies a causal connection between "abnormal parturition" and later physical deformity. In this regard, Shakespeare seems to have predated Little by 200 years in associating "abnormal parturition" with "deformities of human frame."

Acknowledgments: The author sincerely thanks Kristine M. McCulloch, MD, for helping during the preparation of the manuscript.

References

1. Kail AC: *The Medical Mind of Shakespeare.* Williams and Wilkins, ADIS Party, Limited, Balgowlha, Australia, 1986, p 101.
2. Byrne R: *In 1911 Best Things Anybody Ever Said.* Fawcett, Columbine, NY, 1988, p 128.
3. American Academy of Pediatrics and American College of Obstetricians and Gynecologists: *Guidelines for Perinatal Care.* 3rd ed. American Academy of Pediatrics, Elk Grove Village, IL, 1992, pp 221–224.
4. Little WJ: Courses of lectures on the "Deformities of the Human Frame." Lancet 1843–44;1:5–7, 38–44, 70–74, 209–212, 230–233, 257–260, 290–293, 318–320, 346–349, 350–354.
5. MacKeith RC, Mackenzie ICK, Polani PE: The Little Club memorandum on the terminology and classification of "Cerebral Palsy." Cereb Palsy Bull 1959;2:27–35.
6. Polani PE: 1. Classification of cerebral palsy: yesterday and today. Cereb Palsy Bull 1959;2:36–39.
7. Grisoni-Coli A: Our point of view on the standardisation of terminology. Cereb Palsy Bull 1959;2:40–58.
8. Cameron HC: Spasticity and the intellect: Dr. Little versus the obstetricians. Cereb Palsy Bull 1958;1:1–5.
9. Neale AV: Was Little right? Cereb Palsy Bull 1958;1:23–25.
10. Beller FK: The cerebral palsy story: a catastrophic misunderstanding in obstetrics. Obstetr Gynecol Surv 1995;50:83.
11. Accardo P: William John Little and cerebral palsy in the nineteenth century. J Hist Med 1989;44:56–71.

12. Bishop WJ: William John Little 1810–1894: a brief biography. Cereb Palsy Bull 1958;1:34.
13. Schoenberg DG, Schoenberg BS: Eponym: William John Little and his large contribution to medicine. Southern Med J 1978;71:1296–1297.
14. Dunn PM: Dr. William Little (1810–1894) of London and cerebral palsy. Arch Dis Child 1995;72:F209–F210.
15. Little WJ: *On the Nature and Course Treatment of Deformities of the Human Frame. Being a Course of Lectures Delivered at the Royal Orthopaedic Hospital in 1843.* London, Longman, Brown, Green, and Longmans.
16. Little WJ: On the influence of abnormal parturition, difficult labours, premature births and asphyxia neonatorum on the mental and physical condition of the child, especially in relation to deformities. Trans Obstetr Soc London 1862;3:293–344.
17. Longo LD, Ashwal S: William Osler, Sigmund Freud and the evolution of ideas concering cerebral palsy. J Hist Neurosci 1993;2:255–282.
18. McHenry LC: William Osler: a Philadelphia neurologist. J Child Neurol 1993;8:416–421.
19. Osler W: *The Cerebral Palsies of Children: A Clinical Study from the Infirmary for Nervous Diseases.* P. Blakiston, Philadelphia, 1889. (Facsimile reprinted: Classics in Developmental Medicine Oxford, Blackwell Scientific. No 1. 1987.)
20. McNutt SJ: Apoplexia neonatorum. Am J Obstet 1885;1:73–81.
21. McNutt SJ: Double infantile spastic hemiplegia, with the report of a case. Am J Med Sci 1885;89:58–79.
22. Sinkler W: On the palsies of children. Am J Med Sci 1875;69:348–365.
23. Sinkler W: The different forms of paralysis met with in young children. Med News (Philadelphia) 1885;51:521–523.
24. Sinkler W: Discussion. In Parvin T: Injuries of the foetus during labor. Med News (Philadelphia) 1885;51:561–580.
25. Gower WR: Birth palsies. Lancet 1888;1:709–711.
26. Accardo P: Freud on diplegia. Am J Dis Child 1982;136:452–455.
27. Collier JS: The pathogenesis of cerebral diplegia. Brain 1928;47:1–21.
28. Cameron HC: Intracranial birth injuries. Lancet 1922;2:1292–1295.
29. Phelps WM: The etiology and diagnostic classification of cerebral palsy. Nerv Child 1950;7:10.
30. Apgar V: A proposal for a new method of evaluation of the newborn infant. Anesth Analg 1953;32:260–267.
31. Nelson KB, Ellenberg JH: Apgar scores as predictors of chronic neurological disability. Pediatrics 1981;68:36–41.
32. Bax M, Nelson KB: Birth asphyxia and the neonatal brain. What do we know and when do we know it? Clin Perinatol 1993;20:327–344.
33. Nelson KE, Grether JK: Causes of cerebral palsy. Curr Opin Pediatr 1999;11:487–491.
34. Fermor S: *The Raphael Tapestry Cartoons: Narrative Decoration and Design.* Scala Books and Victoria and Albert Museum, London, 1996, p 67.
35. Norwich JJ: King Richard III [1471–1485]. In: *Shakespeare's Kings: The Great Plays and the History of England in the Middle Ages. 1337–1485.* Scribner, NY, 1999, pp 355–388.
36. Accardo PJ: Deformity and character: Dr. Little's diagnosis of Richard III. JAMA 1980;244:2746–2747.

CHAPTER 2

The Relationship of Birth Asphyxia to Later Motor Disability

Michael P. Collins, Nigel S. Paneth

Introduction

For almost a century and a half, medicine and popular superstition have overlapped in the belief that events in the perinatal period are determinants of certain kinds of childhood disabilities (see Chapter 1). The observations, published in 1862, of William John Little,[1] a physician who specialized in childhood deformities, were very influential. In a detailed review of the birth histories of children with what he termed "spastic paresis of the newborn" (well illustrated by the [then] "new" technique of photography), Little noted striking similarities. Children with cerebral palsy (CP) were frequently born prematurely, had had difficult deliveries, and exhibited delayed spontaneous respiration.

Sigmund Freud, in his early career as a neurologist, was a recognized authority on CP. In his monograph, *Infantile Cerebral Paralysis,* the most comprehensive review of CP of its time, Freud acknowledged the association between prematurity and CP. He also argued that some preexisting condition might predispose to both disorders.[2]

It was not until the early 1950s that investigations were undertaken to establish firm epidemiologic and physiologic relationships between neurologic abnormalities of childhood and the events of labor. Lilienfeld and others, in a series of reports, used the case control method to assess the frequency of abnormalities of pregnancy and labor in children with CP and mental retardation, compared to their frequency in children free of such disorders.[3,4] In general, their results supported the notion that phenomena associated with oxygen deprivation, as opposed to those capable of causing mechanical injury, were associated with these disabilities. At about the same time, Windle began a series of landmark studies of the effects of experimental birth

From Donn SM, Sinha SK, Chiswick ML (eds): *Birth Asphyxia and the Brain: Basic Science and Clinical Implications.* © 2002, Futura Publishing Co., Inc., Armonk, NY.

asphyxia on primate neurodevelopment. Like Lilienfeld, Windle also concluded that birth asphyxia might be an important cause of neuro-developmental abnormalities.[5]

Since that time, the scientific community has devoted consider-able effort and substantial journal space to clarifying the role of birth-related asphyxia as a potential cause of neurodevelopmental disor-ders. Concepts of fetal oxygenation under conditions of normal labor, the frequency of abnormalities in the availability of respiratory gases to the fetus, and the contribution of these abnormalities to the burden of neurodevelopmental disorders have all evolved over time. This chapter will address the following: (1) biochemical and functional def-initions of asphyxia; (2) asphyxia at birth; (3) the association between birth asphyxia and CP; (4) the association between birth asphyxia and other neurodevelopmental disorders; and (5) *significant* birth asphyxia, i.e., birth asphyxia severe enough to significantly elevate the risk of CP or other neurodevelopmental disorders.

Biochemical and Functional Definitions of Asphyxia

The terms "asphyxia," "fetal distress," "hypoxia," "hypoxemia," and "hypoxia-ischemia" have often been used interchangeably, without careful consideration of the precise meanings of these terms. As is true in much of medicine, there is a need to first understand how the words are defined physiologically, and then how the terms are applied oper-ationally in the clinical setting. Operational definitions of these terms depend upon our ability to measure these factors, or correlates of them, in living newborns or fetuses.

The central defect that characterizes the clinical situations described by the terms listed above is diminished oxygen delivery to the tissues. It is intracellular hypoxia, leading to anaerobic metabo-lism, metabolic acidosis, other metabolic changes, and ultimately cell death, that is the deleterious outcome of decreased oxygen delivery. The brain is particularly sensitive to the effects of tissue hypoxia and the cascade of metabolic derangements that may follow (see Chapter 3), and dead neurons, in general, are not replaced; thus, brain damage is characteristic of severe degrees of these processes.

Tissue hypoxia can be produced either by lowered oxygen concen-trations within the blood, termed hypoxemia, and/or by limited blood flow to the tissues, termed ischemia. "Asphyxia" refers specifically to impairment in blood gas exchange resulting from either or both of these mechanisms, typically resulting in hypoxemia, hypercapnia, *and* acidosis. Prior to birth, asphyxia may result from a defect in the placental function of oxygenating fetal blood, and may result in metabolic acidosis as cells are forced to metabolize anaerobically. After birth, asphyxia in the newborn most commonly reflects a problem in the lungs' ability to oxygenate the blood and/or to remove carbon dioxide molecules, with concomitant respiratory acidosis.

In response to hypoxia, neural tissues generally experience increasing blood flow, as a redistribution of blood flow tends to preserve oxygen delivery to the brain and other "core" organs.[6–9] This mechanism is apparently protective over a wide margin of hypoxic insult. When the hypoxia is more intense and/or prolonged, however, and particularly when hypotension, either systemic or localized to the brain, adds ischemia to the existing hypoxemia and hypercapnia, this mechanism may fail and brain damage may result.[10–12] For reasons not yet entirely clear, developing white matter is commonly the site of the resulting neuropathology and most typically produces CP, as a neurodevelopmental consequence.[13,14]

The increased cerebral blood flow associated with asphyxia is apparently a direct response to both hypoxemia and hypercapnia, as either alone is capable of regulating cerebral blood flow.[15–23] Blood pH, on the other hand, apparently does not directly regulate cerebral blood flow[1]; and acidosis, though it is often monitored clinically as a marker of "fetal distress" (assumed, incorrectly, to be secondary to asphyxia), correlates poorly with neurologic sequelae.[24] Several investigators have found birth acidemia to be only weakly related to neonatal neurologic pathology,[25] or not related at all.[26–28] Longitudinal studies show a similar lack of association of birth acidemia with long-term neurodevelopmental sequelae,[29–31] and in one study acidemia even appeared slightly protective.[32] Indeed, there are mechanisms by which acidemia, within limits, may be protective against ischemic brain injury.[33–35]

Acidosis found in a newborn thought to have suffered birth asphyxia can be of either respiratory, metabolic, or mixed origin. Respiratory acidosis derives directly from the retention of carbon dioxide, while metabolic acidosis is the result of anaerobic cellular metabolism, with a buildup of lactic acid. The two are best distinguished by calculation of the base excess from blood gas results, as low values (i.e., a greater negative number, also referred to as the base deficit) of this quantity reflect higher levels of buffer base consumption, indicative of metabolic acidosis. Some studies have shown that the metabolic component of a newborn's acid-base status is more closely correlated with neonatal neurologic complications than is either the pH itself or the respiratory component of acidosis.[12,36–38]

Asphyxia is a condition of impaired gas exchange which, when significant, leads to hypoxemia, hypercapnia, and metabolic acidosis, best measured clinically by base excess levels. Low's definition of fetal asphyxia is probably the best clinical definition available: "A condition of impaired blood gas exchange leading to progressive hypoxemia and hypercapnia with a significant metabolic acidosis."[39]

Asphyxia at Birth

The definition of asphyxia at birth by base excess values has only recently been prominent in the literature; historically, papers exploring exposure to intrapartum asphyxia ("birth asphyxia") have defined this condition using other criteria. Measures of neurologic depression at birth have been commonly used, including 1- and 5-minute Apgar scores (in U.S.A. medical literature), or time to spontaneous respiration (in European studies), or necessity for resuscitation. It is now clear, however, that birth depression is not always synonymous with birth asphyxia. Factors other than asphyxia can cause birth depression, and some newborns who are asphyxiated according to blood gas criteria are not clinically depressed. A particular concern arises from the observation that infants exposed to intrauterine infections, accompanying proinflammatory cytokines, and other cellular products may appear depressed at birth. Attribution of low Apgar scores to birth asphyxia should therefore not be made without firm biochemical evidence. Furthermore, though a depressed Apgar score is a statistical risk factor for later neurodevelopmental disability (best shown in the data from the National Institutes of Health National Collaborative Perinatal Project, summarized in Tables 1 through 3), Apgar scores are not usefully specific predictors of neurodevelopmental outcome, except when extremely and persistently low, or perhaps when accompanied by deep acidemia (presumably always with a major metabolic component).[40–43] Even with Apgar scores as low as ≤ 3 at 10 minutes of life, 80% of infants of normal birthweight are free of major disabilities by early school age (see Table 3).[44]

Another presumed measure of asphyxia has been the finding of certain patterns of the fetal heart rate demonstrated on electronic fetal monitoring (EFM). Severe late and variable decelerations and loss of beat-to-beat variability have typically been taken as signs of "fetal distress" presumed to be asphyxial. While probably sensitive to

Table 1

Distribution of 5-Minute Apgar Scores in Children With and Without Later Cerebral Palsy (%)*

	Apgar Score		
Cerebral Palsy	0–3	4–6	7–10
None	1	3	96
Present	15	12	73

*From Nelson and Ellenberg JH,[44] with permisson.

Table 2

Rates of Cerebral Palsy in Surviving Children, by 5-Minute Apgar Score and Birthweight*

	Apgar Score					
	0–3		4–6		7–10	
Birthweight (g)	N	CP rate (%)	N	CP rate (%)	N	CP rate
≤ 2500	95	6.7	346	2.5	3920	0.8
≥ 2501	337	4.7	1010	0.9	42617	0.2

*From Nelson and Ellenberg,[44] with permission.
CP = cerebral palsy.

Table 3

Rates of Cerebral Palsy in Surviving Children, by 10-Minute Apgar Score and Birthweight*

	Apgar Score					
	0–3		4–6		7–10	
Birthweight (g)	N	CP rate (%)	N	CP rate (%)	N	CP rate (%)
≤ 2500	34	3.7	168	3.6	721	1.9
≥ 2501	80	16.7	302	1.6	4291	0.4

*From Nelson and Ellenberg,[44] with permission.
CP = cerebral palsy.

asphyxial processes, this method has been fraught with high interobserver variability, extremely low specificity, and lack of rigorous and consistent definition of terms.[45] Until recently, there has been no consensus of experts about a single definition of abnormality regarding fetal heart rate patterns, and it has been difficult to construct follow-up studies designed to determine the predictive power of this technique.[46] Follow-up studies to date have found abnormal fetal heart rate patterns, as they are now used, to be weakly associated with an increased risk of neurodevelopmental disabilities, and incapable of achieving acceptable positive predictive values.[47–49] Since EFM has been associated with an increase in the rate of operative deliveries, there is considerable controversy over the risk/benefit ratio of this technique. A comprehensive review comparing EFM with intermittent auscultation showed protection only against neonatal seizures.[50] The largest studies, however, are not in agreement even on this conclusion,[51,52] and follow-up of the study in which EFM apparently protected against neonatal seizures showed no difference in rates of CP at 4 years of age.[53] Among premature infants, the prevalence of CP at 18 months of age was actually higher in a group randomized to EFM compared with those monitored by periodic auscultation.[54] Though advocates of EFM continue to insist that only lack of broad expertise prevents EFM from achieving better validity,[55] the limitations of this method in clinical practice have become clear[51] and its routine use has been questioned.[56]

As recently as a decade ago, many clinicians assumed the concept of a "continuum of casualty" to be true – that any degree of true asphyxia (i.e., tissue hypoxia) was bad, and that all infants exposed to asphyxia would suffer some impairment, roughly in proportion to the degree of the asphyxia.[57] More recently, this has been supplanted by a recognition that only severe degrees of asphyxia lead to recognizable long-term morbidity,[58–60] and that such profound asphyxia is likely to be close to the threshold beyond which survival is unlikely.[61,62] The clinical hallmark of severe asphyxia is the appearance in the immediate neonatal period of a set of neurologic signs termed newborn or neonatal encephalopathy, or hypoxic-ischemic encephalopathy (see below).

Newborn encephalopathy is a syndrome that includes a range of neurologic signs appearing within hours or days of birth, classified by Sarnat and Sarnat[63] into three clinical stages, later amplified by Fenichel.[64] Mild newborn encephalopathy includes hyperalertness, hyperreflexia, dilated pupils, and tachycardia, without seizures. Moderate newborn encephalopathy is characterized by lethargy, hyperreflexia, miosis, bradycardia, seizures, hypotonia, and weak Moro and suck responses. Severe newborn encephalopathy includes stupor, flaccidity, poorly reactive pupils, decreased stretch reflexes, hypothermia, and absent Moro and suck responses. The appearance of such a syndrome, and its severity, are predictive of neurodevelopmental outcome in a "dose-response" fashion.[65–70] Asphyxia is apparently not the only potential cause of such encephalopathy,[71] and the point has been well made that it can be misleading to refer to this syndrome as "hypoxic-ischemic encephalopathy."[72,73]

The syndrome is frequently, if not universally, associated with asphyxia. However, several new techniques have demonstrated its correlation with disturbances in oxidative metabolism. The incentive for investigation has largely been the potential for therapies designed to interrupt the progression from mild to severe encephalopathy. Most studies have used methods restricted to research centers, and the number of patients has generally been small. However, as a whole, the studies yield the impression that infants termed "asphyxiated" by the neurologic observations described above are more likely than control infants to show evidence of brain damage. Disturbances measured by these techniques are also correlated with the risk of progression to newborn encephalopathy, and to death or neurodevelopmental impairment.[74]

Proton magnetic resonance spectroscopy (MRS) assesses correlates of oxidative metabolism in the form of cerebral phosphocreatine[75,76] or lactate.[77] Alteration in oxidative metabolism is apparently strongly predictive of survival or disability, though follow-up data are few to date (Table 4). In infants exhibiting metabolic derangement by such measures, elevated cerebral lactate levels apparently persist beyond 1 month of life.[78] Alteration in oxidative metabolism has also been shown through diminished cyclic adenosine monophosphate (cAMP) levels in

Table 4

Overall Neurodevelopmental Status by Phosphocreatine: Inorganic Phosphorus Ratio z Score at 4 Years of Age in Survivors of Birth Asphyxia*

PCr/Pi z Score[†]	No. of Infants Followed	No. with Neurodevelopmental Disability
≥ −1.99	28	5
−2.00 to −3.99	7	5
≤ −4.00	6	5

*From Roth et al,[76] with permission.
[†]Based on normal controls.
PCr = phosphocreatine; Pi = inorganic phosphorus.

cerebrospinal fluid.[79] An elevation in pro-inflammatory cytokines[80] and a decrease in cerebrospinal nerve growth factor[81] within the cerebrospinal fluid of asphyxiated infants have also been reported. The cytokine elevation may implicate infection in some cases of newborn encephalopathy. Elevation of the lactate/creatinine ratio assayed by proton MRS on random urine samples taken within 6 hours of birth appears to discriminate between infants who will develop encephalopathy, and infants with encephalopathy who will have adverse outcomes at 1 year (Table 5).[82] A report of similar findings, based on umbilical cord blood lactate and lactate/pyruvate ratios measured electrochemically,[83] and another in which urinary uric acid/creatinine ratios were calculated,[84] offer the potential of measures of oxidative metabolism that are based on more generally available laboratory tests. Although the emphasis is on the ability to predict encephalopathy among potentially asphyxiated newborns, most of these studies include small control groups. Benign findings in these control groups often support the designation of "asphyxiated" infants (i.e., by Apgar scores or severe fetal heart rate abnormalities) as being at elevated risk for disturbances in oxidative metabolism. An additional caveat, however, is that all of these studies are based on small and highly selected samples of patients seen at tertiary care centers with short-term follow-up. A new generation of studies that extends these findings to larger and more representative samples of infants is necessary before we can be reasonably sure that we have accurate biochemical predictors of long-term neurodevelopmental outcome in encephalopathic or "asphyxiated" newborns.

During the past decade, the American College of Obstetricians and Gynecologists (ACOG) has expressed a justifiable concern regarding the imprecise usage of the diagnostic term "birth asphyxia." Respond-

Table 5

Urinary Lactate/Creatinine Ratios in 58 Normal Infants and 40 Infants Exposed to Asphyxia (means ± SD)*

Sample Time	Normal Infants (N=58)	Asphyxia without NE (N=24)	Asphyxia with NE (N=16)	P†
< 6 hr	0.09 ± 0.02	0.19 ± 0.12	16.75 ± 27.38	< 0.001
48–72 hr	0.09 ± 0.03	0.16 ± 0.17	0.92 ± 1.77	0.008

*From Huang et al.[82]
†Refers to the comparison between asphyxiated infants with and without encephalopathy.
NE = newborn encephalopathy.

ing to this concern, a task force of the World Federation of Neurology Group for the Prevention of Cerebral Palsy and Related Neurological Disorders convened in 1992 to discuss the use of the term. The statement issued by this task force suggests that a newborn's condition should not be attributed to birth asphyxia unless there is specific proof of an asphyxial process, and other possible causes have been ruled out.[85] The statement also reflects skepticism of techniques that assess this process, except for the MRS approach described above, which is not likely to become available outside the research setting. Subsequently, an ACOG Committee opinion strongly supported the concept that "a neonate who has had hypoxia proximate to delivery severe enough to result in hypoxic encephalopathy will show other signs of hypoxic damage, including all of the following: (1) profound metabolic or mixed acidemia (pH <7.0) on an umbilical cord arterial blood sample, if obtained; (2) a persistent Apgar score of 0–3 for longer than 5 minutes; and (3) evidence of neonatal neurologic sequelae (e.g., seizures, coma, or hypotonia), and one or more of the following: cardiovascular, gastrointestinal, hematologic, pulmonary, or renal system dysfunction."[86] In light of the medico-legal climate of this subject for obstetricians, this stance is understandable, but the report does not serve the clinician in need of a reliable and readily available measure of birth asphyxia.

Once infection, organic acidemias, and other conditions have been ruled out, a newborn with a base deficit exceeding 12 mmol/L, measured in arterial blood in the immediate postpartum period, can reasonably be assumed to have experienced a degree of asphyxia that might increase the risk for brain damage.[39,57,87,88] The time of onset and duration of the asphyxia, however, are likely to be unknown. Even infants with this level of metabolic acidosis have a good prognosis, however, if they do not develop the higher grades of newborn encephalopathy.[89] Combining information based on measures of acid-base balance, birth depression, and neonatal neurologic abnormality may ultimately lead to the most useful definition of birth asphyxia.[38,42,90–93] Other commonly applied forms of "evidence" of birth asphyxia, however, such as Apgar scores and fetal heart rate patterns alone, are not specific enough to be reliable.

The Association Between Birth Asphyxia and Cerebral Palsy

Despite major changes over the past two decades in U.S.A. and European obstetric practices dedicated to reducing the incidence of intrapartum asphyxia, with an accompanying drop in neonatal mortality, there has been no "simultaneous" reduction in the prevalence of CP.[94–100] This, in itself, calls into question the strength of any relationship between birth asphyxia and CP.

Evaluation of the literature relating CP to birth asphyxia must be done in the light of the lack of specificity of some of the measures of birth asphyxia, and also in light of the presence of other factors strongly associated with the development of CP. The strong association of CP with premature birth and low birthweight has been recognized for more than a century. Infants weighing 1500–2500 g at birth have a risk of CP that is about three to four times higher than that of larger infants, and the risk for an infant weighing less than 1500 g at birth is about 22 times that of infants of normal birthweight.[101,102] Among low birthweight infants, gestational age is apparently more predictive of survival than it is of the risk of CP,[103] but since low birthweight is associated with low Apgar scores,[104,105] it is likely that some small infants at risk for CP were considered "asphyxiated" only because of their small size. A number of recent studies point to low-grade chorioamnionitis as possibly causative of both premature delivery and of CP.[106–111] Since premature, infected infants are likely to have appeared depressed at birth,[109] their condition may have often been mistakenly interpreted as "birth asphyxia."

Follow-up studies of infants with perinatal risk factors other than the infant's condition at birth have not shown striking associations with CP.[112–119] The use of the biophysical profile (a score including contributions from fetal breathing movements, gross bodily movements, tone, heart rate reactivity, and amniotic fluid volume) has shown that those infants with abnormal scores shortly before delivery are more likely to develop CP by the age of 3 years, but only a third of the cases were detected in this manner, and the false positive rate exceeded 98%.[120]

With regard to intrapartum factors, two studies found an excess of "suboptimal care" in the labors of infants who developed CP,[121,122] but the attributable risk was small, and contrary findings have been reported.[123] In general, adverse factors prior to delivery have not been strongly associated with CP, while postnatal measures, especially the development of neonatal neurologic signs, have a stronger association.[124,125]

As the Apgar score to some extent represents a gross and early newborn neurologic examination, it is not surprising that *severe* depression of the Apgar scores (as well as similar measures, such as time to respiration or need for resuscitation) has been associated with an increased incidence of CP and other neurodevelopmental impairments.[110,115,126,127] Estimates of the proportion of CP attributable to birth asphyxia are in the range of 8–25% among term infants,[53,59,114,118,128] and very likely much less than that in preterm infants,[129] and this estimate must be interpreted in the context of the nonspecific measures of asphyxia commonly used in the past.

Magnetic resonance imaging (MRI) findings in children with CP who were born prematurely tend to differ from those with CP who were born near term. Those who were born prematurely tend to show periventricular damage to the white matter, a pattern that some authors see as suggestive of hypoxic-ischemic damage,[11,130] although others disagree.[99,131] Children with CP from full-term pregnancies show a wider variety of patterns, some of which suggest early intrauterine insults, such as polymicrogyria, or other developmental brain anomalies. In fact, children diagnosed with CP attributed to birth asphyxia, are often found, on MRI or computed tomographic imaging of the brain, to have a developmental malformation that originated in the first or second trimester.[132–134] A subset of term infants with CP also shows periventricular thinning of white matter on MRI scans; it has been suggested that this may represent a brain-damaging event occurring in the late second or early third trimester. The implication is that in some pregnancies an insult that injures the brain leads to premature labor, while in others the fetus remains *in utero* and delivers at term.[132,134]

There is accumulating evidence of an association between chorioamnionitis and later disabilities in children born prematurely.[103,106,108,135] In addition, the "cytokine bath" (see Chapter 4) apparently associated with chorioamnionitis may cause cerebrovascular constriction, which is presumably capable of causing the periventricular white matter damage typically found in premature infants who develop CP.[136–138] This phenomenon may not, however, be restricted to the preterm newborn; Grether and colleagues have reported that newborns later diagnosed with spastic CP, regardless of gestational age at birth, more often had exposure to maternal infection markers,[108] and also had higher cytokine levels at birth, than did control newborns without CP.[139]

A further complicating feature to this association is the subtype of CP, as it appears that some forms of CP are more clearly associated with asphyxia than others. There is a general impression that dyskinetic and quadriplegic forms of CP are more strongly associated with evidence of birth asphyxia, while diplegia is often found in infants who were either premature or small for gestational age and who frequently had unremarkable deliveries. Hemiplegias are seen more commonly in term infants, and are more likely to represent stroke-like vascular syndromes, sometimes occurring long before labor. However, other etiologies of hemiplegia have been proposed.[134]

About 10% of CP is clearly of postnatal origin (e.g., from head trauma or bacterial meningitis). In addition to these forms of postnatal CP, mounting evidence now implicates the immediate postnatal period as a time of occurrence of brain damage, particularly in preterm infants,[140] and especially in relation to therapeutic measures undertaken in the neonatal intensive care unit.[94] The biological plausibility of this idea is supported by the apparent existence of a reperfusion phase following asphyxial injury, possibly lasting days into the neonatal period, which provides a window of time in which brain injury can occur.[11] This impression, however, could also be derived from observing the effects of a delayed response to an earlier asphyxial event.[141] The potential danger of iatrogenic hyperoxemia to immature retinal tissue is well known, and oxygen could be hypothesized to represent a threat to the immature brain as well. Suspicion is mounting that hypocapnia associated with vigorous mechanical ventilation similarly represents a risk factor for brain injury.[142-147] As the depressed, "asphyxiated" newborn is likely to require ventilatory assistance, neonatal factors associated with mechanical ventilation could confound an apparent relationship between asphyxia and CP.

Despite all of these potentially confounding factors, clear evidence persists of at least some association of severe birth asphyxia and CP, if accompanied by neurologic deficits in the neonatal period. Accepting Low's definition of birth asphyxia to include metabolic acidosis, the degree of base deficit is predictive of the risk of newborn encephalopathy.[36,37,87] In turn, the severity of encephalopathy is predictive of the risk of CP, as well as functional disabilities and impaired school performance.[66,68,117] Tables 6 and 7 provide a review of the literature related to the association between newborn encephalopathy, its severity, and CP.

Thus, it appears that the inferences drawn from the recent literature add clarity to two seemingly opposing conclusions regarding the relationship of birth asphyxia to CP. First, it would be imprudent to believe that there is no such relationship at all. Asphyxia, as reflected most clearly by base deficit, somewhat less definitively by measures of depression, and quite tenuously by "ominous" fetal heart rate patterns, is associated with the development of newborn encephalopathy,[148] which, especially when severe, is a risk factor for CP. On the other hand, it seems clear that the bulk of CP is *not attributable* to birth asphyxia,[59,97] and that the concepts of previous decades overemphasized the importance of this factor. It has been calculated that

Table 6

Prevalence of Cerebral Palsy in Infants Who Had Experienced Newborn Encephalopathy

Study	No. of Infants Followed	Proportion with Moderate or Severe Encephalopathy (%)	Prevalence of Cerebral Palsy (%)
De Souza et al[155]	53	60	2
Bergamasco et al[156]	371	37	5
Levene et al[157]	108	29	6
Robertson and Finer[65]	167	60	12
Sarnat and Sarnat[63]	19	100	26
Brown et al[158]	76	≥ 80	30
Fitzhardinge et al[159]	62	100	42

infants qualifying for neuroprotective therapy as a result of birth asphyxia are found only once in 5000[2] to 50,000[119] deliveries (depending on entry criteria) in developed nations.

Assessing the relationship of birth asphyxia to CP retrospectively can be misleading.[149] It is tempting to look back at the perinatal histories of children with CP, to discover "explanatory" antepartum or intrapartum risk factors. Although many children with CP will be found to have experienced such risk factors,[129] a surprisingly similar fraction of unaffected children will also be found to have experienced similar risk factors.[116,150] Nelson and Ellenberg reported some time ago[124] that the data from the National Collaborative Perinatal Project show the risk of CP in normal birthweight infants who had no complications of labor to be identical to the risk in those who had experienced any complication of labor.

The Association Between Birth Asphyxia and Other Neurodevelopmental Disorders

Cerebral palsy appears to be the outcome most specifically associated with measures of birth asphyxia, and white matter damage, whether associated with hypoxia-ischemia or with other pre- and perinatal insults, probably underlies most cases of CP. The motor control areas of the brain are the specific targets of a variety of perinatal insults, including hypoxia-ischemia; mental retardation, in the absence of CP, should not be inferred to result from birth asphyxia.

Table 7

Survival and Prevalence of Major Disability in Infants Who Had Experienced Newborn Encephalopathy, by Severity of Encephalopathy

Study	Location	Mild NE		Moderate NE		Severe NE	
		Death	Disability	Death	Disability	Death	Disability
Levene et al[157]	U.K.	0/77	0/77	1/24	5/23	13/21	3/8
Robertson and Finer[151]	Canada	0/79	0/66	5/119	20/94	21/28	7/7
Thompson et al[66]	S. Africa		0/10		4/14		13/16
Thornberg et al[160]	Sweden	0/36	0/36	1/17	8/16	11/12	1/1
Ellis et al[70]	Nepal	6/35	2/29	11/38	16/27	28/29	0/1

NE = newborn encephalopathy.

Reports that associate asphyxia with measures of neurodevelopment other than CP are often found not to include a sufficient follow-up period to distinguish entirely among the outcomes, or to examine more fully outcomes that were necessarily measured at a very early age. A summary of this literature indicates a general association of severe "asphyxia" with neurologic sequelae, but it is not clear that children are significantly affected in ways other than forms of CP. An exception may be neurosensory deafness, a relatively rare consequence, perhaps associated with birth asphyxia but not with other related neurologic disabilities.[151] With regard to cognitive function, data from the National Collaborative Perinatal Project showed that in a multivariate regression model, all indicators of perinatal asphyxia combined contributed only a tiny fraction of the variance in IQ score at age 7.[152] A follow-up study of survivors of newborn encephalopathy, however, showed that some children who had survived moderate encephalopathy without developing significant motor disabilities did have measurable reductions in later school performance.[153]

Significant Birth Asphyxia

Labor and delivery represent major stresses to even the most optimally supported fetus, and many newborns will show evidence of at least mild "asphyxia" by the various measures that have been discussed. As is the case with many other risk factors for disease that are commonly experienced by the general population, an important task of epidemiologic studies is to determine the relationship of exposure to asphyxia to the risk of CP. Is there a linear relationship, such that the risk of sequelae like CP rises continually with increasing exposure to asphyxia? Or is there a threshold, with increased risk appearing only beyond a certain level of exposure and perhaps increasing linearly thereafter?

Although this question should not be considered resolved, there is, nevertheless, increasing evidence of a threshold relationship. Low and associates, working with a base deficit (which we have considered here to be the best clinical estimate of asphyxia) have concluded that a level of 12 mmol/L is a threshold above which the incidence of encephalopathy increases,[39,87,88] and less markedly affected infants tend to have excellent outcomes.[154] When asphyxia has been assessed by combinations of other less reliable markers, such as the Apgar score, pH, or fetal heart rate patterns, it is also clear that, whatever the marker, the level of asphyxia must be severe for significant neurodevelopmental sequelae to be found. Indeed, when a combination of metabolic acidosis and neonatal neurologic abnormalities exists, the potential for adverse outcomes is most clearly increased. The new measures of oxidative metabolism with which some investigators are characterizing newborns at risk for asphyxia also add to the impression of a threshold, as the difference in findings between brain-injured patients and controls is often very large. Further refinement in the research should add considerably to our understanding of the nature of the relationship between exposure to asphyxia and the risk of CP and other sequelae.

In conclusion, three generalizations can be made about infants who have experienced documented birth asphyxia with apparent subsequent chronic brain impairment:

1. The asphyxia and birth depression are likely to have been very severe.

2. Abnormal neurologic signs were virtually always seen in the neonatal period, such as seizures, uncoordinated feeding, and difficulties with respiratory control, components of the syndrome now termed newborn encephalopathy.

3. The subsequent disability is generally severe and almost always involves the motor system.

The apparent dichotomization of the outcomes of perinatal asphyxia, either normalcy or severe disability, may reflect the considerable recuperative capacities of the developing brain that has been exposed to moderate degrees of birth asphyxia. It could also, however, reflect the limitations of testing for subtle degrees of motor impairment or cognitive dysfunction. Nevertheless, in counseling the parents of asphyxiated infants, an optimistic prognosis can be given unless the asphyxia has been unusually severe and accompanied by at least moderate newborn encephalopathy.

References

1. Little WJ: On the influence of abnormal parturition, difficult labour, premature birth, and asphyxia neonatorum on the mental and physical condition of the child, especially in relation to deformities. Trans Obstet Soc Lond 1862;3:293–344.
2. Freud S: *Infantile Cerebral Paralysis*, Russin LA (trans). University of Miami Press Coral Gables, Florida, 1968, pp 257–259.

3. Lilienfeld AM, Parkhurst E: A study of the association of factors of pregnancy and parturition with the development of cerebral palsy. Am J Hyg 1951;53:262–282.
4. Pasamanick B, Lilienfeld AM: Association of maternal and fetal factors with development of mental deficiency. 1. Abnormalities in the prenatal and perinatal periods. JAMA 1955;119:155–160.
5. Windle WF: *Asphyxia Neonatorum.* Charles C. Thomas Publishers, Springfield, IL, 1950.
6. Peeters LL, Sheldon RE, Jones MD, et al: Blood flow to fetal organs as a function of arterial oxygen content. Am J Obstet Gynecol 1979;135:637–646.
7. Itskovitz J, LaGamma EF, Rudolph AM: Effects of cord compression on fetal blood flow distribution and O_2 delivery. Am J Physiol 1987; 252:H100–H109.
8. Behrman RE, Lees MH, Peterson EN, et al: Distribution of the circulation in the normal and asphyxiated fetal primate. Am J Obstet Gynecol 1970;108:956–969.
9. Jensen A, Roman C, Rudolph AM: Effects of reducing uterine blood flow on fetal blood flow distribution and oxygen delivery. J Dev Physiol 1991; 15:309–323.
10. Volpe JJ: Brain injury in the premature infant: is it preventable? Pediatr Res 1990;27:S28–S33.
11. Volpe JJ: *Neurology of the Newborn.* 3rd ed. W.B. Saunders, Philadelphia, 1995, pp 221–372.
12. Goldstein RF, Thompson RJ, Oehler JM, et al: Influence of acidosis, hypoxemia, and hypotension on neurodevelopmental outcome in very low birth weight infants. Pediatrics 1995;95:238–243.
13. Perlman JM: Intrapartum hypoxic-ischemic cerebral injury and subsequent cerebral palsy: medicolegal issues. Pediatrics 1997;99:851–859.
14. Perlman JM: White matter injury in the preterm infant: an important determination of abnormal neurodevelopment outcome. Early Hum Dev 1998;53:99–120.
15. Shinozuka T, Nemoto EM, Winter PM: Mechanisms of cerebrovascular O_2 sensitivity from hyperoxia to moderate hypoxia in the rat. J Cereb Blood Flow Metab 1989;9:187–195.
16. Omae T, Ibayashi S, Kusuda K, et al: Effects of high atmospheric pressure and oxygen on middle cerebral blood flow velocity in humans measured by transcranial doppler. Stroke 1998;29:94–97.
17. Nijima S, Shortland DB, Levene MI, et al: Transient hyperoxia and cerebral blood flow velocity in infants born prematurely and at full term. Arch Dis Child 1988;63:1126–1130.
18. Rahilly PM: Effects of 2% carbon dioxide, 0.5% carbon dioxide, and 100% oxygen on cranial blood flow of the human neonate. Pediatrics 1980; 66:685–689.
19. Lundstrom KE, Pryds O, Greisen G: Oxygen at birth and prolonged cerebral vasoconstriction in preterm infants. Arch Dis Child 1995;73:F81–F86.
20. Ashwal S, Dale PS, Longo LD: Regional cerebral blood flow: studies in the fetal lamb during hypoxia, hypercapnia, acidosis, and hypotension. Pediatr Res 1984;18:1309–1316.
21. Leahy FAN, Cates D, MacCallum M, et al: Effect of CO_2 and 100% O_2 on cerebral blood flow in preterm infants. J Appl Physiol 1980;48:468–472.

22. Rosenberg AA: Response of the cerebral circulation to hypocarbia in postasphyxia newborn lambs. Pediatr Res 1992;32:537–541.
23. Harkin CP, Schmeling WT, Kampine JP, et al: The effects of hyper- and hypocarbia on intraparenchymal arterioles in rat brain slices. Neuroreport 1997;8:1841–1844.
24. Laptook AR, Peterson J, Porter AM: Effects of lactic acid infusions and pH on cerebral blood flow and metabolism. J Cereb Blood Flow Metab 1988;8:193–200.
25. Dijxhoorn MJ, Visser GH, Huisjes HJ, et al: The relation between umbilical pH values and neonatal neurological morbidity in full term appropriate-for-dates infants. Early Hum Dev 1985;11:33–42.
26. Hibbard JU, Hibbard MC, Whalen MP: Umbilical cord blood gases and mortality and morbidity in the very low birth weight infant. Obstet Gynecol 1991;78:768–773.
27. Goodwin TM, Belai I, Hernandez P, et al: Asphyxial complications in the term newborn with severe umbilical acidemia. Am J Obstet Gynecol 1992;162:1506–1512.
28. King TA, Jackson GL, Josey AS, et al: The effect of profound umbilical artery acidemia in term neonates admitted to a newborn nursery. J Pediatr 1998;132:624–629.
29. Holmqvist P, Plevon H, Svenningsen NW: Vaginally born low-risk preterm infants: fetal acidosis and outcome at 6 years of age. Acta Paediatr Scand 1988;77:638–641.
30. Ruth VJ, Raivio KO: Perinatal brain damage: predictive value of metabolic acidosis the Apgar score. BMJ 1988;297:24–27.
31. Fee SC, Malee K, Deddish R, et al: Severe acidosis and subsequent neurologic status. Am J Obstet Gynecol 1990;162:802–806.
32. Dennis J, Johnson A, Mutch L, et al: Acid-base status at birth and neurodevelopmental outcome at four and one-half years. Am J Obstet Gynecol 1989;161:213–220.
33. Tombaugh GC, Sapolsky RM: Evolving concepts about the role of acidosis in ischemic neuropathology. J Neurochem 1993;61:793–803.
34. Vannucci RC, Towfighi J, Heitjan D, et al: Carbon dioxide protects the perinatal brain from hypoxic-ischemic damage: an experimental study in the immature rat. Pediatrics 1995;95:868–874.
35. Vannucci RC, Brucklacher RM, Vannucci SJ: Effect of carbon dioxide on cerebral metabolism during hypoxia-ischemia in the immature rat. Pediatr Res 1997;42:24–29.
36. Vintzileos AM, Egan JFX, Campbell WA, et al: Asphyxia at birth as determined by cord blood pH measurements in preterm and term gestations: correlation with neonatal outcome. J Matern Fetal Med 1992;1:7–13.
37. Low JA, Panagiotopoulos C, Derrick EJ: Newborn complications after intrapartum asphyxia with metabolic acidosis in the term fetus. Am J Obstet Gynecol 1994;170:1081–1087.
38. Sehdev HM, Stamillo DM, Macones GA, et al: Predictive factors for neonatal morbidity in neonates with an umbilical arterial cord pH less than 7.00. Am J Obstet Gynecol 1997;177:1030–1034.
39. Low JA, Lindsay BG, Derrick EJ: Threshold of metabolic acidosis associated with newborn complications. Am J Obstet Gynecol 1997;177:1391–1394.
40. Dijxhoorn MJ, Visser GHA, Fidler VJ, et al: Apgar score, meconium and

acidaemia at birth in relation to neonatal neurological morbidity in term infants. Br J Obstet Gynaecol 1986;93:217–222.

41. Goldaber KG, Gilstrap LC, Leveno KJ, et al: Pathologic fetal acidemia. Obstet Gynecol 1991;78:1103–1107.

42. Winkler CL, Hauth JC, Tucker JM, et al: Neonatal complications at term as related to the degree of umbilical artery acidemia. Am J Obstet Gynecol 1991;104:637–641.

43. van den Berg PP, Nelen W, Jongsma HW, et al: Neonatal complications in newborns with an umbilical artery pH <7.00. Am J Obstet Gynecol 1996;175:1152–1157.

44. Nelson KB, Ellenberg JH: Apgar scores as predictors of chronic neurologic disability. Pediatrics 1981;68:36–44.

45. Paneth N, Bommarito M, Stricker J: Electronic fetal monitoring and later outcome. Clin Invest Med 1993;16:159–165.

46. NICHD Research Planning Workshop: Electronic fetal heart rate monitoring: research guidelines for interpretation. Am J Obstet Gynecol 1997; 177:1385–1390.

47. Painter MJ, Scott M, Hirsch RP, et al: Fetal heart rate patterns during labor: neurologic and cognitive development at six to nine years of age. Am J Obstet Gynecol 1988;159:854–858.

48. Nelson KB, Dambrosia JM, Ting T, et al: Uncertain value of electronic fetal monitoring in predicting cerebral palsy. N Engl J Med 1996;334: 613–618.

49. Spencer JA, Badawi N, Burton P, et al: The intrapartum CTG prior to neonatal encephalopathy at term: a case-control study. Br J Obstet Gynaecol 1997;104:25–28.

50. Thacker SB, Stroup DF, Peterson HB: Efficacy and safety of intrapartum electronic fetal monitoring: an update. Obstet Gynecol 1995;86:613–620.

51. MacDonald D, Grant A, Sheridan-Pereira M, et al: The Dublin randomized controlled trial of intrapartum fetal heart rate monitoring. Am J Obstet Gynecol 1985;152:524–539.

52. Leveno KJ, Cunningham FG, Nelson S, et al: A prospective comparison of selective and universal electronic fetal monitoring in 34,995 pregnancies. N Engl J Med 1986;315:615–619.

53. Grant A, O'Brien N, Joy MT, et al: Cerebral palsy among children born during the Dublin randomised trial of intraparturn monitoring. Lancet 1989;ii:1233–1235.

54. Shy KK, Luthy DA, Bennett FC, et al: Effects of electronic fetal-heart monitoring, as compared with periodic auscultation, on the neurologic development of premature infants. N Engl J Med 1990;322:588–593.

55. Cibils LA: On intraparturn fetal monitoring. Am J Obstet Gynecol 1996; 174:1382–1389.

56. Kaczorowski J, Levitt C, Hanvey L, et al: A national survey of use of obstetric procedures and technologies in Canadian hospitals: routine or based on existing evidence? Birth 1998;25:11–18.

57. Low JA, Galbraith RS, Muir DW, et al: Motor and cognitive deficits after intrapartum asphyxia in the mature fetus. Am J Obstet Gynecol 1988; 158:356–361.

58. Ounsted M: Causes, continua and other concepts. I. The 'continuum of reproductive casualty'. Paediatr Perinat Epidemiol 1987;1:4–9.

59. Blair E, Stanley FJ: Intrapartum asphyxia: a rare cause of cerebral palsy. J Pediatr 1988;112:515–519.
60. Palmer L, Blair E, Pettersen B, Burton P: Antenatal antecedents of moderate and severe cerebral palsy. Paediatr Perinat Epidemiol 1995;9:171–184.
61. Myers RE: Two patterns of perinatal brain damage and their conditions of occurrence. Am J Obstet Gynecol 1972;112:246–276.
62. Myers RE: Experimental models of perinatal brain damage: relevance to human pathology. In Gluck L (ed): *Intrauterine Asphyxia and the Developing Fetal Brain.* Year Book Medical Publishers, Inc, Chicago, 1977, pp 37–97.
63. Sarnat HB, Sarnat MS: Neonatal encephalopathy following fetal distress. Arch Neurol 1976;33:696–705.
64. Fenichel JM: Hypoxic-ischemic encephalopathy in the newborn. Arch Neurol 1983;40:261–266.
65. Robertson C, Finer N: Term infants with hypoxic-ischemic encephalopathy: outcome at 3.5 years. Dev Med Child Neurol 1985;27:473–484.
66. Thompson CM, Puterman AS, Linley LL, et al: The value of a scoring system for hypoxic ischaemic encephalopathy in predicting neurodevelopmental outcome. Acta Paediatr 1997;86:757–761.
67. Sorensen LC, Borch K: Prediction of outcome following perinatal asphyxia: a retrospective study based on 54 asphyxiated mature newborns. Ugesky Laeger 1999;161:3094–3098.
68. Gonzalez de Dios J, Moya M: Perinatal asphyxia, hypoxic-ischemic encephalopathy, and neurologic sequelae in full-term infants. II. Descriptions and interrelationships. Rev Neurol (Barc) 1996;24:969–976.
69. Bréart G, Rumeau-Rouquette C: Cerebral palsy and perinatal asphyxia in term neonates. Arch Pediatr 1996;3:70–74.
70. Ellis M, Manandhar N, Shrestha PS, et al: Outcome at 1 year of neonatal encephalopathy in Kathmandu, Nepal. Dev Med Child Neurol 1999; 41:689–695.
71. Hull J, Dodd K: What is birth asphyxia? Br J Obstet Gynaecol 1991;98: 953–955.
72. Leviton A, Nelson KB: Problems with definitions and classifications of newborn encephalopathy. Pediatr Neurol 1991;8:85–90.
73. Edwards AD, Nelson KB: Neonatal encephalopathies. BMJ 1998; 317:1537–1538.
74. Patel J, Edwards AD: Prediction of outcome after perinatal asphyxia. Curr Opin Pediatr 1997;9:128–132.
75. Reynolds EOR, Hamilton PA: Magnetic resonance spectroscopy of the brain and early neurodevelopmental outcome. In Kubli F, Patel N, Schmidt W, Linderkamp O (eds): *Perinatal Events and Brain Damage in Surviving Children.* Springer-Verlag, Berlin, 1988, pp 245–253.
76. Roth SC, Baudin J, Cady E, et al: Relation of deranged neonatal cerebral oxidative metabolism with neurodevelopmental outcome and head circumference at 4 years. Dev Med Child Neurol 1997;39:718–725.
77. Hanrahan JD, Cox IJ, Azzopardi D, et al: Relation between proton magnetic resonance spectroscopy within 18 hours of birth asphyxia and neurodevelopment at 1 year of age. Dev Med Child Neurol 1999;41:76–82.
78. Hanrahan JD, Cox IJ, Edwards AD, et al: Persistent increases in cerebral lactate concentration after birth asphyxia. Pediatr Res 1998;44:304–311.
79. Pourcyrous M, Bada HS, Yang W, et al: Prognostic significance of cere-

brospinal fluid cyclic adenosine monophosphate in neonatal asphyxia. J Pediatr 1999;134:90–96.

80. Siivman K, Blennow M, Gustafson K, et al: Cytokine response in cerebrospinal fluid after birth asphyxia. Pediatr Res 1998;43:746–751.

81. Riikonen RS, Korhonen LT, Lindholm DB: Cerebrospinal nerve growth factor: a marker of asphyxia? Pediatr Neurol 1999;20:137–141.

82. Huang CC, Wang ST, Chang YC, et al: Measurement of the urinary lactate: creatinine ratio for the early identification of newborn infants at risk for hypoxic-ischemic encephalopathy. N Engl J Med 1999; 341:328–335.

83. Chou YH, Yau KIT, Wang PJ: Clinical application of the measurement of cord plasma lactate and pyruvate in the assessment of high-risk neonates. Acta Paediatr 1998;87:764–768.

84. Akisij M, Kijlttirsay N: Value of the urinary uric acid to creatinine ratio in term infants with perinatal asphyxia. Acta Paediatr Japonica 1998; 40:78–81.

85. Bax M, Nelson KB: Birth asphyxia: a statement. Dev Med Child Neurol 1993;35:1015–1024.

86. Committee on Obstetric Practice: Inappropriate use of the terms fetal distress and birth asphyxia. Int J Gynecol Obstet 1998;61:309–310.

87. Low JA, Galbraith RS, Muir DW, et al: Mortality and morbidity after intrapartum: asphyxia in the preterm fetus. Obstet Gynecol 1992;80:57–61.

88. Low JA: Intrapartum fetal asphyxia: definition, diagnosis, and classification. Am J Obstet Gynecol 1997;176:957–959.

89. Low JA, Galbraith RS, Muir DW, et al: Factors associated with motor and cognitive deficits in children after intrapartum fetal hypoxia. Am J Obstet Gynecol 1984;148:533–539.

90. Gilstrap LC, Leveno KJ, Burris J, et al: Diagnosis of birth asphyxia on the basis of fetal pH, Apgar score, and newborn cerebral dysfunction. Am J Obstet Gynecol 1989;161:825–830.

91. Portman RJ, Carter BS, Gaylord MS, et al: Predicting neonatal morbidity after perinatal asphyxia: a scoring system. Am J Obstet Gynecol 1990; 162:174–182.

92. Carter BS, McNabb F, Merenstein GB: Prospective validation of a scoring system for predicting neonatal morbidity after acute perinatal asphyxia. J Pediatr 1998;132:619–623.

93. Perlman JM, Risser R: Can asphyxiated infants at risk for neonatal seizures be rapidly identified by current high-risk markers? Pediatrics 1996;97:456–462.

94. Hagberg B, Hagberg G, Olow I: Gains and hazards of intensive neonatal care: an analysis from Swedish cerebral palsy epidemiology. Dev Med Child Neurol 1982;24:13–19.

95. Jarvis SN, Holloway JS, Hey EN: Increase in cerebral palsy in normal birthweight babies. Arch Dis Child 1985;60:1113–1121.

96. Pharoah POD, Cooke T, Cooke RWI, et al: Birthweight specific trends in cerebral palsy. Arch Dis Child 1990;65:602–606.

97. Stanley FJ, Blair E: Why have we failed to reduce the frequency of cerebral palsy? Med J Aust 1991;154:623–626.

98. Escobar GJ, Littenberg B, Petitti DB: Outcome among surviving very low birthweight infants: a meta-analysis. Arch Dis Child 1991;66:204–211.

99. Stanley FJ, Watson L: Trends in perinatal mortality and cerebral palsy in Western Australia, 1967 to 1985. BMJ 1992;304:1658–1663.
100. Pharoah POD, Cooke T, Johnson MA, et al: Epidemiology of cerebral palsy in England and Scotland, 1984–1989. Arch Dis Child Fetal Neonatol Ed 1998;79:F21–F25.
101. Stanley FJ: Survival and cerebral palsy in low birthweight infants: implications for perinatal care. Paediatr Perinat Epidemiol 1992;6:298–310.
102. Kuban KCK, Leviton A: Cerebral palsy. N Engl J Med 1994;330:188–195.
103. Spinillo A, Capuzzo E, Orcesi S, et al: Antenatal and delivery risk factors simultaneously associated with neonatal death and cerebral palsy in preterm infants. Early Hum Dev 1997;48:81–91.
104. Chandra S, Ramji S, Thirupuram S: Perinatal asphyxia: multivariate analysis of risk factors in hospital births. Indian Pediatr 1997;34:206–212.
105. Ramin SM, Gilstrap LC, Leveno KJ, et al: Umbilical artery acid-base status in the preterm infant. Obstet Gynecol 1989;74:256–258.
106. Murphy DJ, Sellers S, MacKenzie IZ, et al: Case-control study of antenatal and intrapartum risk factors for cerebral palsy in very preterm singleton babies. Lancet 1995;346:1449–1454.
107. Murphy DJ, Johnson A: Placental infection and risk of cerebral palsy in very low birth weight infants. J Pediatr 1996;129:776–778.
108. Grether JK, Nelson KB: Maternal infection and cerebral palsy in infants of normal birth weight. JAMA 1997;278:207–211.
109. Damman O, Leviton A: Infection remote from the brain, neonatal white matter damage, and cerebral palsy in the preterm infant. Sem Pediatr Neurol 1998;5:190–201.
110. O'Shea TM, Klinepeter KL, Meis PJ, et al: Intrauterine infection and the risk of cerebral palsy in very low-birthweight infants. Paediatr Perinat Epidemiol 1998;12:72–83.
111. Leviton A, Paneth N, Reuss ML, et al: Maternal infection, fetal inflammatory response, and brain damage in very low birthweight infants. Pediatr Res 1999;46:566–575.
112. Nelson KB, Ellenberg JH: Obstetric complications as risk factors for cerebral palsy or seizure disorders. JAMA 1984;251:1843–1848.
113. Stanley FJ, English DR: Prevalence of and risk factors for cerebral palsy in a total population cohort of low-birthweight (<2000 g) infants. Dev Med Child Neurol 1986;28:559–568.
114. Nelson KB, Ellenberg JH: Antecedents of cerebral palsy: multivariate analysis of risk. N Engl J Med 1986;315:81–86.
115. Stanley F: The changing face of cerebral palsy? Dev Med Child Neurol 1987;29:258–270.
116. Kitchen WH, Doyle LW, Ford GW, et al: Cerebral palsy in very low birthweight infants surviving to 2 years with modern perinatal intensive care. Am J Perinatol 1987;4:29–35.
117. Emond A, Golding J, Peckham C: Cerebral palsy in two national cohort studies. Arch Dis Child 1989;64:848–852.
118. Torfs CP, van den Berg BJ, Oechsii FW, et al: Prenatal and perinatal factors in the etiology of cerebral palsy. J Pediatr 1990;116:615–619.
119. Nelson KB, Grether JK: Selection of neonates for neuroprotective therapies. Arch Pediatr Adolesc Med 1999;153:393–398.
120. Manning FA, Bondagji N, Harman CR, et al: Fetal assessment based on

the fetal biophysical profile score: relationship of last BPS result to subsequent cerebral palsy. J Gynecol Obstet Biol Reprod (Paris) 1997; 26:720–729.

121. Gaffney G, Sellers S, Flavell V, et al: Case-control study of intrapartum care, cerebral palsy, and perinatal death. BMJ 1994;308:743–750.

122. Westgate JA, Gunn AJ, Gunn TR, et al: Antecedents of neonatal encephalopathy with fetal acidaemia at term. Br J Obstet Gynaecol 1999; 106:774–782.

123. Niswander K, Henson G, Elbourne D, et al: Adverse outcome of pregnancy and the quality of obstetric care. Lancet 1984;ii:827–831.

124. Nelson KB, Ellenberg JH: The asymptomatic newborn and risk of cerebral palsy. Am J Dis Child 1987;141:1333–1335.

125. Freeman JM, Nelson KB: Intrapartum asphyxia and cerebral palsy. Pediatrics 1988;82:240–249.

126. Dite GS, Bell R, Reddihough DS, et al: Antenatal and perinatal antecedents of moderate and severe spastic cerebral palsy. Aust NZ J Obstet Gynecol 1998;38:377–383.

127. Sciberras C, Spencer N: Cerebral palsy in Malta 1981 to 1990. Dev Med Child Neurol 1999;41:508–511.

128. Naeye RL, Peters E, Bartholomew M, et al: Origins of cerebral palsy. Am J Dis Child 1989;143:1154–1161.

129. Yudkin P, Johnson A, Clover LM, et al: Assessing the contribution of birth asphyxia to cerebral palsy in term singletons. Paediatr Perinatal Epidemiol 1995;9:156–170.

130. Vannucci RC, Palmer C: Hypoxia-ischemia: pathogenesis and neuropathology. In Fanaroff AA, Martin RJ (eds): *Neonatal-Perinatal Medicine.* Mosby, Philadelphia, 1997, pp 856–877.

131. Paneth N, Rudelli R, Kazam E, Monte W: White matter damage: terminology, typology, pathogenesis. Clin Dev Med 1994;131:117–118.

132. Truwitt CL, Barkovich AJ, Koch TK, et al: Cerebral palsy: MR findings in 40 patients. Am J Neuroradiol 1992;13:67–78.

133. Sugimoto T, Woo M, Nishida N, et al: When do brain abnormalities in cerebral palsy occur? An MRI study. Dev Med Child Neurol 1995;37:285–292.

134. Wiklund LM, Uverbrant P, Flodmark O: Computed tomography as an adjunct in etiologic analysis of hemiplegic cerebral palsy. II. Children born at term. Neuropediatrics 1991;22:121–128.

135. Alexander JM, Gilstrap LC, Cox SM, et al: Clinical chorioamnionitis and the prognosis for very low birth weight infants. Obstet Gynecol 1998; 91:725–729.

136. Damman O, Leviton A: Maternal intrauterine infection, cytokines, and brain damage in the preterm newborn. Pediatr Res 1997;42:1–8.

137. Damman O, Leviton A: Does prepregnancy bacterial vaginosis increase a mother's risk of having a preterm infant with cerebral palsy? Dev Med Child Neurol 1997;39:836–840.

138. Yoon BH, Jun JK, Romero R, et al: Amniotic fluid inflammatory cytokines (interleukin-6, interleukin-I beta, and tumor necrosis factor-alpha), neonatal brain white matter lesions, and cerebral palsy. Am J Obstet Gynecol 1997;177:19–26.

139. Grether JK, Nelson KB, Dambrosia JM, Phillips TM: Interferons and cerebral palsy. J Pediatr 1999;134:324–332.

140. Murphy DJ, Hope PL, Johnson A: Neonatal risk factors for cerebral palsy in very preterm babies: case control study. BMJ 1997;314:404–408.
141. Lorek A, Takei Y, Cady EB, et al: Delayed ("secondary") cerebral energy failure after acute hypoxia-ischemia in the newborn piglet: continuous 48-hour studies by phosphorus magnetic resonance spectroscopy. Pediatr Res 1994;36:699–706.
142. Greisen G, Munck H, Lou H: Severe hypocarbia in preterm infants and neurodevelopmental deficit. Acta Paediatr Scand 1987;76:401–404.
143. Ikonen RS, Janas MO, Koivikko MJ, et al: Hyperbilirubinemia, hypocarbia and periventricular leukomalacia in preterm infants: relationship to cerebral palsy. Acta Paediatr 1992;81:802–807.
144. Graziani LJ, Spitzer AR, Mitchell DG, et al: Mechanical ventilation in preterm infants: neurosonographic and developmental studies. Pediatrics 1992;90:515–522.
145. Fujimoto S, Togari H, Yamaguchi N, et al: Hypocarbia and cystic periventricular leukomalacia in premature infants. Arch Dis Child 1994; 71:F107–F110.
146. Wiswell TE, Graziani LJ, Kornhauser MS, et al: Effects of hypocarbia on the development of cystic periventricular leukomalacia in premature infants treated with high-frequency jet ventilation. Pediatrics 1996; 98:918–924.
147. Salokorpi T, Rajantie I, Viitala J, et al: Does perinatal hypocarbia play a role in the pathogenesis of cerebral palsy? Acta Paediatr 1999;88:571–575.
148. Badawi N, Kurinczuk JJ, Keogh JM, et al: Intrapartum risk factors for newborn encephalopathy: the western Australian case-control study. BMJ 1998;317:1554–1558.
149. Ekert P, Perlman M, Steinlin M, et al: Predicting the outcome of postasphyxial hypoxic-ischemic encephalopathy within 4 hours of birth. J Pediatr 1997;131:613–617.
150. Nelson KB, Grether JK: Potentially asphyxiating conditions and spastic cerebral palsy in infants of normal birth weight. Am J Obstet Gynecol 1998;179:507–513.
151. Robertson CMT, Finer NN: Long-term follow-up of term neonates with perinatal asphyxia. Clin Perinatol 1993;20:483–500.
152. Broman S: Perinatal anoxia and cognitive development in early childhood. In Field TM, Sostek AM, Goldberg S, Shuman HH (eds): Infants Born at Risk. Spectrum Books, New York, 1979, pp 29–52.
153. Robertson CMT, Finer NN, Grace MGA: School performance of survivors of neonatal encephalopathy associated with birth asphyxia at term. J Pediatr 1989;114:753–760.
154. Handley-Derry M, Low JA, Burke SO, et al: Intrapartum fetal asphyxia and the occurrence of minor deficits in 4- to 8-year-old children. Dev Med Child Neurol 1997;39:508–514.
155. De Souza SW, Black P, Cadman J, et al: Umbilical venous pH: a useful aid in the diagnosis of asphyxia at birth. Arch Dis Child 1981; 56:245–252.
156. Bergamasco B, Benna P, Ferrero P, Gavinelli R: Neonatal hypoxia and epileptic risk: a clinical prospective study. Epilepsia 1984;25:131–136.
157. Levene MI, Sands C, Grindulis H, et al: Comparison of two methods of predicting outcome in perinatal asphyxia. Lancet 1986;i:67–68.

158. Brown JK, Purvis RJ, Forfar JO, et al: Neurological aspects of perinatal asphyxia. Dev Med Child Neurol 1974;16:567–580.
159. Fitzhardinge PM, Flodmark O, Fitz CR, et al: The prognostic value of computed tomography as an adjunct to assessment of the term infant with postasphyxial encephalopathy. J Pediatr 1981;99:777–781.
160. Thornberg E, Thiringer K, Odeback A, et al: Birth asphyxia: incidence, clinical course and outcome in a Swedish population. Acta Paediatr 1995;84:927–932.

PART II

Basic Science

CHAPTER 3

The Biochemical Neurotoxic Cascade in Hypoxic-Ischemic Injury

Michael V. Johnston, Akira Ishida, Wako Nakajima,
William Trescher

Introduction

The fetal brain is resistant to injury from hypoxemia because it is adapted to the relatively hypoxic intrauterine environment, and because compensatory increases in cerebral blood flow can usually maintain oxygen delivery.[1–4] Positron emission tomographic (PET) studies of human fetuses and infants indicate that brain oxygen consumption is minimal and below the threshold for brain viability in adults.[5] However, the brain can become vulnerable to severe hypoxemia when cerebral blood flow is also reduced beyond a critical threshold. In contrast to the adult brain, which is far more vulnerable to hypoxemia than other organs, the fetal brain's vulnerability is comparable to that of the heart and kidneys. Asphyxia that is severe enough to injure the brain reduces cerebral perfusion by impairing myocardial function and systemic blood pressure.[6] It has been difficult to produce experimental brain injury in mature fetuses using exposure to pure nitrogen or complete asphyxia because these conditions often cause death from cardiac arrest.[6] Early demise from cardiac failure precludes survival times long enough for a brain insult to produce neuropathologic changes. However, conditions that combine hypoxemia with critical reductions in cerebral blood flow produce brain injuries in animals that resemble those in human infants.[1] It is likely that virtually all damage to human infants from asphyxia results from tissue hypoxia-ischemia: the synergistic effects of severe hypoxemia combined with reduced cerebral blood flow.[1–3]

From Donn SM, Sinha SK, Chiswick ML (eds): *Birth Asphyxia and the Brain: Basic Science and Clinical Implications.* © 2002, Futura Publishing Co., Inc., Armonk, NY.

51

Hypoxic-Ischemic Encephalopathy Includes Prominent Signs of Brain Excitation

Hypoxia-ischemia triggers a cascade of neurotoxic biochemical events within the brain that extends over a number of days and is manifested by the clinical syndrome of hypoxic-ischemic encephalopathy (HIE).[2] Neonatal HIE that is severe enough to be associated with permanent brain injury is characterized by prominent signs of excessive neuronal excitability including seizures and paroxysmal electroencephalographic (EEG) activity.[7] There is a direct link between the severity of clinical signs of neonatal HIE and the likelihood of permanent brain injury.[8] In the National Institutes of Health (NIH) Collaborative Perinatal Project, neonatal seizures were one of the strongest predictors of later cerebral palsy, raising the relative risk of cerebral palsy 71 times.[9] The onset of seizures associated with HIE is delayed by approximately 12 hours, with the vast majority delayed between 6 and 36 hours.[10] In their clinical studies of neonatal encephalopathy, Sarnat and Sarnat[7] reported that seizures began in the first or second day after asphyxia with bursts of sharp and slow wave paroxysmal activity emerging on the second day. Using a model of severe cerebral ischemia in fetal sheep, Williams et al[11] found that seizure activity recorded by EEG was delayed until about 8 hours after the insult, and then increased and diminished again over a period of about 28 hours. In a nonhuman primate model of perinatal asphyxia, seizures were delayed by 12–18 hours.[3] Both animal and human studies indicate that energy production from oxidative phosphorylation fails after a considerable delay following its restoration during resuscitation.[10] The physiologic changes parallel the delayed sequence of morphologic changes that can be monitored using histopathologic and imaging techniques.[12–15] These observations indicate that severe asphyxia can trigger the delayed onset of a prolonged sequence of events in the brain that supports neuronal excitability. This series of neurochemical events has been referred to as the excitotoxic cascade because of evidence that it is triggered and sustained by excessive stimulation of excitatory amino acid neurotransmitter receptors.[16,17]

Early Synaptic Dysfunction in HIE

Dysfunction of synaptic connections between neurons, especially excitatory synapses, appears to play an important early role in triggering HIE in near-term infants.[2] A majority of synapses in the brain utilize the excitatory amino acid glutamate as their neurotransmitter.[2] Elevated extracellular levels of the excitatory neurotransmitters glutamate and glycine accumulate as part of the initial hypoxic-ischemic insult in animal models, and elevated cerebrospinal fluid levels of these transmitters have also been reported in cerebrospinal fluid of infants with severe HIE.[18–23] Early elevations in synaptic glutamate levels during severe experimental asphyxia are probably related to impairment of peri-synaptic glial sodium-dependent glutamate reuptake pumps.[24] These synaptic pumps are responsible for maintaining low synaptic levels of neurotransmitters.[24] Recent studies of neuronal physiology suggest that failure of glucose delivery to the hypoxic-ischemic brain could be primarily responsible for the failure of glutamate reuptake and elevations in glutamate levels.[25] These studies indicate that anaerobic glycolysis, not oxidative metabolism, provides the major power for glutamate reuptake pumps. Experimental studies of insulin-induced hypoglycemia indicate that glucose levels low enough to cause brain injury are associated with high levels of extracellular glutamate.[26] EEG monitoring in this model during profound hypoglycemia shows a suppressed pattern resembling the very early phases following asphyxia. This suggests that reduced glucose delivery during ischemia could contribute to elevated levels of excitatory amino acids observed in experimental hypoxia-ischemia.

Another observation pointing to dysfunction of glutamate synapses in HIE is that regions of the neonatal brain with special vulnerability to asphyxia are relatively enriched in functional glutamate synapses.[27] For example, in the clinical syndrome of acute "total or near-total" asphyxia in full-term human newborns, the putamen in the basal ganglia, the thalamus, and the cerebral cortex, especially the peri-Rolandic cortex, are selectively vulnerable to damage.[28–32] These regions contain important glutamatergic excitatory connections, such as the reciprocal thalamocortical and corticothalamic circuits, and corticostriate projections to the basal ganglia.[33] Receptor autoradiographic studies comparing postmortem human newborn brains with adults demonstrate that these regions are already endowed with glutamate receptors at birth.[34] PET studies of human newborns indicate that these same regions have relatively high rates of regional cerebral glucose metabolism at birth.[35] Studies of brain activation indicate that more than 80% of the brain's glucose metabolism is linked to the activity of neuronal synapses, primarily glutamate synapses.[25] The major trigger for glucose metabolism in the brain appears to be activation of energy-consuming glutamate reuptake pumps that react to glutamate release from pre-synaptic nerve terminals.[25] PET studies of newborns several days after severe asphyxia indicate that the glucose metabolic rate is elevated in the basal ganglia and peri-Rolandic cortex in infants who sustained permanent brain injury.[36] If glucose metabolism is coupled to glutamate turnover in this situation, the results indicate that glutamate release and reuptake are elevated in these vulnerable regions during HIE. Immunohistochemical studies in a piglet asphyxia model do show reduced levels of glutamate transporters in the vulnerable basal ganglia.[37] Therefore, studies in animal models and in human newborns suggest that synaptic dysfunction in excitatory amino acid-containing neuronal circuits contribute to focal damage and signs of hyperexcitability in HIE.

The Activation of NMDA Glutamate Receptor During HIE

Elevated levels of glutamate and glycine in severe asphyxia can contribute to the activation of the N-methyl-D-aspartate (NMDA) receptor, which appears to be the most important excitatory amino acid receptor for mediating brain damage in the newborn.[2,6–18] The NMDA-type glutamate receptor is quite important in brain development, and is unique in requiring simultaneous occupancy by both glutamate and glycine as well as membrane depolarization for channel opening.[38] Observations that point to the importance of this glutamate receptor in HIE include the ability of the potent NMDA receptor channel blocker MK-801 (dizocilpine) and related compounds to block hypoxic-ischemic damage if given prior to or shortly after experimental asphyxial insults.[39–42] Magnesium, a natural blocker of the NMDA channel, can also block excitotoxic injury if given prior to the insult.[43,44]

The central role that the NMDA receptors play in triggering brain injury from HIE in newborns is related in part to their enhanced physiologic activity in the immature brain.[16,45] The receptor plays an important role in activity-dependent neuronal plasticity, the process through which synaptic connections are sculpted in response to neuronal activity.[16] For example, NMDA receptors are thought to play a role in the process through which visual input into the visual cortex from one eye enlarges its territory of dominance if input from the other eye is impaired. NMDA receptors have also been reported to play a role in pruning excess synaptic connections in the developing cerebellum.[46] In the immature brain, the subunit composition of NMDA receptors is programmed to construct a receptor that transmits more physiologic activity than in adults.[47] Immature NMDA receptor channel complexes stay open longer, are more readily activated by glycine, have a higher calcium flux, and are blocked less easily by magnesium than adult channels.[48] The enhanced function of these receptors, especially their ability to allow calcium to flood into neurons, probably contributes to the enhanced ability of NMDA and ischemia to injure the neonatal brain.[45–49] Although other glutamate receptors contribute to damage from HIE, the NMDA receptor appears to be a primary mediator through which hypoxia-ischemia triggers HIE.

The NMDA receptor channel complex at excitatory synapses impaired by severe asphyxia may become involved in a vicious cycle that perpetuates injury as well as prolongs clinical signs of HIE.[50] NMDA receptor channel opening is dependent upon membrane potential, which in turn is influenced by neuronal energy state.[51] Hypoxia can contribute to NMDA channel opening by reducing energy available for oxidative phosphorylation in mitochondria.[52,53] Energy deficiency reduces power to ionic pumps that maintain neuronal membrane potential by restoring ionic gradients to normal levels following neuronal depolarization. Neuronal depolarization, mediated in part by activation of α-amino-3-hydroxy-5-methyl-4-isoxazole propionate-type (AMPA) glutamate receptors during normal neuronal activity and during seizures, can consume energy and passively open NMDA channels.[50] This cycle of oxidative stress, membrane depolarization, and NMDA channel opening could contribute to the seizures and paroxysmal EEG activity seen in HIE.[54] Supporting evidence for the role of NMDA receptor overstimulation in neonatal encephalopathy is provided by studies of infants with nonketotic hyperglycinemia (NKH), a genetic disorder in which glycine is elevated in the cerebrospinal fluid.[55] NKH is associated with seizures, encephalopathy, and burst-suppression EEG abnormalities resembling those that are seen following asphyxia. These abnormalities improve after the reduction of glycine plasma levels and administration of the NMDA antagonist dextromethorphan.[55]

A Model for Understanding the Interactions Between Hypoxia and Ischemia in HIE

A model for understanding the interactions between severe hypoxia and ischemia that cause synaptic dysfunction in HIE is shown in Figure 1. Hypoxia and ischemia can act at two different but intersecting components of the glutamate synapse to synergistically enhance the opening of the NMDA receptor channel. Severe hypoxemia can impair mitochondrial function and enhance the chances for NMDA channels

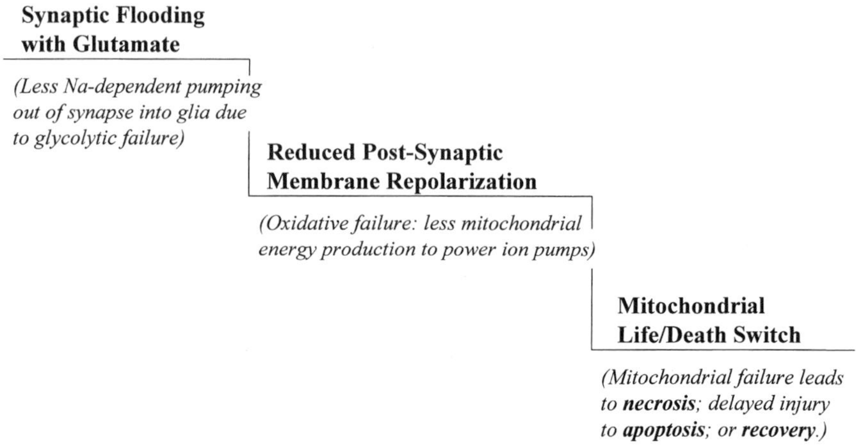

**Synaptic Flooding
with Glutamate**

*(Less Na-dependent pumping
out of synapse into glia due
to glycolytic failure)*

**Reduced Post-Synaptic
Membrane Repolarization**

*(Oxidative failure: less mitochondrial
energy production to power ion pumps)*

**Mitochondrial
Life/Death Switch**

*(Mitochondrial failure leads
to **necrosis**; delayed injury
to **apoptosis**; or recovery.)*

Figure 1. Brain energy failure; synergistic effects of hypoxia and ischemia on developing glutamate synapses. Schematic diagram of potential intersecting effects of hypoxemia and ischemia on developing synapses in hypoxic-ischemic encephalopathy (HIE). Oxidative failure tends to depolarize neuronal membranes, passively opening N-methyl-D-aspartate (NMDA) receptors and increasing the release of glutamate. This effect is modest as long as regional cerebral blood flow can increase to compensate, delivering adequate glucose to power glutamate reuptake pumps. However, when ischemia is superimposed on severe hypoxemia, both glycolytic and aerobic metabolism fail, adding increased levels of synaptic amino acids to produce maximal opening of depolarized post-synaptic NMDA receptors. This can provide the substrate for synergism between hypoxemia and ischemia that triggers HIE.

to open as a consequence of membrane depolarization.[51] However, this effect alone probably does not injure the brain without additional stimulation provided by elevated levels of glutamate and glycine. As described above, synaptic glutamate levels are expected to remain low in the presence of hypoxia with preserved cerebral blood flow because glutamate reuptake pumps are powered anaerobically by glucose.[25] However, ischemia superimposed on hypoxemia elevates synaptic glutamate levels by restricting the delivery of glucose, the primary fuel for the glutamate reuptake pumps. With this additional ischemic insult, elevated glutamate and glycine levels can enhance the opening of the depolarized NMDA receptors, causing maximal channel opening, neuronal depolarization, and calcium flooding into neurons. The model illustrates that hypoxemia and ischemia can synergize because they act independently on pre- and post-synaptic components of excitatory synapses, overlapping at the NMDA receptor. The synergy is based on the NMDA receptor's unique physiology, which requires simultaneous receptor occupancy by the neurotransmitter amino acids, glutamate and glycine, as well as membrane depolarization for channel opening. Under normal conditions, this special feature allows the NMDA receptor to integrate signals from multiple neuronal synapses.[16] The genetically programmed, enhanced physiologic function of the NMDA receptor-channel complex, which is required for expression of synaptic plasticity in the postnatal period, creates a virtual "Achilles heel" for rapidly developing neuronal circuits.

The Role of Calcium in Mediating a Delayed Neurotoxic Cascade

Dysfunction of glutamate synapses and excessive stimulation of NMDA receptors provide major triggers for HIE, but downstream events in the cascade take on a life of their own within a few hours (Figure 2). The initial period of intense hypoxia-ischemia may temporarily stimulate and depolarize NMDA and non-NMDA receptors maximally, causing them to be "locked open," effectively silencing electrophysiologic activity transiently.[56] Large amounts of calcium that flood depolarized neurons through NMDA receptor-operated channels, as well as voltage-sensitive calcium channels, can trigger a delayed chain of events which manifests as HIE and results in permanent brain injury.[57]

Calcium is an essential, multifaceted mediator in brain metabolism, and activation of several calcium-sensitive enzymes, including proteases and lipases, could mediate some of its neurotoxic actions.[57] The exact role of calcium overload in the neurotoxic cascade of HIE is still unclear, but accumulation of calcium within mitochondria has been shown to play an essential role in neuronal death in some experimental models.[58] Elevated intramitochondrial calcium levels may disrupt mitochondrial ionic gradients as well as stimulate production of reactive oxygen species from the electron transport chain.[58] Restoration of oxygen delivery to the brain in the face of elevated intracellular calcium may enhance the formation of oxygen free radicals (see Chapter 8).[58] Oxygen itself, in the form of either nitric oxide or reactive oxygen species has been proposed as a toxin for cells that have suffered a calcium flood.[59] This may contribute to the evolution of delayed signs of HIE after oxidative metabolism is transiently restored following resuscitation.[53,54]

In Figure 2, three potential pathways by which calcium overload may extend HIE are shown. For some neurons, overwhelming calcium flooding leads to implosion of mitochondrial ionic gradients and cellu-

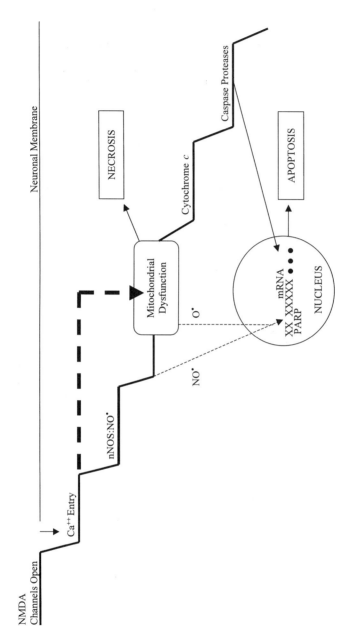

Figure 2. Overview of the excitotoxic cascade triggered in HIE. Synaptic dysfunction triggers a prolonged series of downstream biochemical events that is manifested by clinical signs of HIE. Two major pathways are shown, one leading to relatively quick necrotic death from overwhelming calcium overload, and the other to more protracted events. Events that unfold over several days during HIE can result in either survival or death by apoptosis or necrosis as described in the text. NMDA = N-methyl-D-aspartate; Ca = calcium ions; nNOS = neuronal nitric oxide synthase; NO = nitric oxide; O = oxygen free radicals; PARP = poly(ADP-ribose) polymerase; mRNA = messenger RNA.

lar membranes, irreversible energy failure, and necrosis. For neurons that escape such a severe assault, calcium-mediated activation of neuronal nitric oxide synthase (nNOS), and oxygen free radicals such as superoxide, may set in motion a more prolonged, subacute injury.[60,61] Nitric oxide and superoxide produced through oxidative stress in mitochondria can combine to form the toxic intermediate peroxynitrite, which is damaging for cell membranes and DNA.[60,61] The link between calcium and nNOS is particularly interesting in HIE, because the calcium that stimulates this enzyme is preferentially fluxed through the NMDA channel.[62]

The Role of Neuronal Nitric Oxide Synthase

This neurotransmitter free radical gas plays several roles in brain physiology, including the enhancement of neuronal activity and the dilation of blood vessels.[60,62] Several investigators have shown that nonspecific inhibitors of several isoforms of NOS can reduce injury in models of neonatal HIE.[63–66] Ferriero and colleagues showed that neonatal transgenic mice with reduced levels of nNOS had smaller areas of encephalomalacia than controls following carotid artery ligation combined with hypoxia[67] (see Chapter 8). The authors' studies found that a dose of the nNOS inhibitor 7-nitroindazole, sufficient to inhibit catalytic activity in cerebral cortex over 9 hours after the insult, produced a potent neuroprotective effect in 7-day-old rats. However, neuronal culture studies suggest that the NO-mediated mechanism is more important for mild to moderate NMDA-mediated injuries than for severe injuries. Injury mediated by nNOS is probably confined to the periphery or penumbra of an ischemic lesion, rather than its epicenter where few neurons survive.[60]

Nitric oxide and its toxic derivatives, including peroxynitrite, impair neuronal metabolism in part by causing damage to DNA, which in turn triggers DNA repair mechanisms (Figure 3).[68,69] Activation of the DNA repair enzyme poly(ADP-ribose) polymerase (PARP) is thought to play an important role in nitric oxide (NO)-mediated damage in neuronal culture and in adult stroke models. PARP is activated when DNA strands are broken by exposure to nitric oxide and peroxynitrite. PARP-mediated addition of adenosine diphosphate (ADP)-ribose units to nuclear proteins consumes mitochondrial nicotinamide adenine dinucleotide (NAD), which is needed to produce ADP. A deficiency of NAD impairs mitochondrial energy metabolism, producing further impairment in membrane potentials, and potentially con-

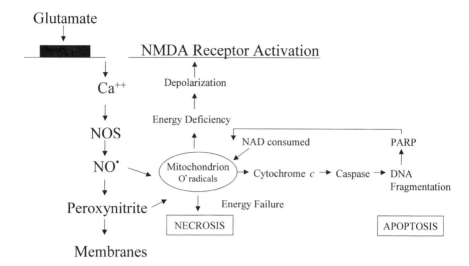

Figure 3. Schematic representation of feedback of mitochondrial dysfunction on the NMDA receptor, showing possible role of NO in effecting mitochondrial dysfunction in HIE. NO and peroxynitrite in the face of calcium overload can directly attack and depolarize the mitochondria. In addition, DNA breaks caused by NO and its derivatives can trigger activation of PARP, which can reduce NAD equivalents, further compromising mitochondrial energy metabolism. Mitochondrial dysfunction can lead to apoptosis by activation of caspase enzymes through release of proteins like cytochrome c. Severe mitochondrial dysfunction can enhance NMDA receptor channel opening and cause necrosis. NMDA = N-methyl-D-aspartate; Ca = calcium ions; NOS = nitric oxide synthase; NO = nitric oxide; NAD = nicotinamide adenine dinucleotide; PARP = poly(ADP-ribose) polymerase; DNA = deoxyribonucleic acid.

tributing to the opening of NMDA receptors.[51] These studies suggest that there could be a direct link between NMDA-mediated stimulation of nNOS activity and prolonged impairment of mitochondrial function during the period of HIE (Figure 2).

Continued production of NO and other reactive oxygen species after an asphyxial injury could contribute to the excitatory signs of encephalopathy in HIE because they can enhance pre-synaptic release of glutamate and cause prolonged mitochondrial dysfunction.[51,54,56,59,63] Our immunohistochemical studies indicate that nNOS-containing neurons proliferate processes for several days after an insult in injured brain regions such as the cortex and thalamus. Although it is unclear at this point how much of a contribution these nNOS-dependent mechanisms make to injury in clinical HIE, the experimental observations illustrate the kinds of sustained processes that could contribute to HIE.

The Role of Mitochondria as a Determinant of Whether Neurons Live or Die

The condition of mitochondria may play a decisive role in determining whether neurons survive or die during the period of HIE (Figures 2 and 3). A disorder of mitochondrial energy metabolism probably underlies the delayed energy failure observed using spectroscopy in both animal models of asphyxia and in asphyxiated human infants.[12] Persistent elevations of brain lactic acid in experimental models and in human infants during and after HIE also point to persistent mitochondrial dysfunction.[70] Defects in cerebral mitochondrial metabolism have been observed in the carotid artery ligation/hypoxia model of HIE in 7-day-old rats, and mitochondrial function improved following NMDA receptor blockade.[52] Ankarcrona et al demonstrated in neuronal cell culture that early or late mitochondrial failure could be produced by low- or high-dose exposure to NMDA.[54] High-dose NMDA exposure produced prompt collapse of the intramitochondrial membrane potential, loss of energy production, and cellular necrosis. On the other hand, low-dose exposure to NMDA caused delayed mitochondrial failure associated histologically with signs of apoptosis. In many cellular models, release of proteins such as cytochrome c from mitochondria provides an important trigger to activate cysteine protease enzymes involved in apoptosis.[71]

Apoptosis in Experimental HIE

Activation of cellular programs intended to fragment DNA and delete cells that are redundant or damaged is known as apoptosis (see Chapter 7). Recognition that apoptosis is a significant and potentially modifiable death pathway in the developing brain has stimulated great interest.[72–75] The relative contribution of apoptosis versus necrosis appears to depend on several factors such as age, brain region, temperature, and the type of insult. Neuronal cell culture studies suggest that immature neurons may be more prone to death by apoptosis.[76] It is noteworthy that in an experimental model of brain trauma, apoptotic neuronal death was far more prominent in the first week of life than at later times.[77] This is consistent with the observation that NMDA-mediated injury reaches a peak at this age and that apoptosis occurs naturally in many areas of the brain during the first weeks of life.[45,49] In rodents, this mechanism is used to "prune" unneeded neurons. Treatment of 7-day-old rats with drugs that inhibit caspase enzymes involved in apoptosis has been shown to provide substantial neuroprotection against damage from HIE,[78] suggesting that this extension of the excitotoxic cascade is important in HIE (Figure 2).

Histopathologic study of excitotoxic cell death in the developing brain suggests that apoptosis and necrosis form a continuum of death options rather than a strict dichotomy.[79] Electron microscopic studies of neonatal rodents following intracerebral injections of excitatory amino acid agonists indicate that cells fitting the criteria for both apoptosis and necrosis, as well as hybrid cells, can be seen. In the 7-day-old rat unilateral carotid artery ligation/hypoxia model, the authors found large populations of apoptotic cells (Figure 4). Many cells with necrotic patterns had a fragmented nuclear pattern suggesting broken DNA. The authors followed the tempo of necrosis and apoptosis in this model and found two distinct patterns. In areas such as the thalamus, a wave of apoptotic cell death was completed within

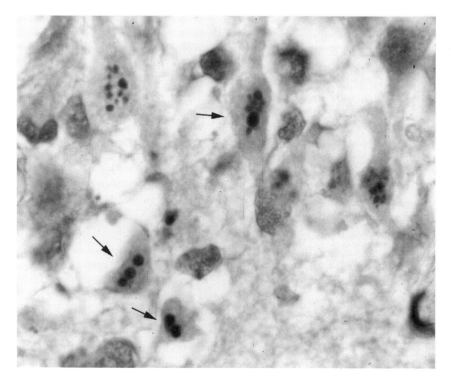

Figure 4. Apoptosis in 7-day-old hypoxic-ischemic rat cortex. Apoptotic nuclei visualized on Nissl staining in the cerebral cortex 48 hours after ipsilateral carotid artery ligation plus hypoxia (8% oxygen) at 7 days of age.

2 to 3 days, while in other areas such as the cerebral cortex, populations of cells with apoptotic morphology persisted for a week or more. These findings are consistent with the hypothesis that the mode of death in the apoptosis/necrosis continuum is influenced by the location of neurons in the brain and the intensity of the excitotoxic insult.[27]

Brain temperature appears to influence the balance between apoptosis and necrosis in the neuropathology of HIE.[80] Deep hypothermia (see Chapter 14) can markedly reduce injury when circulatory arrest is used to support complicated heart surgery in infants.[68,81] A similar period of cardiac arrest at normothermia produces extensive brain damage with marked cerebral edema and necrosis. When brain injury does occur with hypothermic circulatory arrest, the encephalopathy is often delayed for several hours after recovery from anesthesia, and injury is often focal rather than generalized. In an experimental model of hypothermic injury, injury is also quite selective and apoptosis is prominent.[81] Apoptosis in this model is associated with activation of NO production over several hours following reperfusion, and treatment with either MK-801 or nNOS inhibitors can block apoptosis. This suggests that the delayed encephalopathy seen in some infants after cardiac surgery may be related to delayed triggering of apoptotic death programs. Mild post-insult hypothermia can markedly prolong the time over which cell death occurs in the 7-day-old rat unilateral carotid artery ligation/hypoxia model. This may also be related to its ability to modify the relative contributions of necrosis and apoptosis as well as the time over which they evolve.[80]

Modification of the Neurotoxic Cascade in Human HIE

Research on HIE demonstrates important parallels between the clinical disorder in human infants and experimental models (Table 1). The human and animal experimental data are consistent with the current concept of HIE as a prolonged cascade of biochemical events triggered by an initial excitotoxic insult. Although many of the details based on experimental models have yet to be confirmed in humans, a number of key events suggest important parallels. For example, the selective vulnerability of the cerebral cortex, putamen, and thalamus to hypoxic-ischemic injuries in newborns is very similar in rats, piglets, and humans. Elevations in extracellular glutamate levels and delayed onset of seizures that persist over several days during HIE are seen in human infants and animal models. Delayed energy failure as

Table 1

Parallels Between HIE in Human Infants and Experimental Models

- Selective vulnerability of cortex, thalamus, and putamen to severe asphyxial injury in rats, piglets, and humans.
- Elevations in extracellular or cerebral spinal fluid glutamate and glycine in HIE.
- Delayed energy failure, prolonged elevations in lactate concentration in human infants and experimental models.
- Delayed onset of seizures, and evolution of EEG changes in humans and animal models.
- Delayed, prolonged evolution of histologic and imaging changes in brain.
- Neuroprotective effect of hypothermia to delay cascade in human infants undergoing cardiac surgery and in animal models.
- Apoptosis and necrosis identified in human postmortem tissue and in animal models of HIE.

EEG = electroencephalogram; HIE = hypoxic-ischemic encephalopathy.

well as persistent elevations in cerebral lactate concentrations are also present in both experimental models and infants, suggesting that mitochondrial dysfunction plays a key role in determining the outcome of human HIE. Postmortem studies, although limited, suggest that apoptosis also plays a prominent role together with necrosis in human infants. These studies point to multiple newly recognized downstream events, such as caspase activity and programmed cell death, that could potentially be blocked or impeded to salvage brain tissue when given at longer intervals after the initial insult.

Although progress in understanding the pathogenesis of HIE makes it plausible that effective therapies can be developed to salvage brain tissue in human infants, a number of factors make this a challenging endeavor. Current difficulties in making a specific diagnosis and assessing severity and duration of asphyxia prior to birth are impediments to designing effective treatment protocols. The medical instability of infants with HIE, who usually have multiorgan dysfunction, is another concern when administering therapies with potential systemic side effects. The paucity of approved drugs with actions on specific targets is also a problem. However, the authors' current concept of the HIE neurotoxic cascade extending over several days after a severe insult provides a framework for the investigation of effective therapies. This conceptual framework suggests that protocols that combine inhibition of multiple, e.g., mild hypothermia, glutamate blockade, and caspase inhibition, might provide synergistic protective effects.[82–84]

Table 2 provides one possible therapeutic "cocktail" for hypoxic-ischemic injury, as well as probable mechanisms of action and poten-

Table 2

Potential Therapeutic "Cocktail" for Salvaging Hypoxic-Ischemic Brain Injury in the Neonate

Intervention	Mechanism	Potential Drawback
Brain cooling	Reduces glutamate release; inhibits proteolysis; slows cascade, lengthens interventions	Systemic effects; local head cooling may not reach core Window for downstream effects
NMDA receptor blockade by infusion: ketamine or dextromethorphan	Inhibits excitoxicity, calcium overload	? Enhanced apoptosis
GABA receptor stimulation: high-dose barbiturate or benzodiazepine	? Synergistic with NMDA blockade; anticonvulsant	Ventilatory support
Caspase inhibitor	Blocks caspase execution of apoptosis	Current peptides not approved, do not cross into brain

NMDA = N-methyl-D-aspartate; GABA = gamma aminobutyric acid.

tial drawbacks of the therapy. It is anticipated that, in the future, these interventions might be monitored using new techniques such as near-infrared spectroscopy, continuous EEG, magnetic resonance spectroscopy and, possibly, intracerebral microdialysis and temperature monitoring. Better indicators of the status of brain metabolism are needed to assess how much intervention is warranted, as well as to monitor its efficacy. If surface cooling of the head is used to induce hypothermia, monitoring of regional intracerebral brain temperature may be particularly important. Recent studies using a model of the human head suggests that surface cooling may not reach into deep regions such as the basal ganglia.[85]

References

1. Vannucci RC, Perlman JM: Interventions for perinatal hypoxic-ischemic encephalopathy. Pediatrics 1997;100:1004–1014.
2. Johnston MV, Trescher WH, Taylor GA: Hypoxic and ischemic central nervous system disorders in infants and children. Adv Pediatr 1995;42:1–45.
3. Myers RE: Experimental models of perinatal brain damage: relevance to

human pathology. In Gluck L (ed): *Intrauterine Asphyxia and the Developing Fetal Brain.* Year Book Medical Publishers, Chicago, 1977, pp 37–97.

4. Himwich WA, Beneron HB, Tucker BE, et al: Metabolic studies of the perinatal human brain. J Appl Physiol 1959;14:873–877.

5. Altman DI, Perlman JM, Volpe JJ, et al: Cerebral oxygen metabolism in newborns. Pediatrics 1993;92:99–104.

6. Vannucci RC: Experimental biology of cerebral hypoxia-ischemia: relation to perinatal brain damage. Pediatr Res 1990;27:317–326.

7. Sarnat HB, Sarnat MS: Neonatal encephalopathy following fetal distress. Arch Neurol 1976;33:696–705.

8. Levene MI, Grindulis H, Sands C, Moore JR: Comparison of two methods of predicting outcome in perinatal asphyxia. Lancet 1986;i:67–68.

9. Nelson KB, Ellenberg JH: Neonatal signs as predictors of cerebral palsy. Pediatrics 1979;64:225–232.

10. Perlman JM, Risser R: Can asphyxiated infants at risk for neonatal seizures be rapidly identified by current high-risk markers? Pediatrics 1996;97:456–462.

11. Williams CE, Gunn AJ, Synek B, Gluckman PD: Delayed seizures occurring with hypoxic-ischemic encephalopathy in the fetal sheep. Pediatr Res 1990;27:561–565.

12. Azzopardi D, Wyatt JS, Cady EB, et al: Prognosis of newborn infants with hypoxic-ischemic brain injury assessed by phosphorus magnetic resonance spectroscopy. Pediatr Res 1989;25:445–451.

13. Towfighi J, Zec N, Yager J, et al: Temporal evolution of neuropathological changes in an immature rat model of cerebral hypoxia-ischemia: a light microscopic study. Acta Neuropathologica 1995;90:375–386.

14. Albensi BC, Schweizer MP, Rarick TM, et al: Unilateral hypoxic-ischemic injury in the neonatal rat brain evaluated by in vivo MRI. Invest Radiol 1999;34:249–261.

15. Barkovich AJ, Westmark K, Partridge JC, et al: Perinatal asphyxia: MR findings in the first 10 days. Am J Neuroradiol 1995;16:427–438.

16. McDonald JW, Johnston MV: Physiological and pathophysiological roles of excitatory amino acids during central nervous system development. Brain Res Rev 1990;15:41–70.

17. Delivoria-Papadopoulos M, Mishra OP: Mechanisms of cerebral injury in perinatal asphyxia and strategies for prevention. J Pediatr 1998;132:S30–S34.

18. Hagberg H: Glycine and modulation of the NMDA receptor after severe asphyxia. Acta Pediatr 1999;88:1049–1050.

19. Roldan A, Figueras-Aloy J, Deulofeu R, Jimenez R: Glycine and other neurotransmitter amino acids in cerebrospinal fluid in perinatal asphyxia and neonatal hypoxic-ischemic encephalopathy. Acata Paediatr 1999;88:1137–1141.

20. Silverstein FS, Naik B, Simpson J: Hypoxia-ischemia stimulates hippocampal glutamate efflux in perinatal rat brain: an in vivo microdialysis study. Pediatr Res 1986;30:587–590.

21. Hagberg H, Andersson P, Kjellmer I, et al: Extracellular overflow of glutamate, aspartate, GABA and taurine in the cortex and basal ganglia of fetal lambs during hypoxia-ischemia. Neurosci Letters 1987;78:311–317.

22. Hagberg H, Thornberg E, Blennow M, et al: Excitatory amino acids in the

cerebral spinal fluid of asphyxiated infants: relationship to hypoxic-ischemic encephalopathy. Acta Paediatr 1993;82:925–929.

23. Riikonen RS, Kero PO, Simell OG: Excitatory amino acids in cerebrospinal fluid in neonatal asphyxia. Pediatr Neurol 1992;8:37–40.

24. Silverstein FS, Buchanan K, Johnston MV: Perinatal hypoxia-ischemia disrupts striatal high-affinity [3H] glutamate uptake into synaptosomes. J Neurochem 1986;47:1614–1619.

25. Magistretti PJ, Pellerin DL, Rothman DL, et al: Energy on demand. Science 1999;283:496–497.

26. Ichord RN, Northington FJ, VanWylen D, et al: Brain O_2 consumption and glutamate efflux during hypoglycemic coma in piglets are temperature sensitive. Am J Physiol 1999;276:H2053–H2062.

27. Johnston MV: Selective vulnerability in the developing brain. Ann Neurol 1998;44:155–156.

28. Menkes JH, Curran J: Clinical and MR correlates in children with extrapyramidal cerebral palsy. Am J Neuroradiol 1994;15:451–457.

29. Hoon AH, Reinhardt EM, Kelley RI, et al: Brain MRI in suspected extrapyramidal cerebral palsy: observations in distinguishing genetic-metabolic from acquired causes. J Pediatr 1997;131:240–245.

30. Roland EH, Poskitt K, Rodriguez E, et al: Perinatal hypoxic-ischemic thalamic injury: clinical features and neuroimaging. Ann Neurol 1998; 44:161–166.

31. Maller AI, Hankins LL, Yeakley JW, et al: Rolandic type cerebral palsy in children as a pattern of hypoxic-ischemic injury in the full term infant. J Child Neurol 1998;13:313–321.

32. Martin LJ, Brambrink A, Koehler RC, et al: Primary sensory and fore-brain motor systems in the newborn brain are preferentially damaged by hypoxia-ischemia. J Comp Neurol 1997;377:262–285.

33. Alexander GE, Crutcher MD: Functional architecture of basal ganglia circuits: neural substrates of parallel proceeding. Trends Neurosci 1990; 13:266–271.

34. Greenamyre JT, Penney JB, Young AB, et al: Evidence for a transient perinatal glutamatergic innervation of globus pallidus. J Neurosci 1987; 34:41–50.

35. Chugani HT: Metabolic imaging: a window on brain development and plasticity. Neuroscientist 1999;5:29–40.

36. Blennow M, Ingvar M, Lagercrantz H, et al: Early [18F]FDG positron emission tomography in infants with hypoxic-ischaemic encephalopathy shows hypermetabolism during the postasphyctic period. Acta Paediatr 1995;84:1289–1295.

37. Martin LJ, Brambrink AM, Lehmann C, et al: Hypoxia-ischemia causes abnormalities in glutamate transporters and death of astroglia and neurons in newborn stratus. J Comp Neurol 1997;42:335–348.

38. Kemp JA, Leeson PD: The glycine site of the NMDA receptor five years on. Trends Pharmacol Sci 1993;14:20–25.

39. Hagberg H, Gilland E, Diemer NH, et al: Hypoxia-ischemia in the neonatal rat brain: histopathology after post-treatment with NMDA and non-NMDA receptor antagonists. Biol Newborn 1994;66:206–213.

40. McDonald JW, Silverstein FS, Johnston MV: MK-801 protects the neonatal brain from hypoxic-ischemic damage. Eur J Pharmacol 1987;140:359–361.

41. Hattori H, Morin AM, Schwartz PH, et al: Posthypoxic treatment with MK-801 reduces hypoxic-ischemic damage in the neonatal rat. Neurology 1989;39:713–718.

42. Spandou E, Karkavelas G, Soubasi V, et al: Effect of ketamine on hypoxic-ischemic brain damage in newborn rats. Brain Res 1999;819:1–7.

43. Thordstein M, Bagenholm R, Thiringer K, et al: Scavengers of free oxygen radicals in combination with magnesium sulphate ameliorate perinatal hypoxic-ischemic brain injury in the rat. Pediatr Res 1993;34:23–26.

44. Marret S, Gressens P, Gadisseux J-F, et al: Prevention by magnesium of excitotoxic neuronal death in the developing brain: an animal model for clinical intervention studies. Dev Med Child Neurol 1995;37:473–484.

45. McDonald JW, Silverstein FS, Johnston MV: Neurotoxicity of N-methyl-D-aspartate is markedly enhanced in developing rat central nervous system. Brain Res 1988;459:200–203.

46. Rabacchi S, Bailly Y, Delhaye-Bouchaud N, et al: Involvement of the NMDA receptor in synapse elimination during cerebellar development. Science 1992;256:1823–1825.

47. Sheng M, Cummings J, Rolau LA, et al: Changing subunit composition of heteromeric NMDA receptors during development of rat cortex. Nature 1994;368:144–147.

48. Burgard EC, Hablitz JJ: Developmental changes in NMDA and non-NMDA receptor mediated synaptic potentials in rat neocortex. J Neurophysiol 1993;69:230–240.

49. Ikonomidou C, Mosinger JL, Labruyere J, et al: Sensitivity of the developing rat brain to hypobaric/ischemic damage parallels sensitivity to NMDA neurotoxicity. J Neurosci 1989;9:2809–2818.

50. Strijbos PJLM, Leach MJ, Garthwaite J: Vicious cycle involving Na^+ channels, glutamate release, and NMDA receptors mediates delayed neurodegeneration through nitric oxide formation. J Neurosci 1996;16:5004–5013.

51. Novelli A, Reilly JA, Lysko PG, et al: Glutamate becomes neurotoxic via NMDA receptors when intracellular energy levels are reduced. Brain Res 1988;451:205–212.

52. Gilland E, Puka-Sundvall M, Hillered L, et al: Mitochondrial function and energy metabolism after hypoxia-ischemia in the immature brain: involvement of NMDA receptors. J Cereb Blood Flow Metab 1998;18:297–304.

53. Abe K, Aoki M, Kawagoe J, et al: Ischemic delayed neuronal death, a mitochondrial hypothesis. Stroke 1995;26:1478–1489.

54. Ankarcrona M, Dypbukt JM, Bonfoco E, et al: Glutamate-induced neuronal death: a succession of necrosis or apoptosis depending on mitochondrial function. Neuron 1995;15:961–973.

55. Hamosh A, McDonald JW, Valle D, et al: Dextromethorphan and high dose benzoate therapy for non-ketotic hyperglycinemia in an infant. J Pediatr 1992;121:131–135.

56. Hammond C, Crepel V, Gozlan H, et al: Anoxic LTP sheds light on the multiple facets of NMDA receptors. Trends Neurosci 1994;17:497–503.

57. Kristian T, Siesjo BK: Calcium-related damage in ischemia. Life Sci 1996;59:357–367.

58. Stout AK, Raphael HM, Kanterewicz BI, et al: Glutamate-induced neuron death requires mitochondrial calcium uptake. Nature Neurosci 1998;1:366–373.

59. Keelan J, Vergun O, Duchen MR: Excitotoxic mitochondrial depolarization requires both calcium and nitric oxide in rat hippocampal neurons. J Physiol 1999;520:797–813.
60. Strijbos PJLM: Nitric oxide in cerebral ischemic neurodegeneration and excitotoxicity. Crit Rev Neurobiol 1998;12:223–243.
61. Choi YB, Tenneti L, Le DA, et al: Molecular basis of NMDA receptor-coupled ion channel modulation by S-nitrosylation. Nat Neurosci 2000;3:15–21.
62. Christopherson KS, Hillier BJ, Lim WA, et al: PSD-95 assembles a ternary complex with the NMDA receptor and a bivalent neuronal NO synthase PDZ domain. J Biol Chem 1999;274:67–73.
63. Kara P, Friedlander MJ: Dynamic modulation of cerebral cortex synaptic function by nitric oxide. Prog Brain Res 1998;118:183–198.
64. Ashwal S, Cole DJ, Osborne S, et al: L-NAME reduces infarct volume in a filament model of transient middle cerebral artery occlusion in the rat pup. Pediatr Res 1995;38:652–656.
65. Hamada Y, Hayakawa T, Hattori H, et al: Inhibitor of nitric oxide synthesis reduces hypoxic-ischemic brain damage in the neonatal rat. Pediatr Res 1994;35:10–14.
66. Trifiletti R: Neuroprotective effects of N-nitro-arginine in focal stroke in the 7-day old rat. Eur J Pharmacol 1999;218:197–198.
67. Ferriero DM, Holtzman DM, Black SM, et al: Neonatal mice lacking neuronal nitric oxide synthase are less vulnerable to hypoxic-ischemic injury. Neurobiol Dis 1996;3:652–656.
68. Tseng EE, Brock MV, Lange MS, et al: Neuronal nitric oxide synthase inhibition reduces neuronal apoptosis after hypothermic circulatory arrest. Ann Thorac Surg 1997;64:1639–1647.
69. Eliasson MJL, Sampei K, Mandir AS, et al: Poly (ADP-ribose) polymerase gene disruption renders mice resistant to cerebral ischemia. Nature Med 1997;3:1089–1095.
70. Hanrahan JD, Cox IJ, Edwards AD: Persistent increases in cerebral lactate concentration after birth asphyxia. Pediatr Res 1998;44:304–311.
71. Schulz JB, Weller M, Moskowitz MA: Caspases as treatment targets in stroke and neurodegenerative diseases. Ann Neurol 1999;45:421–429.
72. Beilharz EJ, Williams CE, Dragunow M, et al: Mechanisms of delayed cell death following hypoxic-ischemic injury in the immature rat: evidence for apoptosis during selective neuronal loss. Brain Res Mol Brain Res 1995; 29:1–14.
73. Edwards AD, Mehmet H: Apoptosis in perinatal hypoxic-ischemic cerebral damage. Neuropathol Appl Neurobiol 1996;22:494–498.
74. Edwards AD, Yue X, Cox P, et al: Apoptosis in the brains of infants suffering intrauterine cerebral injury. Pediatr Res 1997;42:684–689.
75. Yue X, Mehmet H, Penrice J, et al: Apoptosis and necrosis in the newborn piglet brain following transient cerebral hypoxia-ischemia. Neuropathol Appl Neurobiol 1997;23:16–25.
76. McDonald JW, Behrens MI, Chung C, et al: Susceptibility to apoptosis is enhanced in immature cortical neurons. Brain Res 1997;759:228–232.
77. Bittigau P, Sifringer M, Pohl D, et al: Apoptotic neurodegeneration following trauma is markedly enhanced in the immature brain. Ann Neurol 1999;45:724–735.
78. Cheng Y, Deshmukh MD, Costa A, et al: Caspase inhibitor affords neuro-

protection after delayed administration in a rat model of neonatal hypoxic-ischemic brain injury. J Clin Invest 1998;101:1992–1999.

79. Martin LJ, Al-Abdulla NA, Brambrink AM, et al: Neurodegeneration in excitotoxicity, global cerebral ischemia, and target deprivation: a perspective on the contributions of apoptosis and necrosis. Brain Res Bull 1998; 46:281–309.

80. Trescher WH, Ishiwa S, Johnston MV: Brief post-hypoxic-ischemic hypothermia markedly delays neonatal brain injury. Brain Dev 1997; 19: 326–338.

81. Kupsky WJ, Drozd MA, Barlow CF: Selective injury of the globus pallidus in children with post-cardiac surgery choreic syndrome. Dev Med Child Neurol 1995;37:135–144.

82. Ma J, Endres M, Moskowitz MA: Synergistic effects of caspase inhibitors and MK-801 in brain injury after transient focal cerebral ischemia in mice. Br J Pharmacol 1998;124:756–762.

83. Zhu FK, Namura S, Shimizu-Sasamata M: Prolonged therapeutic window for ischemic brain damage caused by delayed caspase activation. J Cereb Blood Flow Metab 1998;18:1071–1076.

84. Hicks CA, Ward MA, Swettenham JB, O'Neill MJ: Synergistic neuroprotective effects by combining an NMDA or AMPA receptor antagonist with nitric oxide synthase inhibitors in global cerebral ischaemia. Eur J Pharmacol 1999;381:113–119.

85. Nelson DA, Nunnley SA. Brain temperature and limits on transcranial cooling in humans: quantitative modeling results. Eur J Appl Physiol Occup Physiol 1998;78:353–359.

CHAPTER 4

Inflammation and Neonatal Brain Injury

John D.E. Barks, Faye S. Silverstein

Introduction

In the late 1990s, there was a resurgence of interest in the role of intrauterine infection as a mediator of perinatal brain damage. Recent epidemiologic, clinical, and experimental data implicate inflammatory mediators in the pathogenesis of periventricular white matter injury (periventricular leukomalacia [PVL]) in the neonatal brain. This chapter provides a review of the clinicopathologic syndrome of PVL, the epidemiologic data implicating maternal infection/inflammation as a significant risk factor for PVL, and some of the experimental strategies used to gain insights about this distinctive mechanism of neonatal brain injury.

Periventricular Leukomalacia: Clinicopathologic Correlations

Oligodendroglia are specialized glial cells that form the myelin sheath in the central nervous system (CNS). Oligodendroglial maturation is a relatively late developmental event, and in the normal preterm, and even full-term, infant there is little myelination in the forebrain. In the preterm brain, oligodendroglia exist either as pre-oligodendrocytes (mitotically active cells committed to their fates as oligodendroglia) or as immature oligodendrocytes (post-mitotic, immature oligodendroglia). These cells can be detected based on their morphologies, location in the brain, and expression of developmental stage-specific antigens. Clinicians have long recognized the heightened susceptibility of oligoden-

Supported by U.S. Public Health Service grants Neurologic Sciences 35059 (Faye Silverstein, M.D.) and Neurologic Sciences 37036 (John D.E. Barks, M.D.).
From Donn SM, Sinha SK, Chiswick ML (eds): *Birth Asphyxia and the Brain: Basic Science and Clinical Implications.* © 2002, Futura Publishing Co., Inc., Armonk, NY.

droglia in the developing brain to ischemic injury; yet, the cellular and molecular mechanisms underlying this developmental stage-specific vulnerability of immature oligodendroglia to hypoxia-ischemia are unknown.

Neuropathology

Periventricular leukomalacia is a distinctive pattern of subcortical white matter injury first recognized neuropathologically over a century ago. In 1962, Banker and Larroche provided a classic report of the major neuropathologic features, and the three phases of this disorder.[1] Even though there is very little myelin in the neonatal brain, it is possible to identify the acute neuropathologic lesions of PVL. Yet, it is also important to emphasize that the lesion evolves, and in some respects becomes more pronounced over time, as the deficits in myelination become more apparent with CNS maturation.

Acutely, focal lesions are characterized by areas of coagulative necrosis, i.e., loss of all cellular elements in the core (astrocytes, oligodendroglia, and axons), with nuclear pyknosis and tissue spongiosis. Also seen are "axonal spheroids," a consequence of focal disruption of axons in the lesion core. Subsequently, in postmortem tissue samples evaluated 1–10 days after an acute insult, a prominent feature is an inflammatory response characterized by infiltration of microglia-macrophages, astrocytic hypertrophy and proliferation, and then, neovascularization. Later, the lesions evolve either to cysts surrounded by gliosis or noncystic gliotic scars. In long-term survivors, periventricular cysts or *ex vacuo* ventriculomegaly are grossly apparent. Microscopically, loss of myelin in PVL lesions is readily discerned using myelin-specific stains (e.g., Luxol-Fast Blue). The neuroanatomic distribution and severity of white matter injury varies considerably in surviving infants; lesions may be restricted to periventricular regions and/or extend into the subcortical white matter.[1,2]

Ultrasonography

With the advent of ultrasonography, it became feasible to diagnose PVL *in vivo*. Sonographic correlates of the acute PVL lesion include detection of increased echogenicity superolateral to the lateral ventricles, a finding that is neither particularly sensitive nor specific.[3,4] More chronic lesions include cysts in the periventricular white matter, superolateral to the lateral ventricles.[5] Another imaging pattern that is sometimes considered a variant of PVL is an expansion of the ventricular system, in the absence of cysts, or periventricular scarring. Whether this, in fact, represents a lesion in the continuum of the PVL spectrum, or a distinct pattern of perinatal white matter injury, is an important unanswered question.[6]

Clinical Syndrome

It is well recognized in clinical practice that premature infants are at highest risk for the development of the form of cerebral palsy (CP) known as spastic diplegia, a static motor encephalopathy characterized predominantly by weakness and spasticity of the both legs. The upper extremities are often also affected, but to a lesser degree. In the past 10 years, magnetic resonance imaging (MRI) has enabled stronger delineation of the association between chronic periventricular white matter injury and spastic diplegia.[7-9] It is also now apparent that the vulnerability of immature white matter to ischemic injury extends to term newborns and young infants. For example, a recent MRI-based study revealed unexpected white matter abnormalities in a group of infants with congenital heart disease.[10] The radiologic identification of periventricular white matter injury in infants born at term, who had no identifiable perinatal difficulties, has also raised questions about the timing of the insult that resulted in this pattern of brain injury. It has been hypothesized that, in term infants with no identified perinatal adverse events, evidence of white matter injury implicates a prenatal insult.[11]

The neurodevelopmental deficits associated with PVL are complex, variable, and often difficult to predict accurately in preschool children. Little is known about the potential range of adaptive responses of injured oligodendroglia in the immature brain. Yet, it is readily apparent that, particularly in infants born prematurely, periventricular white matter injury is strongly associated with long-term neurodevelopmental abnormalities leading to significant health care costs.

Epidemiology

The first epidemiologic study that provided some important information about PVL was the National Institutes of Health National Collaborative Perinatal Project. In some infants from this cohort who underwent postmortem examination, there was evidence of PVL.[12] In this group, significant associations with PVL included prematurity

(28–31 weeks), bacteremia (9-fold increased risk), maternal urinary tract infection (2.5-fold increased risk), and maternal urinary tract infection with fever (420-fold increased risk). Another independent analysis of the National Collaborative Perinatal Project data revealed some similar trends; prolonged rupture of the membranes and chorioamnionitis were associated with an increased risk of CP, independent of their contribution to low birthweight.[13,14] Subsequently, conflicting data emerged regarding the relationship between maternal infection and the risk for PVL. One postmortem study reported an association between PVL and gram-negative bacteremia,[15,16] whereas another found no association between either sepsis or hypotension, and PVL.[17]

Through the 1980s and early 1990s, the focus of attention shifted to the evaluation of cardiovascular factors (e.g., hypotension, hypocarbia-induced cerebral vasoconstriction) that were implicated in the pathogenesis of PVL.[18–22] This emphasis stemmed from analysis of the vascular supply of the periventricular white matter and the interpretation that this region was in an end-arterial border zone in premature infants. This vascular pattern was developmental stage-specific, and provided an attractive potential mechanism to explain the susceptibility of the premature fetus/newborn to PVL.[23,24] During this period, reports of an association between infection and PVL were infrequent.[25]

In the 1990s, there was a resurgence of interest in the role of maternal infection in the pathogenesis of neonatal white matter injury. Several studies reported an association between evidence of intrauterine infection and either PVL or CP. Of particular interest with respect to the relationship between neonatal white matter injury and intrauterine infection, several studies reported an association between evidence of intrauterine infection and subsequent risk of spastic diplegia; this association was also discerned in term infants.[26–36]

Tables 1 and 2 highlight important trends that have emerged from these recent studies. A retrospective cohort study reported that prolonged rupture of the membranes and chorioamnionitis were predictive of bilateral cystic PVL in infants with a birthweight of less than 1750 g.[26] Remarkably, most of these infants had relatively benign neonatal courses, without episodes of hypotension. Similarly, analysis of a cohort of preterm infants, of 24–32 weeks gestation, revealed a very high risk of cystic PVL (22%) in infants with histories of both premature rupture of the membranes and intrauterine infection.[27] In contrast, intrauterine growth retardation or preeclampsia were seldom associated with PVL. In a study of 500–1500 g infants, chorioamnionitis was associated with an increased risk of PVL, as well as grade 3 or 4 intraventricular hemorrhage (IVH) and neonatal

Table 1

Evidence for an Association Between Intrauterine Infection or Inflammation and Periventricular Leukomalacia

Gestation or Birthweight	N	Risk Factor (n)	Percent with Risk Factor Having Cystic PVL	Incidence of PVL in Entire Cohort	Ref. No.
< 1750 g	632	PPROM (38)	29%	2.3%	26
		Chorioamnionitis (24)	21%		
24–32 wk	753	PPROM (144)	17%	9%	27
		Intrauterine infection (202)	19%		
		PPROM + intrauterine infection (98)	22%		
500–1500 g, ≥ 24 wk	1367	Chorioamnionitis (95)	11%	3.5%	28
25–33 wk	349	Maternal UTI (58)	16%	5.7%	29
500–1500 g	1078	Fetal vasculitis, membrane inflammation, <1 hr ROM (82)	15% (late PVL, detected after day 14)	2.8%	30

PVL = periventricular leukomalacia; PPROM = prolonged preterm rupture of membranes; UTI = urinary tract infection; ROM = rupture of membranes.

seizures.[28] In another investigation examining a group of infants of 25–33 weeks gestation, maternal urinary tract infection, and all maternal infections combined, were associated with an increased risk of bilateral cystic PVL.[29] In a multi-institution study in which placental and membrane pathology was evaluated in all cases, fetal vasculitis was strongly associated with periventricular echolucencies, particularly those detected late, (i.e., more than 2 weeks after birth).[30] In a population-based case-control study of infants born at less than 32 weeks gestation who developed CP, antenatal or intrapartum factors associated with an increased risk of CP were chorioamnionitis, prolonged rupture of the membranes, and maternal bacterial infection other than chorioamnionitis[31]; intrauterine growth retardation, however, was not associated with CP, and preeclampsia was associated with a reduced risk. In another case-control study, chorioamnionitis

Table 2

Evidence for an Association Between Intrauterine Infection or Inflammation and Cerebral Palsy

Gestation or Birthweight	N	Risk Factor	Odds Ratio (95% CI)	Method	Ref. No.
<32 wk	59 cases 235 controls	Chorioamnionitis PPROM Maternal infection	3.9 (1.3–11)* 2.3 (1.2–4.2)* 2.3 (1.2–4.5)*	Case-control	31
<1500 g	42 cases 75 controls	Chorionitis (with birth >5 hr after admission)	4.3 (1.1–13)	Case-control	32
24–33 wk	363	PPROM (>48 hr)	2.88 (1.22–6.83)*	Cohort	33
≤1500 g	312	POL or PROM	2.7 (1–7.3)*	Cohort	34
500–1500 g	62 cases 124 controls	Chorioamnionitis	2.6 (1.1–6.0)*	Case-control	35
<33 wk	203	PPROM PPROM with POL	4.3 (1.6–11.8)* 7.5 (2.2–26.2)*	Cohort	36

*Adjusted odds ratio.
CI = confidence interval; PROM = prelabor rupture of membranes; PPROM = prolonged preterm rupture of membranes; POL = preterm onset of labor.

was associated with CP within the subgroup of mothers who delivered more than 5 hours after hospital admission; this association was strengthened if neonatal seizures ensued.[32] In a report of 24–33 weeks gestation infants in which survivors were followed to 2 years corrected age, prolonged (>48 hr) rupture of the membranes was associated with CP.[33] Other studies also support the association of either chorioamnionitis, preterm rupture of the membranes, or prolonged preterm rupture of the membranes with CP (Table 2). Of note, in several of the cited studies, the associated cases of CP were predominantly of the spastic diplegia subtype.[32,34,35]

The association of intrauterine infection/inflammation and CP is apparently not unique to premature infants. In a case-control study of infants identified from a population-based register using the criteria of a diagnosis of CP and a birthweight ≤ 2500 g, maternal fever and clinically diagnosed chorioamnionitis were both associated with the subsequent diagnosis of CP.[37]

Inflammation and Neonatal Brain Injury

Clinical Evidence Linking Cytokines with Perinatal Brain Injury

The reports cited in Tables 1 and 2 raise compelling questions about the underlying mechanisms that could link maternal infection with fetal/neonatal brain injury. The majority of infants with PVL and a history of potential exposure to intrauterine infection had neither bacteremia nor meningitis. This led several investigators to hypothesize that soluble inflammatory mediators could be involved, such as cytokines derived from the maternal circulation, and that the immaturity of the blood-brain barrier might facilitate transport of potentially toxic inflammatory mediators into the brain.

Cytokines are soluble proteins produced in many tissues, which can act locally and/or circulate and exert their effects at remote sites. Their cellular targets and signaling mechanisms are complex and incompletely understood. Within the CNS, cytokines play physiologic and pathologic roles, and their effects may vary depending on the cellular target (e.g., oligodendroglia or neurons) and maturational stage. It is often particularly difficult experimentally to detect the pathogenetic role of a specific cytokine because these signaling molecules interact in many complex direct and indirect ways.

In the 1990s, refinement of the analytical methods for measurement of pro-inflammatory cytokines in human tissue samples or body fluids provided the impetus to study their roles in preterm birth, as well as in contributing to the adverse respiratory and CNS sequelae of prematurity. Table 3 summarizes some important trends that emerged from these reports.

The work of Yoon, Romero, and collaborators provided data linking premature labor with evidence of an intrauterine inflammatory cytokine response, and implicated overt or subclinical chorioamnionitis as the inciting event.[38] In addition, these investigators found strong associations between the intrauterine cytokine response and a subsequent diagnosis of PVL.

Among the cytokines most strongly linked to premature labor and chorioamnionitis were tumor necrosis factor alpha (TNF-α), interleukin-1 beta (IL-1β), and interleukin-6 (IL-6). In a group of women who underwent clinically indicated amniocentesis prior to full term and who delivered within 72 hours after the procedure, elevated amniotic fluid levels of IL-1β and IL-6 were associated with two adverse outcomes, an early sonographic diagnosis of PVL, and a subsequent diagnosis of CP.[39] Yet, highlighting the complexity of the pathogenesis of

Table 3

Evidence Linking Pro-Inflammatory Cytokines with Perinatal Brain Injury

Gestation or Birthweight	N (Study Type)	Associated Cytokine(s) (Fluid or Tissue)	Outcome of Interest	Result or Odds Ratio (95% CI)	Ref. No.
25–36 wk	172 (cohort)	IL-6 ≥ 400 pg/mL (cord blood)	PVL-associated lesions*	6.2 (2–19.1)	40
26–35 wk	94 (cohort)	IL-6 ≥ 2.95 pg/mL IL-1β ≥ 32 pg/mL (amniotic fluid)	PVL-associated lesions*	5.7 (1.3–14.4) 4.4 (1.1–17.0)	39
28–41 wk (cases) 28–41 wk (controls)	17 PVL cases 17 controls	TNF-α, IL-1β, or IL-6 immunoreactivity (autopsy)	Cytokine expression in PVWM	15/17 cases 3/17 controls	41
23–27 wk (cases) 21–28 wk (controls)	13 PVL cases 9 controls	TNF-α immunoreactivity (autopsy)	Cytokine expression in PVWM	9/13 cases 0/9 controls	42
Mostly term	31 CP cases 65 controls	Immunoaffinity chromatography, multiple cytokines, chemokines, coagulation factors (blood spots)	CP	Il-1β, IL-6, IL-8, IL-9, IL-13, TNF-α in CP cases exceeded controls	43
Mostly term	31 CP cases 65 controls	Immunoaffinity chromatography, interferons-α, -β, and -γ (blood spots)	CP	14/31 cases, IFNs exceeded controls, with elevated cytokines; 17/31 cases IFNs in control range; 13/17 with pro-coagulation factor elevations	44

*PVL-associated lesions defined as either: periventricular white matter cysts; localized ventriculomegaly adjacent to area of increased white matter echogenicity; persistent abnormally increased periventricular echogenicity; or autopsy findings of PVL.
PVWM = periventricular white matter; CP = cerebral palsy; PVL = periventricular leukomalacia; IL-6 = interleukin-6; IL-1β = interleukin-1 beta; TNF-α = tumor necrosis factor alpha; IFNs = interferons.

spastic diplegia, it should be noted that cytokine expression did not predict which of the infants with early PVL later developed CP.

The same group also found that in a series of consecutive preterm (25–36 weeks) births, elevation of cord blood levels of IL-6 occurred more frequently in infants with sonographic evidence of PVL.[40] In a related case-control postmortem study of premature infants, TNF-α, IL-1β, or IL-6 were localized to reactive microglia or astrocytes in the periventricular white matter by immunohistochemistry in 15 of 17 (88%) of PVL cases versus 3 of 17 (18%) non-PVL cases.[41] Other investigators have reported similar findings.[42]

Nelson et al used a novel approach to evaluate the relationship between cytokines and neonatal brain injury.[43] These investigators developed a large number of ultramicro-immunoassays and evaluated archived newborn screen blood samples for expression of multiple cytokines (including IL-1β, IL-6, TNF-α, and interferon-γ [IFN-γ]) and coagulation factors. One of the most robust trends that emerged from their analyses was that in a group of 31 children in whom spastic diplegia was subsequently diagnosed (most were born at term), levels of multiple cytokines and chemokines in neonatal blood samples were much higher than in controls. This correlation was not evident in those children who developed hemiparetic CP. Grether et al subsequently found that in the 31 children with spastic CP, there were 14 with concentrations of interferons that were higher than in any child in the control group, whereas in the other 17 the values were similar to those in controls.[44] In those 14 of 31, other cytokine levels tended to be markedly elevated as well, while levels of complement components were low (presumably reflecting consumption). A distinct subgroup of patients was also identified in whom there was an association between abnormalities of coagulation factors and CP; these cases did not overlap with the pro-inflammatory cytokine cases.

Thus, compelling epidemiologic data now link maternal infection and pro-inflammatory mediators in the neonatal systemic circulation with an increased risk of PVL and/or spastic diplegia. Yet, these data provide no insights about the underlying pathophysiologic mechanisms by which cytokines could injure immature oligodendroglia. The following hypotheses have been raised: (1) induction of hypotension and subsequent hypoperfusion in the watershed periventricular regions of the neonatal brain; (2) induction of a pro-inflammatory phenotype in the cerebral microvasculature, which would increase susceptibility to other inflammatory stimuli; (3) stimulation of production of other potentially deleterious inflammatory mediators in the fetal/neonatal circulation; (4) disruption of the blood-brain barrier, allowing greater exposure to toxic mediators; and (5) initiation or amplification of a CNS inflammatory response initiated by other forms of brain injury (e.g., ischemia). Currently, there is no evidence to support any of these hypotheses. Yet, one factor that provides a strong impetus for the investigation of the roles of inflammatory mediators in the pathogenesis of neonatal brain injury is the potential for therapeutic intervention with a rapidly expanding range of anti-inflammatory agents.

Experimental Evidence

Research to address the influence of inflammation on the expression of neonatal brain injury has incorporated several complementary approaches. Studies have been done to determine if inflammatory mediators could cause brain injury or modulate the progression of tissue injury, and also to examine injury-initiated inflammatory responses in the brain.

Do Inflammatory Mediators Cause Brain Injury?

Some of the earliest experimental evidence for an inflammatory etiology of PVL comes from the work of Gilles et al.[45] These investigators developed animal models of endotoxin-induced "perinatal telencephalic leukoencephalopathy" in the 1970s. Striking pathologic similarities to PVL were described, especially in their feline model, but there was also some evidence of white matter injury in monkeys and rats.[5]

One important challenge has been to develop relevant animal models for examining how a pro-inflammatory milieu could alter vulnerability to hypoxic-ischemic injury *in utero*. One of the first encouraging strategies was developed by Yoon et al.[46] These researchers evaluated the impact of intrauterine inoculations of *E. coli* in pregnant rabbits on fetal neuropathology and were able to discern white matter lesions in some surviving fetuses 5 to 6 days later. The pathology included increased karyorrhexis in the periventricular white matter consistent with coagulation necrosis in 10 of 12 and focal rarefaction and disorganization of periventricular white matter in 2 of 12. The variable outcome and high intercurrent fetal mortality were limitations of this approach.

In a recent study, Cai et al treated pregnant rats with the potent pro-inflammatory stimulus lipopolysaccharide (derived from gram-negative bacteria cell wall).[47] These authors documented increases in cytokine gene expression in fetal rat brain and subtle evidence of altered glial responses in early postnatal life (increased expression of glial fibrillary acidic protein and decreased expression of myelin basic protein). Whether these changes reflect long-lasting white matter injury remains to be determined, but the data lend credence to the notion that maternally derived systemic pro-inflammatory signaling can influence postnatal brain integrity.

Similarly, a study by Dommergues et al provided complementary experimental evidence that circulating cytokines could damage developing white matter.[48] In this study, performed in neonatal mice, 5-day-old animals received intracerebral injections of ibotenate, an excitatory amino acid agonist. This procedure elicits an age-dependent lesion, which at 5 days involves both cortex and white matter along injection sites. The investigators administered several different cytokines, by repeated systemic injection prior to intracerebral injection of ibotenate, and evaluated the extent of brain injury in comparison with vehicle-injected controls. Pretreatment with several pro-inflammatory cytokines (including IL-1β, IL-6, IL-9, or TNF-α) resulted in more extensive cortical and white matter damage. Of note, the cytokines alone did not elicit overt brain injury. These trends suggested that certain pro-inflammatory cytokines could alter tissue responses to excitotoxins. There are considerable data that pathophysiologic insults such as cerebral ischemia result in marked release of the endogenous excitotoxin glutamate. Thus, this experimental paradigm may be relevant for modeling the effects of antecedent and concurrent exposure to pro-inflammatory stimuli at the time of a perinatal hypoxic-ischemic insult.

Several pro-inflammatory cytokines can exert deleterious effects on oligodendroglia. Studies performed in the context of understanding the pathogenesis of immune-mediated demyelination (e.g., in experimental autoimmune encephalitis) have highlighted the pathogenetic role of cytokines and chemokines in demyelination.[49] Immature oligodendroglia have distinctive patterns of responsiveness to pro-inflammatory cytokines, which could contribute to their patterns of vulnerability to injury. For example, the cytotoxic effects of TNF-α and IFN-γ are greatest in immature oligodendroglia.[50,51]

Does Hypoxic-Ischemic Brain Injury Elicit Inflammation?

Studies performed in a neonatal rodent stroke model have provided important insights about the inflammatory response initiated by acute hypoxic-ischemic brain injury in the immature brain. In addition, these studies have also provided some evidence that anti-inflammatory interventions could attenuate tissue injury. In 7-day-old rats, carotid ligation followed by 1.5–3 hours of exposure to 8% oxygen (O$_2$) elicits ipsilateral forebrain ischemic injury.[52] During hypoxia, cerebral blood flow declines ipsilaterally (<10% baseline); normal cerebral blood flow returns when animals again breathe room air (i.e., this model incorporates both focal cerebral ischemia and reperfusion).[53,54] The original description of histopathology in this model emphasized the distinctive white matter vulnerability of the immature brain to ischemia.[52] White matter necrosis, originating in and spreading from myelinogenic foci, is a prominent feature. Thus, although this model does not precisely replicate human neonatal neuropathology, it can be used to generate relevant information about developmental stage-specific mechanisms. In this model, hypoxic-ischemic brain injury elicits an acute inflammatory response characterized by increased expression of pro-inflammatory cytokines including chemokines,[55–57] a rapid microglial/monocyte response,[58,59] and gliosis.[60] Some features of inflammation persist for at least 5 weeks.[57] This neonatal stroke model has also been successfully adapted for neonatal mice.[61,62]

Many cell types, both resident brain cells and blood-derived leukocytes, contribute to acute and chronic inflammation in brain pathology. Microglia, resident macrophages that constitute 5–10% of brain cells, play important pathophysiologic roles in the brain's responses to diverse forms of injury.[63] In human neuropathology, microglia are implicated in the pathophysiology of CNS acquired immunodeficiency syndrome (AIDS), multiple sclerosis, and Alzheimer's disease.[63] In P7 rat brain, hypoxic-ischemic injury elicits a rapid and intense microglial response.[58,59]

Activated microglia have the potential to exert both adverse and beneficial effects in the recovery period after CNS injury, and the factors that determine their predominant effects in the setting of brain injury are incompletely understood. In fact, in the context of understanding the impact of inflammation on the ultimate expression of brain injury, a frequent theme is that a specific mediator may have the potential to amplify injury and/or to induce repair. The predominant mode of action may depend on a multitude of factors, including: maturational stage; the cell types that are injured and recruited to the area of injury; the combination of mediators secreted; and the expression of specific receptors for these mediators on diverse cells in the territory of injury. Although relatively little is known about microglial function in human infant brain, there is indirect evidence that microglia in the newborn could generate inflammatory mediators; *in vitro* studies have shown that human fetal microglia produce and respond to a broad range of cytokines and chemokines.

Interleukin (IL)-1β was one of the first pro-inflammatory cytokines implicated in the pathogenesis of ischemic brain injury.[64] Its role in the setting of acute ischemic brain injury is complex. Recent studies to evaluate the impact of administration of exogenous IL-1β or of an IL-1 receptor antagonist in adult stroke models have shown that both the timing of administration (before or after the ischemic event) and the injection site (cortex or striatum) determine whether IL-1β contributes predominantly to tissue damage or to neuroprotection mechanisms.[65] IL-1β is produced as an inactive precursor "pro-IL-1"; IL-1-converting enzyme (ICE), a member of the cysteine protease "caspase" family, plays a critical role in production of mature IL-1β. ICE-deficient mice are resistant to ischemic brain injury, both as newborns and as adults. This trend is consistent with a role for IL-1β in worsening ischemic brain injury.[62,66] It should also be noted that ICE has additional substrates, including pro-IL-1β, also known as IFN-γ-inducing factor, so it could also be conceivable that resistance to ischemic brain injury reflected reduced IFN-γ production. Another potential confounding factor in analysis of the mechanisms that account for reduced vulnerability to ischemic injury in ICE-deficient animals is that members of the caspase enzyme family regulate apoptosis. Although there is currently no evidence that ICE regulates neuronal apoptosis, the possibility that these animals are relatively resistant to injury-induced apoptosis has not been fully excluded.

Several pharmacologic agents with complex modes of action that include attenuation of specific components of the inflammatory cascade have also been shown to confer neuroprotection in this model. Of particular clinical relevance, some of these agents retain therapeutic efficacy even when administered after the hypoxic-ischemic insult. For example, post-hypoxia-ischemia treatment with BN 52021, a drug that acts as an antagonist of the pro-inflammatory lipid mediator platelet-activating factor, substantially decreased the incidence of cerebral infarction.[67]

Future Directions for Research

Future research will focus on an increased understanding of the following processes: (1) how inflammation initiated by acute brain injury influences the ultimate expression of tissue damage; (2) how perinatal stressors such as maternal infection can induce a pro-inflammatory milieu and thus amplify inflammatory responses to brain injury; and (3) how critical components of this inflammatory response can be modulated to improve neurologic outcome. The degree to which inflammatory mediators cause injury and/or contribute to ultimate tissue repair is poorly understood. Yet, the data highlighted in this chapter provide strong support for the hypothesis that, in the brain, as in other organs, induction of inflammatory mechanisms does contribute to tissue injury. A greater understanding of these mechanisms may enable therapeutic modulation after the onset of injury in order to attenuate the deleterious effects and, perhaps, to amplify intrinsic recovery mechanisms.

In addition, studies are needed that incorporate both experimental work in relevant animal models and clinical data to answer the following questions: (1) Do cytokines derived from the maternal circulation, the placenta, or the fetus, in response to infection or other stimuli, reach the fetal brain (perhaps because of immaturity of the blood-brain barrier)? (2) Are cytokines directly toxic to the immature brain and/or do they alter susceptibility to other agents or insults? (3) Are there maturational-stage-determined vulnerabilities of distinct cell types to specific pro-inflammatory cytokines? (4) Do present anti-inflammatory strategies represent an effective therapeutic modality in newborns at high risk for adverse neurodevelopmental outcome?

References

1. Banker BQ, Larroche JC: Periventricular leukomalacia of infancy: a form of neonatal anoxic encephalopathy. Arch Neurol 1962;7:386–410.
2. Rorke LB: *Pathology of Perinatal Brain Injury*. Raven Press, New York, 1982.
3. Carson SC, Hertzberg BS, Bowie JD, Burger PC: Value of sonography in the diagnosis of intracranial hemorrhage and periventricular leukomalacia: a postmortem study of 35 cases. Am J Roentgenol 1990;155:595–601.
4. DiPietro MA, Brody BA, Teele RL: Peritrigonal echogenic "blush" on cranial sonography: pathologic correlates. Am J Roentgenol 1986;146:1067–1072.
5. Bowerman RA, Donn SM, DiPietro MA, et al: Periventricular leukomalacia in the pre-term newborn infant: sonographic and clinical features. Radiology 1984;151:383–388.
6. Leviton A, Gilles F: Ventriculomegaly, delayed myelination, white matter hypoplasia, and "periventricular" leukomalacia: how are they related? Pediatr Neurol 1996;15:127–136.
7. de Vries LS, Eken P, Groenendaal F, et al: Correlation between the degree of periventricular leukomalacia diagnosed using cranial ultrasound and MRI later in infancy in children with cerebral palsy. Neuropediatrics 1993;24:263–268.
8. Olsen P, Paakko E, Vainionpaa L, et al: Magnetic resonance imaging of periventricular leukomalacia and its clinical correlation in children. Ann Neurol 1997;41:754–761.
9. Okumura A, Kato T, Kuno K, et al: MRI findings in patients with spastic

cerebral palsy. II. Correlation with type of cerebral palsy. Dev Med Child Neurol 1997;39:369–372.

10. du Plessis AJ: Mechanisms of brain injury during infant cardiac surgery. Semin Pediatr Neurol 1999;6:32–47.

11. Truwit CL, Barkovich AJ, Koch TK, Ferriero DM: Cerebral palsy: MR findings in 40 patients. Am J Neuroradiol 1992;13:67–78.

12. Leviton A, Gilles FH: Acquired perinatal leukoencephalopathy. Ann Neurol 1984;16:1–8.

13. Nelson KB, Ellenberg JH: Obstetric complications as risk factors for cerebral palsy or seizure disorders. JAMA 1984;251:1843–1848.

14. Nelson KB, Ellenberg JH: Predictors of low and very low birth weight and the relation of these to cerebral palsy. JAMA 1985;254:1473–1479.

15. Leviton A, Gilles FH: An epidemiologic study of perinatal telencephalic leucoencephalopathy in an autopsy population. J Neurol Sci 1973;18: 53–66.

16. Leviton A, Gilles F, Neff R, Yaney P: Multivariate analysis of risk of perinatal telencephalic leucoencephalopathy. Am J Epidemiol 1976;104:621–626.

17. Shuman RM, Selednik LJ: Periventricular leukomalacia: a one-year autopsy study. Arch Neurol 1980;37:231–235.

18. Donn SM, Bowerman RA: Association of paroxysmal supraventricular tachycardia and periventricular leukomalacia. Am J Perinatol 1986;3:50–52.

19. Calvert SA, Hoskins EM, Fong KW, Forsyth SC: Etiological factors associated with the development of periventricular leukomalacia. Acta Paediatr Scand 1987;76:254–259.

20. de Vries LS, Regev R, Dubowitz LM, et al: Perinatal risk factors for the development of extensive cystic leukomalacia. Am J Dis Child 1988; 142:732–735.

21. Watkins AM, West CR, Cooke RW: Blood pressure and cerebral haemorrhage and ischaemia in very low birthweight infants. Early Hum Dev 1989;19:103–110.

22. Graziani LJ, Spitzer AR, Mitchell DG, et al: Mechanical ventilation in preterm infants: neurosonographic and developmental studies. Pediatrics 1992;90:515–522.

23. Wigglesworth JS, Pape KE: An integrated model for haemorrhagic and ischaemic lesions in the newborn brain. Early Hum Dev 1978;2:179–199.

24. Takashima S, Tanaka K: Development of cerebrovascular architecture and its relationship to periventricular leukomalacia. Arch Neurol 1978; 35:11–16.

25. Faix RG, Donn SM: Association of septic shock caused by early-onset group B streptococcal sepsis and periventricular leukomalacia in the preterm infant. Pediatrics 1985;76:415–419.

26. Perlman JM, Risser R, Broyles RS: Bilateral cystic periventricular leukomalacia in the premature infant: associated risk factors. Pediatrics 1996; 97:822–827.

27. Zupan V, Gonzalez P, Lacaze-Masmonteil T, et al: Periventricular leukomalacia: risk actors revisited. Dev Med Child Neurol 1996;38:1061–1067.

28. Alexander JM, Gilstrap LC, Cox SM, et al: Clinical chorioamnionitis and the prognosis for very low birth weight infants. Obstet Gynecol 1998; 91:725–729.

29. Spinillo A, Capuzzo E, Stronati M, et al: Obstetric risk factors for periven-

tricular leukomalacia among preterm infants. Br J Obstet Gynaecol 1998;105:865–871.
30. Leviton A, Paneth N, Reuss ML, et al: Maternal infection, fetal inflammatory response, and brain damage in very low birth weight infants. Pediatr Res 1999;46:566–575.
31. Murphy DJ, Sellers S, MacKenzie IZ, et al: Case-control study of antenatal and intrapartum risk factors for cerebral palsy in very preterm singleton babies. Lancet 1995;346:1449–1454.
32. Grether JK, Nelson KB, Emery ES III, Cummins SK: Prenatal and perinatal factors and cerebral palsy in very low birth weight infants. J Pediatr 1996;128:407–414.
33. Spinillo A, Capuzzo E, Orcesi S, et al: Antenatal and delivery risk factors simultaneously associated with neonatal death and cerebral palsy in preterm infants. Early Hum Dev 1997;48:81–91.
34. Dammann O, Allred EN, Veelken N: Increased risk of spastic diplegia among very low birth weight children after preterm labor or prelabor rupture of membranes. J Pediatr 1998;132:531–535.
35. O'Shea TM, Klinepeter KL, Meis PJ, Dillard RG: Intrauterine infection and the risk of cerebral palsy in very low-birthweight infants. Paediatr Perinat Epidemiol 1998;12:72–83.
36. Burguet A, Monnet E, Pauchard JY, et al: Some risk factors for cerebral palsy in very premature infants: importance of premature rupture of membranes and monochorionic twin placentation. Biol Neonate 1999; 75:177–186.
37. Grether JK, Nelson KB: Maternal infection and cerebral palsy in infants of normal birth weight. JAMA 1997;278:207–211.
38. Romero R, Gomez R, Ghezzi F, et al: A fetal systemic inflammatory response is followed by the spontaneous onset of preterm parturition. Am J Obstet Gynecol 1998;179:186–193.
39. Yoon BH, Jun JK, Romero R, et al: Amniotic fluid inflammatory cytokines (interleukin-6, interleukin-1β, and tumor necrosis factor-α), neonatal brain white matter lesions, and cerebral palsy. Am J Obstet Gynecol 1997; 177:19–26.
40. Yoon BH, Romero R, Yang SH, et al: Interleukin-6 concentrations in umbilical cord plasma are elevated in neonates with white matter lesions associated with periventricular leukomalacia. Am J Obstet Gynecol 1996;174:1433–1440.
41. Yoon BH, Romero R, Kim CJ, et al: High expression of tumor necrosis factor-alpha and interleukin-6 in periventricular leukomalacia. Am J Obstet Gynecol 1997;177:406–411.
42. Deguchi K, Oguchi K, Takashima S: Characteristic neuropathology of leukomalacia in extremely low birth weight infants. Pediatr Neurol 1997; 16:296–300.
43. Nelson KB, Dambrosia JM, Grether JK, Phillips TM: Neonatal cytokines and coagulation factors in children with cerebral palsy. Ann Neurol 1998;44:665–675.
44. Grether JK, Nelson KB, Dambrosia JM, Phillips TM: Interferons and cerebral palsy. J Pediatr 1999;134:324–332.
45. Gilles FH, Averill DR Jr, Kerr CS: Neonatal endotoxin encephalopathy. Ann Neurol 1977;2:49–56.

46. Yoon BH, Kim CJ, Romero R, et al: Experimentally induced intrauterine infection causes fetal brain white matter lesions in rabbits. Am J Obstet Gynecol 1997;177:797–802.
47. Cai Z, Pan Z-L, Pang Y, et al: Cytokine induction in fetal rat brains and brain injury in neonatal rats after maternal lipopolysaccharide administration. Pediatr Res 2000;47:64–72.
48. Dommergues MA, Patkai J, Renauld JC, et al. Proinflammatory cytokines and IL-9 exacerbate excitotoxic lesions of the newborn murine neopallium. Ann Neurol 2000;47:54–63.
49. Hartung HP, Jung S, Stoll G, et al: Inflammatory mediators in demyelinating disorders of the CNS and PNS. J Neuroimmunol 1992;40:197–210.
50. Andrews T, Zhang P, Bhat NR: TNF alpha potentiates IFN gamma-induced cell death in oligodendrocyte progenitors. J Neurosci Res 1998;54:574–583.
51. Baerwald KD, Popko B: Developing and mature oligodendrocytes respond differently to the immune cytokine interferon-gamma. J Neurosci Res 1998;52:230–239.
52. Rice JE, Vannucci RC, Brierley JB: The influence of immaturity on hypoxic-ischemic brain damage in the rat. Ann Neurol 1981;9:131–141.
53. Vannucci RC, Lyons DT, Vasta F: Regional cerebral blood flow during hypoxia-ischemia in immature rats. Stroke 1988;19:245–250.
54. Mujsce DJ, Christensen MA, Vannucci RC: Cerebral blood flow and edema in perinatal hypoxic-ischemic brain damage. Pediatr Res 1990;27:450–453.
55. Szaflarski J, Burtrum D, Silverstein FS: Cerebral hypoxia-ischemia stimulates cytokine gene expression in perinatal rats. Stroke 1995;26:1093–1100.
56. Hagberg H, Gilland E, Bona E, et al: Enhanced expression of interleukin (IL)-1 and IL-6 messenger RNA and bioactive protein after hypoxia-ischemia in neonatal rats. Pediatr Res 1996;40:603–609.
57. Bona E, Andersson AL, Blomgren K, et al: Chemokine and inflammatory cell response to hypoxia-ischemia in immature rats. Pediatr Res 1999;45:500–509.
58. McRae A, Gilland E, Bona E, Hagberg H: Microglia activation after neonatal hypoxic-ischemia. Dev Brain Res 1995;84:245–252.
59. Ivacko JA, Sun R, Silverstein FS: Hypoxic-ischemic brain injury induces an acute microglial reaction in perinatal rats. Pediatr Res 1996;39:39–47.
60. Burtrum D, Silverstein FS: Hypoxic-ischemic brain injury stimulates glial fibrillary acidic protein mRNA and protein expression in neonatal rats. Exp Neurol 1994;126:112–118.
61. Ferriero DM, Holtzman DM, Black SM, Sheldon RA: Neonatal mice lacking neuronal nitric oxide synthase are less vulnerable to hypoxic-ischemic injury. Neurobiol Dis 1996;3:64–71.
62. Liu XH, Kwon D, Schielke GP, et al: Mice deficient in interleukin-1 converting enzyme are resistant to neonatal hypoxic-ischemic brain damage. J Cereb Blood Flow Metab 1999;19:1099–1108.
63. Gonzalez-Scarano F, Baltuch G: Microglia as mediators of inflammatory and degenerative diseases. Annu Rev Neurosci 1999;22:219–240.
64. Rothwell NJ, Relton JK: Involvement of interleukin-1 and lipocortin-1 in ischaemic brain damage. Cerebrovasc Brain Metab Rev 1993;5:178–198.
65. Stroemer RP, Rothwell NJ: Exacerbation of ischemic brain damage by

localized striatal injection of interleukin-1beta in the rat. J Cereb Blood Flow Metab 1998;18:833–839.

66. Schielke GP, Yang GY, Shivers BD, Betz AL: Reduced ischemic brain injury in interleukin-1β converting enzyme-deficient mice. J Cereb Blood Flow Metab 1998;18:180–185.

67. Liu XH, Eun BL, Silverstein FS, Barks JDE: The platelet-activating factor antagonist BN 52021 attenuates hypoxic-ischemic brain injury in the immature rat. Pediatr Res 1996;40:797–803.

CHAPTER 5

Glucose, Acidosis, and the Developing Brain

Robert C. Vannucci, Susan J. Vannucci

Introduction

Normal cerebral development and consequent function requires that an adequate amount of metabolizable substrate be supplied to the brain during the perinatal period. It has long been known that glucose is the primary energy substrate for the adult brain, and investigations indicate that glucose is also the predominant cerebral fuel for fetal and newborn animals under normal physiologic conditions.[1-5] Presumably, glucose is an obligate source of energy for the fetal and newborn human brain, although studies have been limited to older infants and children.[6] However, under conditions of starvation, suckling, and hypoglycemia, other organic substrates are capable of supplementing glucose in infants, children, and adults.[6,7] The most prominent alternate cerebral fuels include the ketone bodies, β-hydroxybutyrate and acetoacetate, and lactic acid.[8-11] Furthermore, these substrates are present in biologically significant concentrations in the blood of newborn and suckling infants.[12-14]

Of additional importance to normal cerebral development and function is the maintenance of an optimal intracellular pH of brain, including neurons and glial elements. Alterations in Pco_2 of blood will translate immediately to alterations in brain intracellular pH, owing to the diffusibility of carbon dioxide (CO_2) across the blood-brain barrier. Alteration in the blood bicarbonate (HCO_3^-) does not acutely change brain intracellular pH, although chronic metabolic acidemia or alkalemia will ultimately lead to similar changes in brain and cere-

This work has been supported by the National Institute of Child Health and Human Development (Program Project HD30704; RCV and SJV), and the American Heart Association, the American Diabetes Association, and the United Cerebral Palsy Foundation (RCV).

From Donn SM, Sinha SK, Chiswick ML (eds): *Birth Asphyxia and the Brain: Basic Science and Clinical Implications.* © 2002, Futura Publishing Co., Inc., Armonk, NY.

brospinal fluid.[15,16] Accordingly, it is necessary that brain intracellular pH remains tightly controlled for normal function to proceed.

Hyperglycemia and Perinatal Hypoxic-Ischemic Brain Damage

Research conducted many years ago demonstrated that pretreatment of perinatal animals with glucose prolongs their survival when subjected to systemic hypoxemia, asphyxia, or cerebral ischemia,[17–19] and might reduce permanent brain damage as well.[20,21] In contrast to the apparent increased hypoxic-ischemic resistance of glucose-treated immature animals, more recent experiments in juvenile and adult animals have shown that glucose supplementation actually accentuates hypoxic-ischemic brain damage. Accordingly, a paradox exists regarding the effect of glucose on hypoxic-ischemic brain damage; specifically, glucose prolongs hypoxic-ischemic survival of immature animals while increasing brain damage in adults.

Myers and Yamaguchi were the first investigators to champion the proposal that glucose pretreatment accentuates hypoxic-ischemic brain damage. These investigators subjected juvenile rhesus monkeys (aged 2–4 years) to total cerebral ischemia produced by circulatory arrest. All of the animals had been food-deprived for 12–24 hours, but three of ten animals received a glucose infusion shortly prior to circulatory arrest. All of the monkeys were successfully resuscitated following cardiopulmonary arrest. Two of the three glucose-treated monkeys exhibited severe to profound neurologic deficits following resuscitation, and neuropathologic examination revealed extensive brain damage with widespread necrosis involving the cerebral cortex, basal ganglia, brainstem, and cerebellum. In the majority of animals not receiving glucose, neuropathologic analysis revealed little or no brain damage. Based on their investigation, Myers and Yamaguchi speculated that glucose supplementation prior to circulatory arrest "augments the severity of brain injury and alters its distribution."[22]

Experiments from several other research laboratories have confirmed and extended the original observation that glucose pretreatment of mature animals accentuates hypoxic-ischemic brain damage.[23–29] Furthermore, genetically diabetic db/db mice and pancreatectomized diabetic dogs, both with associated hyperglycemia, exhibit more extensive brain damage arising from cerebral hypoxia-ischemia than normoglycemic control animals.[30,31] Clinical studies of adult human stroke patients also support the notion that hyperglycemia with or without antecedent diabetes mellitus accentuates ischemic neuronal injury.[32–34]

The pathophysiologic mechanism(s) by which glucose accentuates brain damage in juvenile and adult animals has, in large part, been related to an excessive production of tissue lactic acid or to an associated derangement in pH homeostasis of the brain.[35–38] In this regard, it has been shown that the injection of lactic acid into the cerebral cortex of adult rats leads to histologic alterations resembling ischemic infarction, an injury that does not occur following injection of other organic acids of comparable pH.[39–41] It has been proposed that excessive lactic acid production during hyperglycemic cerebral hypoxia-ischemia results from a greater acceleration of anaerobic glycolytic flux than that which occurs when the circulating glucose concentration is not increased. Furthermore, glial elements, specifically astrocytes, appear to be a primary buffer of cellular pH in the brain. Kraig and associates have shown that astrocytes are capable of achieving and maintaining an extremely low pH (approximately 6.0) during ischemia, suggesting that these cells act to buffer excess hydrogen ions produced by anaerobic glycolysis.[42,43] With hyperglycemia superimposed upon cerebral ischemia, tissue acidosis exceeds the astrocytic buffering capacity, leading to both glial and neuronal death, i.e., infarction.[24]

Given the apparent paradox that glucose prolongs hypoxic-ischemic survival of immature animals while increasing brain damage in adults, a series of experiments were performed on a rat model of perinatal hypoxic-ischemic brain damage developed in the authors' laboratory 20 years ago.[44] In this model, 7-day postnatal rats are subjected to unilateral common carotid artery ligation followed thereafter by exposure to hypoxia (8% oxygen), an insult that produces permanent injury to the cerebral hemisphere ipsilateral to the carotid artery occlusion in the vast majority of animals. The 7-day-old rat was chosen for study because at this age the rat's brain roughly corresponds to that of a 32–34 week gestation human fetus or newborn infant; specifically, cerebral cortical layering is complete, the germinal matrix is involuting, and white matter is beginning to myelinate. Tissue injury is characterized by either selective neuronal death (necrosis or apoptosis) or infarction of selected structures of the cerebral hemisphere including cerebral cortex, hippocampus, striatum, and subcortical and periventricular white matter. Hypoxia-ischemia of 1.0–1.5 hours duration typically results in selective neuronal death, while longer durations of hypoxia-ischemia are associated with infarction.[44–46] The end-stage lesions closely mimic the neuropathologic entities of ulegyria and porencephaly observed in human fetuses and newborn infants subjected to cerebral hypoxia-ischemia.[47–49]

A preliminary study was conducted to confirm previous reports that glucose prolongs the hypoxic survival of developing animals.[50] Immature rats received a 0.1 mL subcutaneous injection of either 50% glucose or normal saline. The glucose injection was associated with a near threefold increase in blood glucose concentrations for up to 90 minutes, decreasing thereafter into the normoglycemic range. Hyperglycemia did not occur in the saline-treated controls. Fifteen minutes following the glucose injections, the rat pups were exposed to hypoxia produced by the inhalation of 8% oxygen. The animals were examined at 15-minute intervals, and the time when death occurred was recorded. The glucose-supplemented rats survived more than twice as long as their control litter mates. Specifically, the duration of hypoxia required to kill 50% of the saline-treated animals (LD_{50}) was 3.5 hours compared with an LD_{50} of 8 hours for the glucose-treated rat pups.

More recently, the authors undertook a neuropathologic analysis of glucose- and saline-treated immature rats exposed to the same duration (2 hours) of hypoxia-ischemia.[51] Seven-day postnatal rats received 0.2 mL 50% glucose at the onset of hypoxia-ischemia, followed by 0.15 mL 25% glucose 1 hour later to maintain glucose concentrations in the range of 400–600 mg/dL for the entire hypoxic-ischemic interval (Figure 1). Control rat pups received equivalent volumes of normal saline at the same intervals. Following recovery from hypoxia-ischemia, the immature rats were reared with their dams until a postnatal age of 30 days, at which time they underwent neuropathologic analysis. The findings showed a dramatic protection afforded to the glucose-supplemented animals to the extent that little or no brain damage occurred with hyperglycemia, while the normoglycemic animals exhibited major tissue injury, with infarction seen in the majority (Figure 2). Accordingly, moderate hyperglycemia superimposed upon cerebral hypoxia-ischemia is highly protective to the perinatal brain.

Further experiments were conducted to ascertain the cerebral metabolic responses of hyperglycemic and normoglycemic immature rats to cerebral hypoxia-ischemia.[53] The same concentrations of glucose or normal saline as for the neuropathologic experiment were injected into immature rats subjected to 2 hours of cerebral hypoxia-ischemia. Cerebral hemispheric glucose utilization was determined, using a modification of the Sokoloff technique, with ^{14}C-2-deoxyglucose as the radioactive tracer.[54] Cerebral glucose utilization increased from a control value of 7.1 to 20.2 µmol/100 g/min in the hyperglycemic rat pups during the first hour of hypoxia-ischemia, 79% greater than the rate for the saline-injected animals at the same interval. Calculated

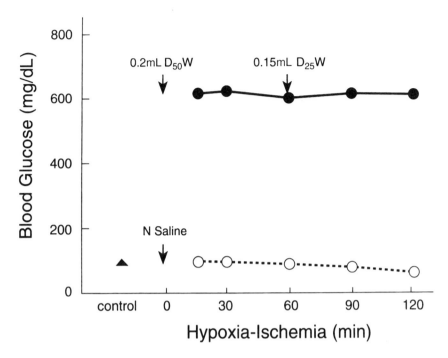

Figure 1. Blood glucose concentrations during hypoxia-ischemia in hyperglycemic and normoglycemic immature rats. The rat pups to be rendered hyperglycemic received 0.2 mL of 50% glucose ($D_{50}W$) at the onset of hypoxia-ischemia, followed by 0.15 mL of 25% glucose ($D_{25}W$) 1 hour later. Control litter mates received equivalent volumes of normal saline (N Saline) at the same intervals. From Vannucci and Vannucci,[52] with permission.

brain intracellular glucose concentrations were approximately 4.0 mmol/kg in the hyperglycemic rat pups at both 1 and 2 hours of hypoxia-ischemia, respectively, while the glucose levels were near negligible in the saline-treated animals at the same intervals (Figure 3). Brain intracellular lactate concentrations averaged 13.4 and 23.3 mmol/kg in the hyperglycemic animals at 1 and 2 hours of hypoxia-ischemia, respectively, more than twice the concentrations estimated for the saline-treated litter mates. Despite the higher concentrations of intracellular lactate in the hyperglycemic animals during hypoxia-ischemia, calculated intracellular pH decreased to comparable levels in the experimental and control animals. Phosphocreatine and adenosine triphosphate (ATP) decreased in both groups, but the high-energy metabolites were preserved to a greater extent in the hyperglycemic animals (Figure 4). It appears that anaerobic glycolytic flux is

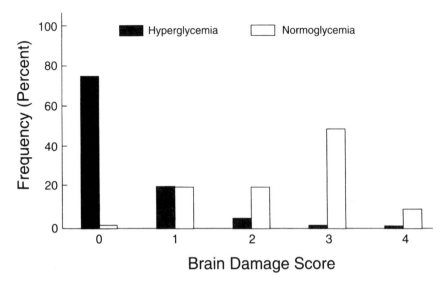

Figure 2. Severity of brain damage in rats previously subjected to hyperglycemia versus normoglycemia (control) during cerebral hypoxia-ischemia at 7 days of postnatal age. The severity of brain damage was graded as follows: grade 0 = normal; grade 1 = mild brain atrophy; grade 2 = moderate brain atrophy; grade 3 = atrophy with cystic cavitation < 3 mm; grade 4 = atrophy with cystic cavitation ≥ 3 mm. From Vannucci and Vannucci,[52] with permission.

increased to a greater extent in the hyperglycemic immature rats than in normoglycemic litter mates subjected to cerebral hypoxia-ischemia, and that the enhanced glycolysis leads to a greater intracellular lactate accumulation. Despite the cerebral lactic acidosis, energy reserves are better preserved in the hyperglycemic animals than in the saline-treated controls, thus accounting for the greater resistance of the hyperglycemic immature rats to hypoxic-ischemic brain damage.

Additional biochemical support for the finding that glucose supplementation is beneficial rather than deleterious to immature rat brain exposed to hypoxia-ischemia stems from other investigations in the authors' laboratory. Yager et al subjected immature rats to cerebral hypoxia-ischemia, during and following which their brains were prepared for the determination of cytosolic and mitochondrial oxidation-reduction (redox) states.[55,56] As anticipated, the cytosolic redox state was reduced relative to control throughout the hypoxic-ischemic interval. In contrast, an early mitochondrial reduction occurred followed by reoxidation during the course of hypoxia-ischemia (Figure 5). Concurrent measurements of brain glucose, pyruvate, α-ketoglutarate, gluta-

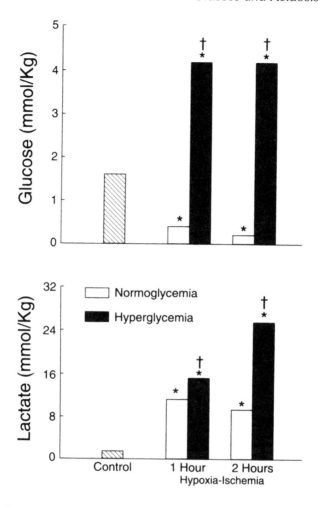

Figure 3. Brain intracellular glucose (top) and lactate (bottom) concentrations during hypoxia-ischemia in hyperglycemic and normoglycemic immature rats. Columns represent mean concentrations. Asterisks indicate p<0.01 compared with controls. Daggers indicate p<0.001 compared with normoglycemia at the same interval. From Vannucci and Vannucci,[52] with permission.

mate, acetoacetate, and β-hydroxybutyrate indicated that the secondary mitochondrial oxidation was the result of a limited substrate supply to the mitochondria. The oxidation reflected a partial depletion in reducing equivalents and coincides temporally with the duration of hypoxia-ischemia required to convert selective neuronal death into

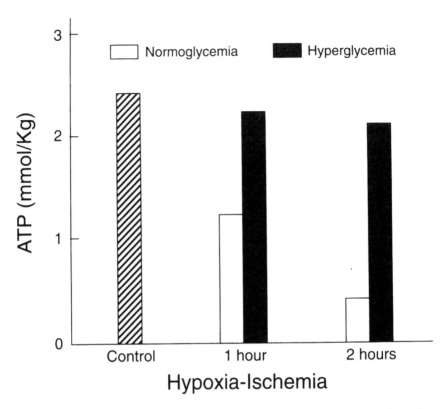

Figure 4. Brain adenosine triphosphate (ATP) concentrations during hypoxia-ischemia in hyperglycemic and normoglycemic immature rats. Columns represent mean tissue concentrations. ATP values in the normoglycemic rat pups at both 1 and 2 hours of hypoxia-ischemia were significantly lower than control and hyperglycemic values at the same intervals (p<0.01). From Vannucci and Vannucci,[52] with permission.

cerebral infarction (approximately 90 minutes). An analogous situation occurs in the adult brain subjected to severe hypoglycemia, during which cellular oxidation is observed.[57] From the findings, the authors concluded that perinatal cerebral hypoxia-ischemia is characterized more by a limitation of substrate than of oxygen supply to the brain, which explains why glucose supplementation of the immature animal during hypoxia-ischemia dramatically improves neuropathologic outcome, in contrast to adults.

Investigations in experimental animals of species other than the rat support the notion that glucose is not deleterious to the immature

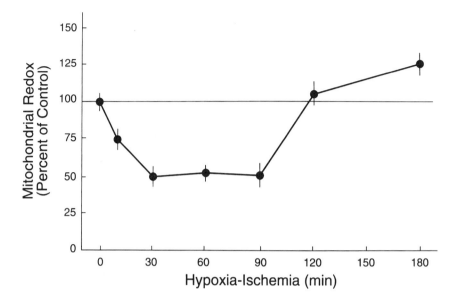

Figure 5. Calculated brain mitochondrial oxidation-reduction (redox) state during hypoxia-ischemia in the immature rat. Symbols represent means ±SE. The redox states were calculated from the acetoacetate/β-hydroxybutyrate coupled reaction. From Vannucci and Vannucci,[52] with permission.

brain undergoing hypoxia-ischemia through the mechanism of enhanced tissue lactate production. Chao et al compared the perturbations in oxidative metabolism that occur during partial cerebral ischemia in near-term fetal sheep under conditions of normoglycemia and hyperglycemia with arterial glucose concentrations of 23 and 45 mg/dL, respectively.[58] No differences in cerebral blood flow, oxygen or glucose consumption, or lactate efflux from the brain were observed during ischemia in the two groups. In a newborn sheep model of cerebral ischemia, Hope et al reported that hyperglycemia has no effect on brain lactate concentrations or tissue pH, measured by magnetic resonance spectroscopy (MRS), despite plasma glucose levels as high as 320 mg/dL[59] (see also reference 60). Young et al subjected hyperglycemic and normoglycemic newborn dogs to total cerebral ischemia produced by cardiac arrest with potassium chloride; these investigators found no difference in the rate of cerebral lactate accumulation, measured by MRS, despite a mean glucose concentration of 418 mg/dL in the hyperglycemic puppies.[61] The combined results of these studies suggest that hyperglycemic cerebral ischemia is not associated with increased glucose utilization via anaerobic glycolysis any more than that observed during normoglycemic ischemia in either the perinatal lamb or dog, unlike the authors' observations in the immature rat.

Hattori and Wasterlain developed a model of severe forebrain ischemia in the immature rat.[62] The model entails the ligation of both carotid arteries in the 7-day postnatal rat, followed by exposure to 8% oxygen for 1 hour. Immediately following the hypoxic-ischemic insult, some rat pups received an intraperitoneal injection of glucose sufficient to increase plasma glucose to 500 mg/dL for over 2 hours; litter mates received normal saline. Brain damage assessed at 3 days of recovery was far less extensive in the glucose-treated animals, with a 63% reduction in infarct volume of the cerebral cortex and nearly complete attenuation of ischemic injury to the striatum and dentate gyrus when compared with the saline-treated controls. The findings suggest that cerebral glucose supplementation immediately following cerebral hypoxia-ischemia also is beneficial in ameliorating the ultimate brain damage in the immature rat. However, using the authors' model of cerebral hypoxia-ischemia in which a single common carotid artery is ligated, Sheldon et al demonstrated that glucose supplementation immediately upon recovery from hypoxia-ischemia actually accentuates the ultimate brain damage compared with normoglycemic litter mates.[63] These findings are noteworthy in light of the authors' data, which indicate that even at normoglycemia, cerebral glucose concentrations are elevated for 24 or more hours during recovery from hypoxia-ischemia in the immature rat.[64,65] The contrasting results of glucose therapy during recovery from cerebral hypoxia-ischemia in two distinct immature rat models merit further investigations to ascertain the effect of glucose on perinatal hypoxic-ischemic brain damage.

A study by LeBlanc et al further complicates the issue of the protective effect of hyperglycemia on perinatal hypoxic-ischemic brain damage.[66] These investigators subjected newborn pigs to cerebral hypoxia-ischemia produced by ligation of both common carotid arteries combined with systemic hypoxemia and hypotension. One-half of the piglets were rendered hyperglycemic with blood glucose concentrations approximating 400 mg/dL during the course of hypoxia-ischemia, while blood glucose concentrations averaged 36 mg/dL in an insulin-treated group. Neurologic examination scores in the glucose-treated piglets at 1 day following cerebral hypoxia-ischemia were significantly worse than those in the insulin-treated animals. In addition, brain damage, determined pathologically, was substantially worse in the hyperglycemic animals compared with the insulin-treated controls. Pathologic alterations were especially apparent in cerebral cortex, hippocampus, and basal ganglia structures. From the data, the investigators concluded that hyperglycemia accentuates hypoxic-ischemic injury in the newborn pig brain.

The contrasting effect of hyperglycemia on hypoxic-ischemic brain damage in the immature rat and newborn pig requires clarification. Obviously, differences exist in the two experimental models to produce hypoxic-ischemic brain damage. The brain of the newborn pig is far more mature both structurally and functionally than that of the 7-day postnatal rat.[67] Indeed, the pig brain at birth is roughly comparable to that of a 6-month-old human infant. The more mature blood-brain transport of glucose and higher rate of cerebral glucose metabolism in both the newborn pig and 6-month-old infant renders them susceptible to the deleterious effect of hyperglycemia during hypoxia-ischemia.[68] The methods to produce brain damage are different in the two models; in the rat, brain damage is limited to one cerebral hemisphere, while, in the piglet, damage is global in nature. Differences in the rates of glucose uptake and metabolism by brain probably exist, as well as differences in the rate of lactate accumulation in brain during hypoxia-ischemia and its clearance from brain during recovery. Clearly, further experimentation in these and other perinatal animal models is required to clarify the issue.

The landmark study of Myers and Yamaguchi suggesting that glucose enhances hypoxic-ischemic brain damage was restricted to juvenile monkeys.[22] Despite generalizations that extended to the fetus and newborn human infant, controlled studies in perinatal animals other than the newborn pig and immature rat specifically correlating blood glucose concentrations with the extent of hypoxic-ischemic brain injury have not been forthcoming.[35,69] Wagner et al elucidated the metabolic alterations occurring during systemic hypoxemia in mid-gestational fetal sheep.[70] This insult generally produces brain damage when hypoxemia accompanies systemic hypotension (blood pressure values below 30 mmHg).[71] Both blood and brain glucose concentrations were actually slightly lower in those sheep fetuses that developed hypotension during hypoxemia (and by inference, brain damage), compared with animals that maintained systemic blood pressures above 30 mmHg. This suggests that glucose served to maintain optimal cardiac function and cerebral blood flow during hypoxemia (see also references 20 and 21). Although tissue concentrations of lactate were higher (16–24 mmol/kg) in the hypoxemic/hypotensive fetuses, little or no correlation existed between lactate levels and the presence and extent of tissue injury in specific structures of brain.

Hypoglycemia and Perinatal Hypoxic-Ischemic Brain Damage

Assuming that hyperglycemia favorably influences neuropathologic outcome resulting from perinatal cerebral hypoxia-ischemia, hypoglycemia might be deleterious to the immature brain undergoing hypoxia-ischemia. Investigations in adult animals suggest a beneficial effect of at least mild reductions in blood glucose concentrations on the extent of hypoxic-ischemic brain damage.[72–74] To determine whether hypoglycemia is protective or deleterious to the perinatal brain subjected to hypoxia-ischemia, Yager et al rendered immature rats hypoglycemic by the subcutaneous injection of insulin or by fasting for 12 hours.[75] Control animals (no insulin or fasting) received subcutaneous injections of normal saline. Mean blood glucose concentrations were 97, 77, and 61 mg/dL for the control, insulin, and fasted animals, respectively. Blood β-hydroxybutyrate concentrations were near identical in the control and insulin-treated animals but more than doubled in the fasted animals (Figure 6). All animals underwent cerebral hypoxia-

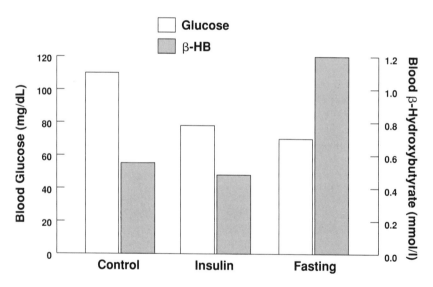

Figure 6. Blood glucose and β-hydroxybutyrate concentrations in insulin-treated and fasted immature rats. Insulin (0.5 U/kg) was injected subcutaneously 90 minutes prior to blood collection. Other rat pups were fasted for 12 hours. All blood samples were obtained from the tail immediately prior to the onset of cerebral hypoxia-ischemia. Data derived from Voll and Auer,[74] with permission.

ventricles, and also in glia. GLUT3 is the neuronal glucose transporter.[82,83] The MCT family has been cloned only within the past few years, and now contains eight members (for review, see reference 84). MCT1 and MCT2 are both expressed in rodent brain.[85–88] MCT1 is the most widely distributed, is detected in cerebral microvessels, and appears to be expressed by all neural cells, whereas MCT2 expression is more restricted and primarily neuronal. Both the GLUTs and the MCTs are developmentally regulated in brain, which may underlie many of the observations discussed above.[89]

The concentrations of the glucose transporter proteins are quite low in the immature rat brain,[90] in keeping with the well-described low rates of cerebral glucose transport into immature rat brain,[78] and increase sharply after the second postnatal week (Figure 9). The observation of greatly reduced brain glucose concentrations during hypoxia-ischemia, at least in the normoglycemic immature rat (Figure 3), provides evidence that the concentration of glucose transporter protein is limiting to cerebral glucose utilization in this age animal. Because the delivery of glucose from the blood to the brain is a function of both the substrate concentration in the blood and the transporter concentration, an increase in substrate concentration produced by glucose supplementation maintains a near normal or even elevated brain glucose level. In addition, although calculated intracellular glucose concentrations in normoglycemic immature rats become very low during hypoxia-ischemia, the level of glucose in the cerebrospinal fluid – as a reflection of the concentration in the brain extracellular compartment – does not decrease.[91] Accordingly, it appears that there is a greater limitation imposed at the level of the neurons and glia than at the blood-brain barrier.

The developmental expression of the MCTs shows the reverse pattern. Rodent milk is very high in fat and suckling pups are naturally ketotic, with circulating levels of β-hydroxybutyrate approaching the millimolar range by the second postnatal week.[89,92] At this time, cerebral ketone body utilization is also maximal,[92] and this is further reflected in the level and extent of the expression of MCT1.[88,89] Thus, the high levels of ketone body transporter in the blood-brain barrier, as well as in neurons and glia, not only facilitate ketone body transport into the brain but can also aid the clearance of the generated lactate.

Clinical Implications Regarding Hyperglycemia and Hypoglycemia

Both hyperglycemia and hypoglycemia are frequently encountered in the sick human fetus and newborn, especially those who are born pre-

ischemia, during which mortality was significantly greater in the insulin-treated animals (30%) than in either the fasted (4%) or control (0%) animals. In the insulin-treated animals, mortality increased as the blood glucose concentration decreased. The fasted animals showed a significant reduction in hypoxic-ischemic brain damage compared with either the insulin-treated or control animals, while the insulin-treated animals exhibited an increased hypoxic-ischemic mortality and an enhanced neuropathologic morbidity (Figure 7). From the data, it may be concluded that: (1) insulin-induced hypoglycemia does not provide a protective effect on hypoxic-ischemic brain damage, as in adults, and is actually deleterious; and (2) fasting adequate to produce hypoglycemia and ketonemia improves neuropathologic outcome.

To further investigate the manner in which fasting protects the perinatal brain from hypoxic-ischemic damage, Yager subjected imma-

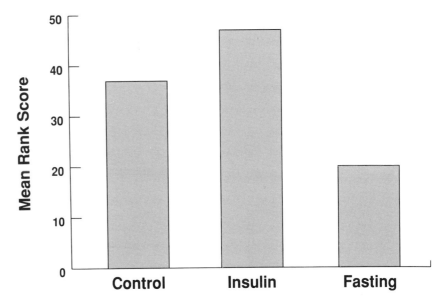

Figure 7. Rank score analysis of hypoxic-ischemic brain damage in insulin-treated and fasted rats previously subjected to cerebral hypoxia-ischemia. Insulin (0.5 U/kg) was injected subcutaneously 90 minutes prior to hypoxia-ischemia. Other rat pups were fasted for 12 hours before hypoxia-ischemia at 7 days of postnatal age. Pathologic analysis was performed at 30 days of postnatal age. The insulin-treated animals were significantly more brain damaged than both the normoglycemic control and hypoglycemic fasted animals ($p<0.05$). The fasted animals were significantly less brain damaged than control animals ($p<0.05$). Data derived from Voll and Auer,[74] with permission.

ture rats to either fasting for 12 hours or to subcutaneous injections of either 2, 5, or 10 mmol/kg of β-hydroxybutyrate; litter mate controls received normal saline.[76] All rat pups then were subjected to 2 hours of hypoxia-ischemia and underwent neuropathologic analysis at 30 days of postnatal age. The results showed that the injection of either 5 or 10 mmol/kg of β-hydroxybutyrate proved as beneficial to neuropathologic outcome as did fasting, when either treatment was compared with control animals undergoing hypoxia-ischemia (Figure 8). The equally beneficial effect occurred despite higher concentrations of brain lactate during hypoxia-ischemia in those immature rats supplemented with the ketone body.

The biochemical mechanism by which ketone bodies might protect the brain from hypoxic-ischemic mortality and hypoxic-ischemic brain damage presumably relates to the ability of these alternate substrates to readily enter the immature brain, undergo oxidative decarboxyla-

tion, and provide reducing equivalents for mitochondria, at le conditions of partial ischemia.[28,77] Such protection would not able to the immature brain subjected to total cerebral isch occurs with cardiac arrest, when no oxygen is available to the

To elucidate more specifically the biochemical mechanism b fasting or ketone body supplementation improves neuropatholo come, at least in immature rats, concentrations of the high-energy phate reserves were measured at specific intervals during hy ischemia in fasted and non-fasted immature rats.[79] As was antici the fasted rat pups exhibited a substantial preservation of the energy reserves, including phosphocreatine and ATP, compared to trols. Presumably, the mechanism for the energy preservation relate the increased availability of ketone bodies to brain tissue for oxida decarboxylation to produce reducing equivalents to mitochondria energy production. The ready utilization of ketone bodies to prote immature rat brain from hypoxic-ischemic damage contrasts with tl brain of the newborn pig, which appears to consume glucose exclusivel This species difference might explain, at least in part, the species differ ence in the effect of glucose on perinatal hypoxic-ischemic brain damage.

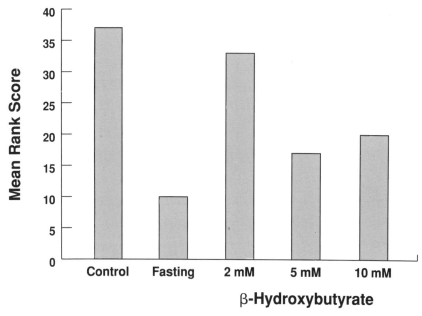

Figure 8. Rank score analysis of the severity of brain damage in rats previously supplemented with β-hydroxybutyrate or fasted prior to hypoxia-ischemia. The ketone body was injected subcutaneous 90 minutes prior to hypoxia-ischemia. Other rat pups were fasted for 12 hours before hypoxia-ischemia. The fasted animals and those which received 5 or 10 mM β-hydroxybutyrate were the least damaged (p<0.05 compared to control and 2 mM). Data derived from Yager,[76] with permission.

Glucose and Monocarboxylic Acid Transporters

The beneficial effects of both hyperglycemia and ketosis in the immature brain can be partially explained by differences in the expression of the transporter proteins for these substrates. Blood-borne nutrients such as glucose and monocarboxylic acids, i.e., lactate and ketone bodies, cannot readily cross the blood-brain barrier but require integral membrane proteins for transport. These integral membrane proteins now comprise two distinct families, the facilitative glucose transporter proteins, GLUTs, and the monocarboxylic acid proteins, MCTs, which mediate proton-coupled co-transport. GLUT1 was cloned in 1985,[80] and there are now five proteins, GLUTs1–5, with distinct tissue distribution and kinetic characteristics (for a review, see reference 81). Although all of these proteins have been detected in mammalian brain, GLUT1 and GLUT3 are the isoforms primarily involved with cerebral glucose uptake and utilization.[82] The initial transport of glucose across the endothelial cells of the blood-brain barrier is mediated by a heavily glycosylated form of GLUT1, 55 kDa GLUT1; a less glycosylated product of the same gene, 45 kDa GLUT1, is highly concentrated in choroid plexus, the ependymal lining of the

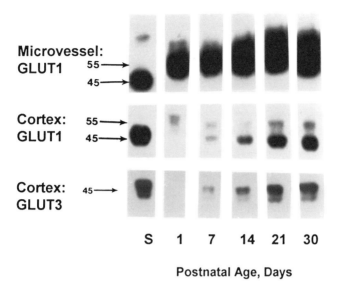

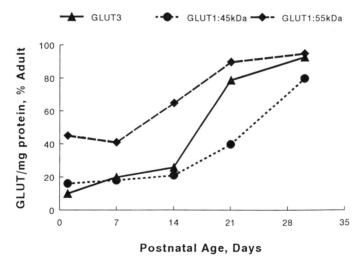

Figure 9. Brain glucose transporter proteins during development in the immature rat. Isolated microvessels and cortical membranes were prepared from postnatal rats between birth and 30 days of age, and adults. GLUT1 and GLUT3 content per milligram membrane protein was determined by Western blot analysis with specific antipeptide antisera to GLUT1 and GLUT3 and ^{125}I-protein. Representative autoradiograms are depicted in the upper part of the figure. S = brain microsomal membrane "standard" included in all blots for purposes of interblot comparisons and quantification. The lower part of the figure represents the quantification of 4–6 animals/age, expressed as a percent of the adult value. From Vannucci and Vannucci,[52] with permission.

maturely and those who have undergone prior or concurrent metabolic stress, e.g., respiratory distress syndrome, sepsis, or asphyxia.[48,93–96] Hyperglycemia in the fetus also occurs secondary to maternal diabetes mellitus.[96] Perinatal hyperglycemia, defined as a blood glucose concentration in excess of 125 mg/dL, results from glucose intolerance in association with increased endogenous glucose production (glycogenolysis or gluconeogenesis) or intravenous glucose supplementation.[97] Clinical investigations suggest an association between persistently elevated blood glucose levels and increased infant mortality,[97,98] although an independent study comparing the mortality of hyperglycemic and normoglycemic stressed newborn infants does not suggest such a relationship.[99] The effect of transient, iatrogenically induced hyperglycemia on fetal and neonatal systemic homeostasis is presently unknown.

Premature infants and those who are small for gestational age, as well as offspring of diabetic mothers, are prone to hypoglycemia.[48,96] An additional frequent cause of hypoglycemia is asphyxia, during which glucose is rapidly consumed anaerobically in an attempt to preserve cellular energy stores in all tissues of the body, including the brain.[48,49,96] The question remains as to whether or not fetuses or newborn infants subjected to asphyxia should receive intravenous glucose therapy adequate to produce hyperglycemia. The currently available animal studies are conflicting in this regard, and as suggested by LeBlanc et al,[66] controlled clinical trials in humans are necessary to determine whether hyperglycemia or hypoglycemia is beneficial or deleterious to the perinatal brain undergoing metabolic stress. Clinical investigations also are warranted to determine whether an infusion of ketone bodies would protect the perinatal brain from hypoxic-ischemic injury.

Carbon Dioxide and Perinatal Hypoxic-Ischemic Brain Damage

There are two forms of acidosis that occur in both perinatal experimental animals and human fetuses and newborn infants suffering asphyxia, metabolic and respiratory. Respiratory alkalosis (hypocapnia) also occurs in premature infants who require mechanical ventilation to prevent or minimize hypoxemia arising from respiratory distress syndrome. Several clinical investigations have now demonstrated that premature infants who are rendered hypocapnic during the course of ventilator care are at increased risk for the development of periventricular leukomalacia.[100–102] The association between hypocapnia and hypoxic-ischemic brain damage in the premature infant is reminiscent of the alterations in systemic acid-base homeostasis that occur in immature rats undergoing hypoxic-ischemic brain damage.[44] When 7-day postnatal rats are exposed to 8% oxygen, the hypoxemia leads to lactic acidemia. The animals spontaneously hyperventilate to an extent that produces hypocapnia, which in turn completely compensates for the metabolic acidemia, and blood pH remains normal. The question remained as to the contribution of the hypocapnia to the severity of the ultimate hypoxic-ischemic brain damage. Accordingly, experiments were conducted whereby immature rats were subjected to cerebral hypoxia-ischemia with or without CO_2 added to the hypoxic gas mixture to which the animals were exposed.[103] As in previous experiments,[44] 7-day postnatal rats underwent unilateral common carotid artery ligation, after which they were subjected to hypoxia at 37°C for 2.5 hours. Varying concentrations of CO_2 were added to the hypoxic gas mixture, specifically 0%, 3%, 6%, or 9% CO_2. There was a minimal mortality rate in all of the rat groups during the hypoxic exposure. The rat pups were returned to their dams following hypoxia-ischemia until 30 days of postnatal age, at which time they were sacrificed and their brains underwent neuropathologic analysis.

CO_2 tensions in blood averaged 26, 42, 54, and 71 mmHg in the 0, 3, 6, and 9% CO_2-exposed immature rats, respectively, during systemic hypoxia. Blood oxygen tensions during hypoxia were not different among the four groups, and averaged 34.7 mmHg. The neuropathologic results showed that 79% of the rats exposed to 3% CO_2 demonstrated either no, or only mild, brain damage compared with 39% of controls (0% CO_2) (Figure 10). Cystic cavitation occurred in only four 3% CO_2-exposed rat pups compared with 14 controls. At 6% CO_2 exposure, all rat pups showed either no damage or mild atrophy compared with controls, while at 9% CO_2 exposure, 83% of rat pups showed no or mild damage compared to controls. The results indicated that in an immature rat model, normocapnic cerebral hypoxia-ischemia is associated with less severe brain damage than in hypocapnic hypoxia-ischemia, and that mild hypercapnia is more protective than normocapnia.

In more recent and as yet unpublished experiments, 7-day postnatal rats were subjected to hypoxia-ischemia during which they inhaled either 12% or 15% CO_2. In these experiments, control animals were subjected to the same interval of hypoxia-ischemia breathing 3% CO_2. No neuropathologic difference was noted in those animals breathing 12% CO_2 compared with controls exposed to 2 hours of hypoxia-ischemia. However, animals who breathed 15% CO_2 showed greater brain damage

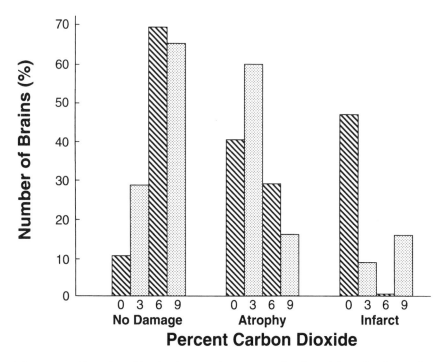

Percent Carbon Dioxide

Figure 10. Severity of brain damage in rats previously subjected to hypoxia-ischemia with or without supplemental CO_2 inhalation. Seven-day postnatal rats underwent unilateral carotid artery ligation followed by inhalation of 0%, 3%, 6%, or 9% CO_2, 8% O_2 and balanced nitrogen. The extent of brain damage in each animal then was determined at 30 days of postnatal age. From Vannucci and Vannucci,[52] with permission.

compared with controls breathing 3% CO_2 and exposed to 1.5 hours of hypoxia-ischemia. In this experiment, no cerebral infarcts were noted in the 3% CO_2-exposed animals, whereas 8 of 14 (57%) of the 15% CO_2 animals exhibited cystic infarcts. Indeed, the severity of the brain damage in the 15% CO_2-exposed animals was comparable to that previously seen in hypocapnic immature rats (Figure 11).

Several physiologic and biochemical mechanisms potentially exist whereby CO_2 protects the immature brain from hypoxic-ischemic damage. Cerebrovascular reactivity is strongly influenced by CO_2. Hypocapnia lowers cerebral blood flow, whereas hypercapnia increases flow. These responses to CO_2 are active in immature animals, albeit less well developed than in adults.[16] It is possible that the anticipated hypoxic dilation of the cerebrovascular bed is attenuated, to some

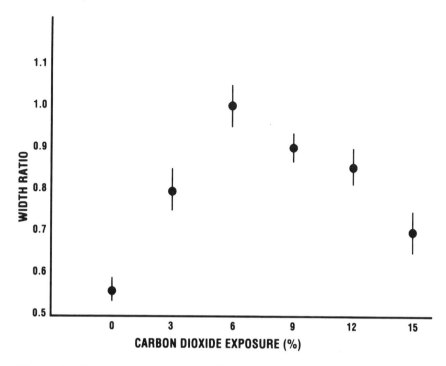

Figure 11. Brain interhemispheric width ratios of rats previously subjected to hypoxia-ischemia at various concentrations of carbon dioxide. Seven-day postnatal rats underwent unilateral common carotid artery ligation followed by hypoxia with 8% O_2. The width ratio was derived from the diameter of the cerebral hemisphere ipsilateral to the arterial occlusion/contralateral hemisphere. The lower the width ratio, the greater the brain damage. Symbols represent means; vertical lines denote ±SE. Data derived from Vannucci et al,[103] with permission, and from unpublished studies.

extent, by the concurrent hypocapnia that occurs in immature rats exposed to 8% oxygen without supplemental CO_2 (hypocapnia). Accordingly, increasing the partial pressure of CO_2 might serve to maximally dilate the cerebrovascular bed in the setting of hypoxia, thereby improving oxygen delivery to the cerebral hemisphere even when its major nutrient artery (common carotid) has been previously ligated.

CO_2 has several actions on cerebral metabolism *per se.* Hypercapnia leads to a generalized suppression of oxidative metabolism, as indicated by an inhibition of cerebral energy utilization and a curtailment of glycolytic flux by inhibition of phosphofructokinase.[104–106] Tissue lactate production is also reduced, at least under physiologic conditions.[107,108] During anoxia in newborn rats, hypercapnia is associated with a greater preservation of high-energy phosphate reserves and energy expenditure than during normocapnic anoxia.[109] The combined effect of enhanced substrate (glucose) delivery and reduced energy demand would serve to maximally protect the vulnerable tissue from energy failure and ultimate damage during hypoxia-ischemia.

To resolve the issue of the effect of CO_2 on perinatal cerebral hypoxia-ischemia, metabolic studies were performed in addition to neuropathologic experiments.[110] Seven-day postnatal rats were subjected to hypoxia-ischemia, during which they were rendered either hypocapnic (0% CO_2 and 8% O_2), normocapnic (3% CO_2 and 8% O_2), or mildly hypercapnic (6% CO_2 and 8% O_2). Cerebral blood flow during hypoxia-ischemia was better preserved in the normo- and hypercapnic rat pups; these animals also exhibited a stimulation of cerebral glucose utilization (Table 1). Brain glucose concentrations were higher and lactate was lower in the normo- and hypercapnic animals, indicating that glucose was consumed oxidatively in these groups rather than by anaerobic glycolysis, as had apparently occurred in the hypocapnic animals. ATP and phosphocreatine were better preserved in the normo- and hypercapnic rats compared with the hypocapnic animals. Cerebrospinal fluid glutamate, a reflection of the brain extracellular fluid concentration, was lowest in the hypercapnic rats at 2 hours of hypoxia-ischemia (Table 2). From the findings, it was concluded that during hypoxia-ischemia in the immature rat, cerebral blood flow is better preserved during normo- and hypercapnia, and the greater oxygen delivery promotes cerebral glucose utilization and oxidative

Table 1

Cerebral Glucose Utilization During Hypoxia-Ischemia with Carbon Dioxide Supplementation*

Variable	CGU (μmol/100 g/min)
Control	15.4
Hypoxia-ischemia	
0% CO_2	17.5
3% CO_2	25.5†
6% CO_2	23.9†

*Values represent means for 5–6 immature rats in each group. The interval of 2-deoxyglucose circulation extended from 40 to 100 minutes of hypoxia-ischemia.
†p<0.05 compared to control.
CGU = cerebral glucose utilization.

Table 2

Cerebrospinal Fluid Glutamate During Hypoxia-Ischemia with Carbon Dioxide Supplementation*

Variable	CSF Glutamate ($\mu mol/100$ g/min)
Control	35
Hypoxia-ischemia (2 hours)	
0% CO_2	58†
3% CO_2	56†
6% CO_2	38

*Values represent means for 6–10 immature rats in each group and 39 control animals. Cerebrospinal fluid (CSF) was obtained from the cisterna magna.
†$p < 0.05$ compared to control and to 6% CO_2.

metabolism for optimal maintenance of tissue high-energy phosphate reserves. An inhibition of glutamate secretion into the synaptic cleft, thereby attenuating post-synaptic receptor activation, would further protect the hypercapnic animal from hypoxic-ischemic brain damage. The effect of higher blood CO_2 tensions on cerebral blood flow and metabolism during hypoxia-ischemia has not been elucidated.

Intrapartum Acidosis and Human Perinatal Hypoxic-Ischemic Brain Damage

Obstetricians have long used blood acid-base status to ascertain the presence or absence of systemic asphyxia in the fetus during the intrapartum period. Early studies found a relatively poor correlation between the presence of acidosis, determined by measurement of either fetal scalp or umbilical cord blood pH, and either neonatal depression (low Apgar scores) or encephalopathy.[111–114] Other early studies found essentially no correlation with long-term neurologic outcome.[115,116] The lack of any correlation between these variables was related, at least in part, to the use of pH values not indicative of severe acidosis or to the failure to discern whether the acidosis was respiratory, metabolic, or mixed in origin. More recent investigations have concentrated on more severe degrees of acidosis than previously reported, and on the extent to which the altered pH reflects an underlying metabolic (lactic) acidosis. In a study by Goldaber et al, 2.5% of full-term newborn infants exhibited an umbilical artery pH of < 7.00, of which 67% had a metabolic component to their acidosis.[117] Significantly more of the severely acidotic newborn infants exhibit low (< 3) 1- and 5-minute Apgar scores compared to infants with higher umbilical artery pH values. In addition, neonatal death is significantly more frequent in the severely acidotic group. Low et al compared 59 term fetuses exhibiting metabolic acidosis with 59 fetuses with normal umbilical blood acid-base status and 51 fetuses exhibiting only a respiratory acidosis at birth.[118] A variety of newborn complications, including encephalopathy, was apparent in 54% of the newborn infants experiencing a metabolic acidosis compared with very low complication rates in those infants with either respiratory acidosis or no acidosis at all (see also references 119 and 120). Furthermore, Low et al previously demonstrated a positive correlation between the severity and duration of intrapartum metabolic acidosis and neurodevelopmental outcome at 1 year of age.[121]

The aforementioned data suggest the following: (1) in order for intrapartum asphyxia to produce neonatal complications, including encephalopathy, the systemic hypoxemia must be severe enough to cause an associated severe metabolic or mixed acidosis; (2) mild respiratory acidosis in association with intrapartum asphyxia does not appear to be deleterious; and (3) the weak correlation between intrapartum acidosis and neonatal complications or adverse neurologic outcome indicates that factors in addition to acidosis are involved in the pathogenesis of perinatal hypoxic-ischemic brain damage.[122] These conclusions are consistent with the observations in experimental animal models that brain damage is always associated with at least tissue metabolic acidosis and that mild respiratory acidosis might actually be neuroprotective. Furthermore, blood lactic acidosis need not indicate tissue acidosis.

Conclusions

In summary, this chapter has focused on current knowledge regarding the effects of hyperglycemia/hypoglycemia and respiratory and metabolic acidosis/alkalosis on cerebral blood flow and metabolism. In addition, a review was also provided of the neuropathologic outcomes arising from cerebral hypoxia-ischemia in perinatal animals, and in human fetuses and newborns. The data regarding glucose supplementation are conflicting and require further animal and human investigation. However, available data do suggest that excessive tissue lactic acid formation does not aggravate hypoxic-ischemic brain damage. Furthermore, hypocapnia is deleterious, while mild respiratory acidosis is probably neuroprotective. These findings in perinatal experimental animals are corroborated to some extent by clinical data in fetuses and newborn human infants undergoing perinatal hypoxia-ischemia.

References

1. Mann LI: Developmental aspects and the effect of carbon dioxide tension on fetal cephalic blood flow. Exp Neurol 1970;26:136–141.
2. Jones MD, Burd LI, Makowski EI, et al: Cerebral metabolism in sheep: a comparative study of the adult, the lamb, and the fetus. Am J Physiol 1975;229:235–239.
3. Levitsky LL, Fisher DE, Paton JB, et al: Fasting plasma levels of glucose, acetoacetate, D-β-hydroxybutyrate, glycerol and lactate in the baboon infant: correlation with cerebral uptake of substrates and oxygen. Pediatr Res 1977;11:298–302.
4. Gregoire NM, Gjedde A, Plum F, et al: Cerebral blood flow and cerebral metabolic rates for oxygen, glucose, and ketone bodies in newborn dogs. J Neurochem 1978;30:63–69.
5. Hernandez MJ, Vannucci RC, Salcedo A, et al: Cerebral blood flow and metabolism during hypoglycemia in newborn dogs. J Neurochem 1980; 35:622–628.
6. Settergren G, Lindblad BS, Persson B: Cerebral blood flow and exchange of oxygen, glucose, ketone bodies, lactate, pyruvate and amino acids in anesthetized children. Acta Pediatr Scand 1980;69:457–465.
7. Owen OE, Morgan AP, Kemp KG, et al: Brain metabolism during fasting. J Clin Invest 1967;46:1585–1589.
8. Hawkins RA, Williamson DH, Krebs HA: Ketone-body utilization by adult and suckling rat brain *in vivo*. Biochem J 1971;122:13–18.
9. Spitzer JJ, Weng JT: Removal and utilization of ketone bodies by the brain of newborn puppies. J Neurochem 1972;19:2169–2173.
10. Hellmann J, Vannucci RC, Nardis EE: Blood-brain barrier permeability to lactic acid in the newborn dog: lactate as a cerebral metabolic fuel. Pediatr Res 1982;16:40–44.
11. Vicario C, Medina JM: Metabolism of lactate in the rat brain during the early neonatal period. J Neurochem 1992;59:32–40.
12. Stemberg ZK, Hodr J: The relationship between the blood levels of glucose, lactic acid and pyruvic acid in the mother and in both umbilical vessels of the healthy fetus. Biol Neonate 1966;10:227–238.
13. Yoshioka T, Roux JF: Correlation of fetal scalp pH, glucose, lactate and pyruvate concentrations with cord blood determinations at the time of delivery and cesarean section. J Reprod Med 1970;5:209–214.
14. Stanley CA, Anday EK, Baker L, et al: Metabolic fuel and hormone responses to fasting in newborn infants. Pediatrics 1979;64:613–619.
15. Siesjö BK: *Brain Energy Metabolism*. Wiley, Chichester, England, 1978.
16. Vannucci RC: Acidosis/alkalosis. In Stevenson DK, Sunshine P (eds): *Fetal and Neonatal Brain Injury*. Oxford University Press, Oxford, 1997, pp 512–526.

17. Himwich HE, Bernstein AO, Herrlich H, et al: Mechanisms for the maintenance of life in the newborn during anoxia. Am J Physiol 1942;135: 387–391.
18. Britton SW, Kline RF: Age, sex, carbohydrate, adrenal cortex and other factors in anoxia. Am J Physiol 1945–46;145:190–202.
19. Stafford A, Weatherall JAC: The survival of young rats in nitrogen. J Physiol (London) 1960;153:457–472.
20. Dawes GS, Hibbard E, Windle WF: The effect of alkali and glucose infusion on permanent brain damage in rhesus monkeys asphyxiated at birth. J Pediatr 1964;65:801–806.
21. Adamsons K, Behrman R, Dawes CS, et al: Resuscitation by positive pressure ventilation and tris-hydroxymethylaminomethane of rhesus monkeys asphyxiated at birth. J Pediatr 1964;65:807–811.
22. Myers RE, Yamaguchi S: Nervous system effects of cardiac arrest in monkeys: preservation of vision. Arch Neurol 1977;34:65–74.
23. Kalimo H, Rehncroná S, Söderfeldt B, et al: Brain lactic acidosis and ischemic cell damage: 2. Histophathology. J Cereb Blood Flow Metabol 1981;1:313–327.
24. Pulsinelli WA, Waldman S, Rawlinson D, et al: Hyperglycemia converts neuronal damage into brain infarction. Neurology 1982;32:1239–1246.
25. Inamura K, Ollsson Y, Siesjö BK: Substantia nigra damage induced by ischemia in hyperglycemic rats: a light and electron microscopic study. Acta Neuropathol 1987;75:131–139.
26. Duverger D, MacKenzie ET: The quantification of cerebral infarction following focal ischemia in the rat: influence of strain, arterial pressure, blood glucose concentration and age. J Cereb Blood Flow Metabol 1988; 8:449–461.
27. Prado R, Ginsberg MD, Dietrich WD, et al: Hyperglycemia increases infarct size in collaterally perfused but not end-arterial vascular territories. J Cereb Blood Flow Metabol 1988;8:186–192.
28. Li P-A, Kristián T, Shamloo M, Siesjö BK: Effects of preischemic hyperglycemia on brain damage incurred by rats subjected to 2.5 or 5 minutes of forebrain ischemia. Stroke 1996;27:1592–1602.
29. Kawai N, Keep R, Betz AL: Hyperglycemia and the vascular effects of cerebral ischemia. Stroke 1997;28:149–154.
30. Sieber FE, Martin EJ, Brown PR, et al: Diabetic chronic hyperglycemia and neurologic outcome following global ischemia in dogs. J Cereb Blood Flow Metabol 1996;16:1230–1235.
31. Vannucci SJ, Willing LB, Rutherford T, et al: The impact of diabetes or gender on hypoxic-ischemic brain damage in the mouse. (Submitted for publication.)
32. Pulsinelli WA, Levy DE, Sigsbee B, et al: Increased damage after ischemic stroke in patients with hyperglycemia with or without diabetes mellitus. Am J Med 1983;74:540–544.
33. Berger L, Hakim AM: The association of hyperglycemia with cerebral edema in stroke. Stroke 1986;17:865–871.
34. Levine SR, Welsh KMA, Helpern JA, et al: Prolonged deterioration of ischemic brain energy metabolism and acidosis associated with hyperglycemia: human cerebral infarction studies by serial ^{31}P NMR spectroscopy. Ann Neurol 1988;23:416–418.

35. Myers RE: A unitary theory of causation of anoxic and hypoxic brain pathology. In Fahn S, Davis JN, Rowland LP (eds): *Cerebral Hypoxia and Its Consequences*. Raven Press, New York, 1979, pp 195–213.

36. Rehncroná S, Rosen I, Siesjö BK: Excessive cellular acidosis: an important mechanism of neuronal damage in the brain? Acta Physiol Scand 1980; 110:435–437.

37. Welsh FA, Ginsberg MD, Reider W, et al: Deleterious effect of glucose pretreatment on recovery from diffuse cerebral ischemia in the cat. II. Regional metabolite levels. Stroke 1980;11:355–363.

38. Rehncroná S, Rosen I, Siesjö BK: Brain lactic acidosis and ischemic cell damage. 1. Biochemistry and neurophysiology. J Cereb Blood Flow Metabol 1981;1:297–311.

39. Kraig RP, Petito CK, Plum F, et al: Hydrogen ions kill brain at concentrations reached in ischemia. J Cereb Blood Flow Metabol 1987;7:379–386.

40. Petito CK, Kraig RP, Pulsinelli WA: Light and electron microscopic evaluation of hydrogen ion-induced brain necrosis. J Cereb Blood Flow Metabol 1987;7:625–632.

41. Goldman SA, Pulsinelli WA, Clarke WY, et al: The effects of extracellular acidosis on neurons and glia *in vitro*. J Cereb Blood Flow Metabol 1989; 9:471–477.

42. Kraig RP, Petito CK: Interrelationship of proton and volume regulation in astrocytes. In Ginsberg MD, Dietrich WD (eds): *Cerebrovascular Diseases, 16th Princeton Research Conference*. Raven Press, New York, 1989, pp 239–246.

43. Kraig RP, Chesler M: Astrocyte acidosis in hyperglycemic and complete ischemia. J Cereb Blood Flow Metabol 1990;10:104–114.

44. Rice JE, Vannucci RC, Brierley JB: The influence of immaturity on hypoxic-ischemic brain damage in the rat. Ann Neurol 1981;9:131–141.

45. Towfighi J, Yager JY, Housman C, et al: Neuropathology of remote hypoxic-ischemic damage in the immature rat. Acta Neuropathol 1991;81:578–587.

46. Towfighi J, Zec N, Yager J, et al: Temporal evolution of neuropathologic changes in an immature rat model of cerebral hypoxia-ischemia: a light microscopic study. Acta Neuropathol 1995;90:375–386.

47. Rorke LB: *Pathology of Perinatal Brain Injury*. Raven Press, New York, 1982.

48. Volpe JJ: *Neurology of the Newborn*. 3rd ed. W.B. Saunders, Philadelphia, 1995.

49. Vannucci RC, Palmer C: Hypoxic-ischemic encephalopathy: pathogenesis and neuropathology. In Fanaroff AA, Martin RJ (eds): *Neonatal-Perinatal Medicine*. 4th ed. Philadelphia, Mosby-Year Book, Inc., 1997, pp 856–877.

50. Voorhies TM, Rawlinson D, Vannucci RC: Glucose and perinatal hypoxic-ischemic brain damage in the rat. Neurology 1986;36:1115–1118.

51. Vannucci RC, Mujsce DJ: The effect of glucose on perinatal hypoxic-ischemic brain damage. Biol Neonate 1992;62:215–224.

52. Vannucci RC, Vannucci SJ: Glucose, acidosis, and perinatal hypoxic-ischemic brain damage. Ment Retard Dev Disab Res Rev 1997;3:69–75.

53. Vannucci RC, Brucklacher RM, Vannucci SJ: The effect of hyperglycemia on cerebral metabolism during hypoxia-ischemia in the immature rat. J Cereb Blood Flow Metabol 1996;16:1026–1033.

54. Vannucci RC, Christensen MA, Stein DT: Regional cerebral glucose uti-

lization in the immature rat: effect on hypoxia-ischemia. Pediatr Res 1989;26:208–214.

55. Yager JY, Brucklacher RM, Vannucci RC: Cerebral oxidative metabolism and redox state during hypoxia-ischemia and early recovery in the immature rat. Am J Physiol 1991;261:H1102–H1108.

56. Yager JY, Brucklacher RM, Vannucci RC: Paradoxical mitochondrial oxidation in perinatal hypoxic-ischemic brain damage. Brain Res 1996; 712:230–238.

57. Bryan RM, Jöbsis FF: Insufficient supply of reducing equivalents to the respiratory chain in cerebral cortex during severe insulin-induced hypoglycemia in cats. J Cereb Blood Flow Metabol 1986;2:286–291.

58. Chao CR, Hohimer AR, Vissonnette JM: The effect of elevated blood glucose on the electroencephalogram and cerebral metabolism during short-term brain ischemia in fetal sheep. Am J Obstet Gynecol 1989;161:221–228.

59. Hope PL, Cady EB, Delpy DT, et al: Brain metabolism and intracellular pH during ischemia: effects of systemic glucose and bicarbonate administration studied by ^{31}P and ^{1}H nuclear magnetic resonance spectroscopy *in vivo* in the lamb. J Neurochem 1988;50:1394–1402.

60. Corbett RJT, Laptook AR, Sterett R, et al: Effect of hypoxia on glucose-modulated cerebral lactic acidosis, agonal glycolytic rates, and energy utilization. Pediatr Res 1996;39:477–486.

61. Young RSK, Petroff OAC, Aquila WJ, et al: Hyperglycemia and the rate of lactic acid accumulation during cerebral ischemia in developing animals: an *in vivo* protron MRS study. Biol Neonate 1991;61:235–239.

62. Hattori H, Wasterlain CG: Posthypoxic glucose supplement reduces hypoxic-ischemic brain damage in the neonatal rat. Ann Neurol 1990;28:122–128.

63. Sheldon RA, Partridge JC, Ferriero DM: Postischemic hyperglycemia is not protective to the neonatal rat brain. Pediatr Res 1992;32:489–493.

64. Palmer C, Brucklacher RM, Christensen MA, et al: Carbohydrate and energy metabolism during the evolution of hypoxic-ischemic brain damage in the immature rat. J Cereb Blood Flow Metabol 1990;10:227–235.

65. Vannucci RC, Yager JY, Vannucci SJ: Cerebral glucose and energy utilization during the evolution of hypoxic-ischemic brain damage in the immature rat. J Cereb Blood Flow Metabol 1994;14:279–288.

66. LeBlanc MH, Huang M, Vig V, et al: Glucose affects the severity of hypoxic-ischemic brain injury in newborn pigs. Stroke 1993;24:1055–1062.

67. Davison A, Dobbing J: The developing brain. In Davison A, Dobbing J (eds): *Applied Neurochemistry*. Blackwell, Oxford, 1968, pp 253–286.

68. Chugani HT, Phelps ME: Maturational changes in cerebral function in infants determined by ^{18}FDG positron emission tomography. Science 1986; 231:840–843.

69. Myers RE: Experimental models of perinatal brain damage: relevance to human pathology. In Gluck L (ed): *Intrauterine Asphyxia and the Developing Fetal Brain*. Year Book Medical Publishers, Chicago, 1977, pp 37–96.

70. Wagner KR, Ting P, Westfall MV, et al: Brain metabolic correlates of hypoxic-ischemic cerebral necrosis in mid-gestational sheep fetuses: significance of hypotension. J Cereb Blood Flow Metabol 1986;6:425–434.

71. Ting P, Yamaguchi S, Bacher JD, et al: Hypoxic-ischemic cerebral necrosis in mid-gestational sheep fetuses: physiopathologic correlations. Exp Neurol 1983;80:227–245.

72. LeMay DR, Gehua L, Zelenock GB, et al: Insulin administration protects neurologic function in cerebral ischemia in rats. Stroke 1988;19:1411–1419.
73. Nedergaard M, Diemer NH: Hypoglycemia reduces infarct size in experimental focal ischemia: the influence of plasma glucose on ischemic brain damage. In Ginsberg MD, Dietrich WD (eds): *Cerebrovascular Diseases, 16th Princeton Research Conference.* Raven Press, New York, 1989, pp 259–264.
74. Voll CL, Auer RN: Effect of post-ischemic blood glucose levels on ischemic brain damage in the rat. Ann Neurol 1988;24:638–646.
75. Yager JY, Heitjan DF, Towfighi J, et al: Effect of insulin-induced and fasting hypoglycemia on perinatal hypoxic-ischemic brain damage. Pediatr Res 1992;31:138–142.
76. Yager JY: Protective effects of fasting and ketone body supplementation on hypoxic-ischemic brain damage in the immature rat. Ann Neurol 1994;36:540. Abstract.
77. Cremer JE, Braun LD, Oldendorf WH: Changes during development in transport processes of the blood-brain barrier. Biochem Biophys Acta 1976;448:633–637.
78. Cremer JE, Cunningham UJ, Pardridge WM, et al: Kinetics of blood-brain barrier transport of pyruvate, lactate and glucose in suckling, weanling and adult rats. J Neurochem 1979;33:439–445.
79. Yager JY: Personal communication.
80. Mueckler M, Caruso C, Baldwin SA, et al: Sequence and structure of a human glucose transporter. Science 1985;229:941–945.
81. Pessin JE, Bell GI: Mammalian facilitative glucose transporter family: structure and molecular regulation. Am Rev Physiol 1992;54:911–930.
82. Vannucci SJ, Maher F, Simpson IA: Glucose transporter proteins in brain: delivery of glucose to neurons and glia. Glia 1997;21:2–21.
83. Maher F, Vannucci SJ, Simpson IA: Glucose transporter proteins in brain. FASEB J 1994;8:1003–1011.
84. Price NT, Jackson VN, Halestrap AP: Cloning and sequencing of four new mammalian monocarboxylate transporter (MCT) homologues confirms the existence of a transporter family with an ancient past. Biochem J 1998; 329:321–328.
85. Gerhart DZ, Enerson BE, Zhdankina OY, et al: Expression of monocarboxylate transporter MCT1 by brain endothelium and glia in adult and suckling rats. Am J Phyiol 1997;273(Endocrinol Metab 36):E207–E213.
86. Gerhart DZ, Enerson BE, Zhdankina OY, et al: Expression of the monocarboxylate transporter MCT2 by rat brain glia. Glia 1998;22:272–281.
87. Koehler-Stec EM, Simpson IA, Vannucci SJ, et al: Monocarboxylate transporter expression in mouse brain. Am J Physiol 1998;275:E516–E524.
88. Pellerin L, Pellegri G, Martin JL, Magistretti PJ: Expression of monocarboxylate transporter mRNAs in mouse brain: support for a distinct role of lactate as an energy substance for neonatal vs. adult brain. Proc Natl Acad Sci 1998;95:3990–3995.
89. Vannucci SJ, Corpe C, Koehler-Stec E, Simpson IA: Developmental expression of the monocarboxylate transporter proteins in rat brain. J Neurochem (Submitted for publication).
90. Vannucci SJ: Developmental expression of GLUT1 and GLUT3 glucose transporters in brain. J Neurochem 1994;62:240–246.

91. Vannucci SJ, Seaman LB, Vannucci RC: Effects of hypoxia-ischemia on GLUT1 and GLUT3 glucose transporters in immature brain. J Cereb Blood Flow Metabol 1996;16:77–81.
92. Nehlig A, Boyet S, Perriera de Vasconcelos A: Autoradiographic measurement of local cerebral β-hydroxybutyrate uptake in the rat during postnatal development. Neuroscience 1991;40:871–878.
93. Vannucci RC: Hypoxic-ischemic encephalopathy. In Fanaroff AA, Martin RJ (eds): *Neonatal-Perinatal Medicine*. 4th ed. Mosby-Year Book Inc, Philadelphia, 1997, pp 877–891.
94. Dweck HS, Cassady G: Glucose intolerance in infants of very low birthweight. Pediatrics 1974;53:189–195.
95. Monaco M, Copen P, Bloom E, et al: Cerebrospinal fluid/blood glucose ratios in premature and full-term infants. Pediatr Res 1978;12:554. Abstract.
96. Cornblath M, Schwartz R: *Disorders of Carbohydrate Metabolism in Infancy*. W.B. Saunders, Philadelphia, 1986.
97. Pildes RS: Neonatal hyperglycemia. J Pediatr 1986;109:905–907.
98. Zarif M, Pildes RS, Vidyasagar D: Insulin and growth hormone responses in neonatal hyperglycemia. Diabetes 1976;25:428–433.
99. Lilien LD, Rosenfield RL, Pildes RS: Hyperglycemia in stressed small premature neonates. J Pediatr 1979;94:454–459.
100. Greisen G, Munck H, Lou H: Severe hypocarbia in preterm infants and neurodevelopmental deficit. Acta Pediatr Scand 1987;76:401–404.
101. Graziani L, Spitzer AR, Mitchell DG, et al: Mechanical ventilation in preterm infants: neurosonographic and developmental studies. Pediatrics 1992;90:515–522.
102. Ikonen RS, Janas MO, Koidikko MJ, et al: Hyperbilirubinemia, hypocarbia and periventricular leukomalacia in preterm infants: relationship to cerebral palsy. Acta Pediatr Scand 1992;81:802–807.
103. Vannucci RC, Towfighi J, Heitjan DF, et al: Carbon dioxide protects the perinatal brain from hypoxic-ischemic damage: an experimental study in the immature rat. Pediatrics 1995;95:868–874.
104. Kogure K, Busto R, Scheinberg P, et al: Dynamics of cerebral metabolism during moderate hypercapnia. J Neurochem 1975;24:471–478.
105. Berntman L, Dehlgren N, Siesjö BK: Cerebral blood flow and oxygen consumption in the rat brain during extreme hypercarbia. Anesthesiology 1979;50:299–305.
106. Miller AL, Corddry DH: Brain carbohydrate metabolism in developing rats during hypercapnia. J Neurochem 1981;36:1202–1210.
107. Granholm R, Siesjö BK: The effects of hypercapnia and hypocapnia upon the cerebrospinal fluid lactate and pyruvate concentrations and upon the lactate, pyruvate, ATP, ADP, phosphocreatine and creatine concentrations of rat brain tissue. Acta Physiol Scand 1969;75:257–266.
108. Folbergrová J, Pontén U, Siesjö BK: Patterns of changes in brain carbohydrate metabolites, amino acids, and organic phosphates at increased carbon dioxide tensions. J Neurochem 1974;22:1115–1125.
109. Vannucci RC, Duffy TE: Cerebral oxidative and energy metabolism of fetal and neonatal rats during anoxia and recovery. Am J Physiol 1976;230:1269–1275.
110. Vannucci RC, Brucklacher RM, Vannucci SJ: Effect of carbon dioxide on

cerebral metabolism during hypoxia-ischemia in the immature rat. Pediatr Res 1997;42:24–29.

111. Bowen LW, Kochenour NK, Rehm NE, et al: Maternal-fetal pH difference and fetal scalp pH as predictors of neonatal outcome. Obstet Gynecol 1986;67:487–495.

112. Page FO, Martin JN, Palmer SM, et al: Correlation of neonatal acid-base status with Apgar scores and fetal heart rate tracings. Am J Obstet Gynecol 1986;154:1306–1311.

113. Vintzileos AM, Gaffney SE, Salinger LM, et al: The relationships among the fetal biophysical profile, umbilical cord pH and Apgar scores. Am J Obstet Gynecol 1987;157:627–631.

114. Winkler CL, Hauth JC, Tucker JM, et al: Neonatal complications at term as related to the degree of umbilical artery acidemia. Am J Obstet Gynecol 1991;164:637–641.

115. Dennis J, Johnson A, Mutch L, et al: Acid-base status at birth and neurodevelopmental outcome for four and one-half years. Am J Obstet Gynecol 1989;161:213–220.

116. Fee SC, Malee K, Deddish R, et al: Severe acidosis and subsequent neurologic status. Am J Obstet Gynecol 1990;162:802–806.

117. Goldaber KG, Gilstrap LC, Leveno KJ, et al: Pathologic fetal acidemia. Obstet Gynecol 1991;78:1103–1107.

118. Low JA, Panagiotopoulos C, Derrick EJ: Newborn complications after intrapartum asphyxia with metabolic acidosis in the term fetus. Am J Obstet Gynecol 1994;170:1081–1087.

119. Perlman JM, Risser R: Severe fetal acidemia: neonatal neurologic features and short-term outcome. Pediatr Neurol 1993;9:277–282.

120. Socol ML, Garcia PM, Riter S: Depressed Apgar scores, acid-base status, and neurologic outcome. Am J Obstet Gynecol 1994;170:991–999.

121. Low JA, Galbraith RS, Muir DW: Factors associated with motor and cognitive deficits in children after intrapartum fetal hypoxia. Am J Obstet Gynecol 1984;148:533–539.

122. Vannucci RC: Experimental biology of cerebral hypoxia-ischemia: relation to perinatal brain damage. Pediatr Res 1990;27:317–326.

CHAPTER 6

Energy Consequences of Cerebral Hypoxia-Ischemia

John S. Wyatt

Introduction

Since glucose and oxygen are the principal substrates for oxidative energy metabolism in the perinatal brain, the interruption of substrate delivery as a result of severe and acute hypoxia-ischemia is accompanied by rapid depletion of the high-energy phosphates adenosine triphosphate (ATP) and phosphocreatine (PCr) within brain cells. The classic experiments of Vannucci and Duffy in the 1970s used postmortem tissue chemical analysis in the newborn puppy exposed to acute asphyxia.[1] They demonstrated that following the onset of asphyxia, PCr rapidly fell to a low concentration, while ATP concentrations were maintained for a brief period as a result of the creatine kinase equilibrium, followed by a subsequent decline. Simultaneously, brain glucose levels declined rapidly and brain tissue lactate concentration rose to very high values as a result of anaerobic glycolysis.[1] Similar changes over a much more prolonged time course have been observed in the immature rat brain exposed to unilateral carotid artery ligation and hypoxia.[2,3]

Although rapid postmortem biochemical analysis of brain tissue continues to have a role in experimental animal models, the development of magnetic resonance spectroscopy (MRS) has allowed *in vivo* assessment of cerebral energy metabolism in both experimental animal models and newborn infants with hypoxic-ischemic encephalopathy. In particular, phosphorus (^{31}P) MRS allows the measurement of intracellular nucleotide triphosphate, mainly ATP, PCr, and inorganic phosphate (Pi), as well as determination of the intracellular pH. Proton (^{1}H) spectroscopy provides measurement of lactate, N-acetyl aspartate (Naa), choline, and creatine-containing compounds.

From Donn SM, Sinha SK, Chiswick ML (eds): *Birth Asphyxia and the Brain: Basic Science and Clinical Implications.* © 2002, Futura Publishing Co., Inc., Armonk, NY.

Secondary Cerebral Energy Failure in Encephalopathic Infants

The first clinical studies with MRS were performed in the early 1980s. Infants were selected because of clinical suspicion of severe intrapartum asphyxia, based on a compatible obstetrical history, lactic acidosis at birth, and signs of early onset encephalopathy. Studies from several groups have shown a consistent pattern of derangement of energy metabolism.[4-7] Phosphorus spectra are frequently normal within the first hours following resuscitation, suggesting that mitochondrial oxidative phosphorylation is sufficiently restored to meet energetic demands. However, after 12–24 hours, a progressive decline in the PCr/Pi ratio is frequently observed.[8,9] In more severely affected infants, a delayed decline in ATP signal can also be detected. The maximum energetic derangements are generally seen at 48–72 hours and in the most severe cases, both the PCr and ATP signals may fall to very low levels. In less severe cases, the PCr/Pi ratio usually returns to approximately normal values within about 7 days. A representative study is shown in Figure 1.

This complex sequence of events has been termed "secondary" or delayed cerebral energy failure to distinguish it from the "primary" rapid changes in ATP and PCr seen during acute ischemia in experimental models. These profound secondary disturbances in cerebral energetics are frequently observed in infants in whom systemic circulatory and metabolic homeostasis has been successfully maintained with conventional intensive care techniques.

The earliest studies used ^{31}P MRS, but later studies using ^{1}H MRS in asphyxiated infants have demonstrated that the delayed decline in PCr and ATP is associated with a rise in cerebral lactate concentration.[10-12] A correlation between the magnitude of the rise in cerebral lactate within the first 18 hours and the subsequent fall in PCr/Pi ratio has been reported.[13] In severely affected infants, cerebral lactate elevation persists and becomes more marked after 24 hours, despite the presence of normal blood lactate; this suggests that anaerobic glycolysis occurs within the brain simultaneously with the delayed derangement in oxidative phosphorylation.[12] Studies using localized ^{1}H MRS, in which spectra are obtained from precisely defined anatomic volumes, enable regional differences to be explored. In one study of encephalopathic infants, lactate elevation was much more marked within the thalamic region compared to the occipito-parietal white matter.[12]

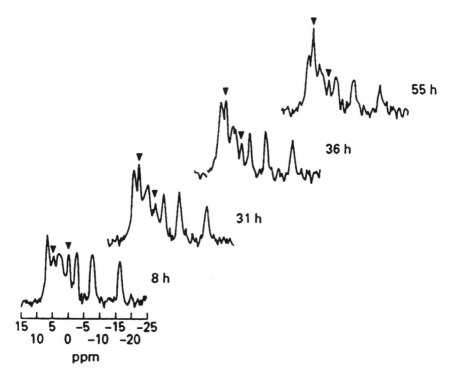

Figure 1. Phosphorus spectra from a baby born at 37 weeks gestation who had sustained severe birth asphyxia. The age at the time of each study is shown. At each age, the peak marked by the left arrow is attributable to inorganic phosphate (Pi), and the right arrow indicates phosphocreatine (PCr). The three major peaks on the right of each spectrum represent the γ, α, and β phosphorous nuclei, respectively, of adenosine triphosphate (ATP). At 8 hours, the spectrum was normal, but PCr/Pi fell to a minimum value at 55 hours, when the ATP/total phosphorous also fell. From Azzopardi et al,[6] with permission.

It is interesting that, despite the marked elevation of cerebral lactate, intracellular pH during secondary energy failure has been found to remain within normal limits or even to show a slight alkalotic shift. This is in marked contrast to the results obtained from experimental models during "primary" energy failure, in which intracellular pH falls markedly.[3,14] A possible explanation for the lack of acidosis despite lactate accumulation during secondary energy failure is that hydrogen ions are transported out of damaged neurons rapidly, whereas the capacity of transmembrane transporters for lactate is limited.

Most MRS studies of asphyxiated infants have used concentration ratios, but recently, absolute quantification (in mmol/kg) of both phosphorus and proton metabolites has become possible. Either external reference solutions or brain water may be utilized as an internal concentration reference.[15–17] The results are broadly consistent with studies using metabolite ratios. In one study, measurements from the thalamic region demonstrated an elevated tissue lactate concentration of a median of 5.4 mmol/kg (compared to 2.8 mmol/kg in control infants), and a reduced Naa of 5.2 mmol/kg (compared to 10.3 mmol/kg).[16] (N-acetyl aspartate is present in high concentrations within the neuronal cytoplasm, although its precise biochemical role remains controversial, and it has also been detected in immature oligodendrocytes.) Phosphocreatine, ATP, and total phosphorus concentrations in the asphyxiated infants were markedly reduced compared with control infants, whereas inorganic phosphate was elevated. The combination of an elevated cerebral lactate concentration with a decrease in phosphorylation potential strongly suggests that there is an increase in the glycolytic rate secondary to a fall in the rate of mitochondrial ATP synthesis.

In asphyxiated infants studied somewhat later (1–3 weeks after delivery), a significant decline in Naa has been observed.[10,11] As Naa is thought to be present primarily within the neuronal cytoplasm, this late decline may provide a quantitative measure of permanent neuronal loss following asphyxia. Recently, the persistence of elevated cerebral lactate together with intracellular alkalosis has been described in a group of infants with early neonatal encephalopathy who were studied by MRS between 1 and 12 months of age.[18] This observation is intriguing in its implications and is an important topic for further research. It is plausible that anaerobic glycolysis persists for many months in regions of injured brain as a result of long-standing mitochondrial dysfunction, and it is conceivable that low-grade cellular injury continues to occur many months after the acute encephalopathic episode.

Prognosis in Intrapartum Asphyxia

The detection of secondary energy failure by MRS has important prognostic implications in encephalopathic newborn infants. Follow-up studies have demonstrated close relationships between minimum PCr:Pi during the first week of life and adverse long-term neurodevelopmental outcome and reduced head growth.[6,9,15,19] Similarly, elevation of lactate:creatine or lactate:Naa ratios after birth is associated with a poor long-term prognosis.[10–12] In one recent study, proton MRS was more predictive of outcome at 1 year of age than a carefully performed neurologic examination after birth.[20] These studies suggest that there is a "dose-response" relationship between the magnitude of the cerebral biochemical disturbance detected in the first week of life and the severity of long-term adverse outcome. They provide supportive evidence that the development of secondary cerebral energy failure following intrapartum asphyxia has a close causal and temporal relationship with brain cell death, and hence with its permanent neurologic and developmental sequelae.

Animal Models of Secondary Energy Failure

The complex biphasic sequence of metabolic and pathophysiologic changes following intrapartum asphyxia has been reproduced in a neonatal piglet model, which used continuous ^{31}P and ^{1}H MRS maintained over a period of more than 48 hours.[21,22] During transient cerebral hypoxia-ischemia, acute "primary" depletion of cerebral PCr and ATP occurred within 60–120 minutes. Following reperfusion and reoxygenation of the brain, phosphorus metabolites rapidly returned to normal. After a few hours, a progressive delay in PCr/Pi ratio and in ATP was observed despite maintenance of cardiorespiratory homeostasis. Cerebral lactate levels in this model demonstrated a similar biphasic pattern, with rapid elevation during the acute hypoxic-ischemic episode and recovery within 1 to 2 hours of resuscitation, followed by progressive elevation during the phase of delayed energy failure.[22] Metabolite spin-spin relaxation times (T2 values) were markedly elevated during delayed energy failure. This may reflect neuronal swelling and increased cytoplasmic water following failure of the ATP-dependent sodium-potassium pump.

The neonatal piglet has particular advantages as a model for investigating secondary energy failure in view of the anatomic similarities between the brains of the piglet and the human newborn, and the possibility of using standard intensive care techniques to maintain cardiorespiratory and metabolic homeostasis. However, studies using ^{31}P MRS in a neonatal rat model have also demonstrated a similar biphasic pattern in cerebral energy metabolism following unilateral carotid artery ligation.[23] In this model, there was a significant relationship between the extent of the delayed reduction in high-energy metabolites and the magnitude of the cerebral infarction.

A fundamental limitation in both ^{1}H and ^{31}P MRS is low spatial resolution. Therefore, it is necessary to collect signals from a substantial volume of tissue to attain an acceptable signal-to-noise ratio. ^{1}H MRS chemical shift imaging has the potential to display spectra that have been collected simultaneously from multiple areas within the tissue of interest. If this technique can be successfully applied to the neonatal brain following intrapartum asphyxia, there is likely to be a substantial improvement in the spatial localization of metabolic derangement. The technical problems are substantial and, to date, no studies on the neonatal brain have been published.

Use of Diffusion-Weighted Imaging to Assess Cerebral Energetics

An alternative approach to provide improved spatial resolution of disturbances in cerebral energetics is to use diffusion-weighted MRI. Several studies have documented an acute reduction in the apparent diffusion coefficient (ADC) of water, which occurs within minutes following the onset of cerebral ischemia.[24] The physical mechanisms underlying this reduction in water diffusion are not fully understood, although there is evidence that it reflects, at least in part, the microscopic redistribution of tissue water from the extracellular to the intracellular compartment. Thus, changes in ADC can provide a sensitive index of cellular membrane integrity and the functioning of the sodium-potassium ATPase enzyme. A very close correlation between decreases in ADC and reductions in the tissue ATP concentration (reflecting the phosphorylation potential of the tissue) has been demonstrated in animal models of focal cerebral ischemia.[25] As a result, two-dimensional mapping of ADC values has the potential to provide information about disturbances in cerebral energetics with a much higher spatial resolution (1 mm or less) than is possible with conventional localized spectroscopy.

Measurements of ADC values during the development of secondary energy failure in the piglet model have shown a progressive decrease that mirrors the decline in ATP and PCr.[26] Of particular interest is the observation that highly localized ADC abnormalities were detected within 12 hours of resuscitation, either in the region of the parasagittal cortex or the thalamus. Over the next 24–48 hours, the ADC abnormalities were observed to have spread across the cerebral hemisphere, leading ultimately to uniform reductions in ADC throughout the hemisphere.[26] A decrease in the anisotropy of water diffusion in both gray and white matter has also been observed with the development of secondary energy failure.[27] At present, these observations are intriguing, but unexplained. They suggest that the development of secondary energy failure is accompanied by a very slow migration of oxidative energetic disturbance across brain tissue. It is interesting that the early ADC abnormalities in the parasagittal cortex coincide with an anatomic vascular watershed zone between the cerebral arteries, and thus this region is particularly prone to ischemic injury. A similar delayed decline in ADC has recently been reported in the neonatal rat brain following middle cerebral artery occlusion.[25]

Magnetic resonance techniques thus have the potential to provide detailed early assessment of the encephalopathic infant and novel insights into the temporal and spatial evolution of cellular injury following an acute hypoxic-ischemic insult. They may allow the anatomic localization and the identification of the severity of permanent cellular injury within the first few days of life. Reductions in Naa may provide a quantitative index of neuronal loss, while increases in Naa T2 may indicate edema and impaired membrane ATPase activity in injured neurons that have not yet undergone autolysis. ^{1}H chemical shift imaging or the measurement of ADC values may provide early detailed definition of the anatomic pattern of injury. It seems likely that a combination of these measurements will lead to marked improvements in the accuracy of early predictions of long-term neurologic impairment or death.

Use of Near-Infrared Spectroscopy to Investigate Cerebral Oxidative Metabolism

Near-infrared spectroscopy (NIRS) has the potential to provide complementary information about cellular energy metabolism in the brain. Changes in oxy- and deoxyhemoglobin concentrations reflect the balance between cerebral oxygen delivery and tissue extraction, and the total hemoglobin concentration. Measurement of changes in the redox state of the copper A center of cytochrome oxidase (Cu_A) reflects oxygen availability and electron flux at the mitochondrial level.

Near-infrared spectroscopy studies in newborn infants with acute encephalopathy following a presumed asphyxial insult have provided insights into the profound hemodynamic changes that usually accompany the development of secondary energy failure. A frequent observation has been the combination of elevated cerebral blood volume and cerebral blood flow together with a diminished response to changing arterial carbon dioxide tension.[28] When the hemodynamic changes in encephalopathic infants are compared to the long-term outcome, elevated cerebral blood volume and cerebral blood flow are associated with an increased risk of adverse outcome.[28] The attenuation of the cerebrovascular response to carbon dioxide suggests that cerebral energy failure is associated with disruption of normal vascular control mechanisms and cerebral arteriolar vasodilation.

Near-infrared spectroscopy studies in the newborn piglet have confirmed the expected changes during acute cerebral hypoxia-ischemia. Marked declines are seen in both cerebral hemoglobin oxygenation and in the Cu_A redox state.[29] In one study, no change in the Cu_A redox state was observed until cerebral oxyhemoglobin had decreased by more than 10 μmol/L, indicating that the Cu_A redox state is maintained until hemoglobin oxygen delivery to the cytochrome oxidase-binding site falls below a critical level.[29] In another study, a close correlation was demonstrated between cerebral high-energy phosphates measured by ^{31}P MRS and cytochrome redox state measured by NIRS.[30]

In the piglet, following resuscitation, cerebral hemoglobin oxygenation and Cu_A signal return rapidly towards normal. However, 12–24 hours later a rise in cerebral hemoglobin oxygenation and blood volume is seen at the same time that progressive depletion of high-energy phosphates occurs. These observations are entirely consistent with those from encephalopathic infants and confirm that secondary cellular energy failure is associated with *increased* tissue oxygenation. Similar findings have been obtained in a fetal sheep model following transient cerebral ischemia.[31] A delayed and progressive increase in cerebral oxygenation coincided with a decline in the redox state of cytochrome oxidase and an increase in cortical impedance, which may reflect cellular swelling.

Preliminary data in the newborn piglet indicate that the increase in cerebral hemoglobin oxygenation represents a combination of increased oxygen tissue delivery resulting from cerebral arteriolar vasodilation and reduced cerebral oxygen extraction secondary to reduced tissue oxygen consumption. Thus, there is little evidence that secondary energy failure is a consequence of impaired substrate delivery. Instead, mitochondrial oxygen consumption must be impaired by an alternative mechanism leading to a reduction in the rate of phosphorylation and progressive depletion of cytoplasmic ATP and PCr levels.

One possible explanation is the action of an inhibitor on the mitochondrial respiratory chain. Nitric oxide (NO) has been shown to be a potent inhibitor of mitochondrial cytochrome oxidase *in vivo* by competing directly at the oxygen-binding site of the enzyme.[32] Since the inhibition acts downstream of the Cu_A center, accumulation of electrons would be anticipated at the Cu_A site, leading to a reduction in its redox level. Preliminary studies in the piglet model have detected a reduction from baseline in Cu_A redox level in the first 12 hours following resuscitation.[33] Studies using electron spin resonance spectroscopy to analyze the presence of Hb-NO in samples taken from the cerebral venous blood are currently under way to confirm whether NO release can be detected.

Mechanisms of Secondary Energy Failure

In the fetal sheep model of delayed cerebral injury, extracellular levels of citrulline (a by-product of NO synthesis measured by microdialysis in the cerebral cortex) are elevated during both the primary and delayed phases of energy failure.[34] It seems plausible, therefore, that the delayed cerebral vasodilation may be related to excessive NO release. This hypothesis is supported by evidence in the fetal sheep model that administration of an NO synthase inhibitor leads to a reduction in the degree of delayed vasodilation,[35] although there is no amelioration in the evidence of secondary energy failure nor in the magnitude of the resultant cellular injury.

In the piglet model of secondary energy failure, a close relationship has been demonstrated between the magnitude of the delayed decline in cerebral ATP and the percentage of brain cells that undergo apoptotic and necrotic cell death.[36] Similarly, clinical studies have demonstrated a dose-response relationship between the decline in cerebral high-energy phosphates and both the long-term neurodevelopmental outcome and the degree of cerebral atrophy.[19] These data indicate the close relationship between derangements of oxidative energy metabolism and brain cell death in this clinical context. The rapidly accumulating evidence of the critical role that mitochondria play in apoptotic cell death is highlighted elsewhere (see Chapter 7). The opening of the mitochondrial permeability transition pore may lead to cell death either by causing an acute decline in cytoplasmic ATP concentration, cellular energy failure, and necrosis, or by the release of cytochrome *c* from mitochondria into the cytoplasm leading to caspase activation and apoptotic execution. Thus, detection of a decline in cytoplasmic ATP concentration *in vivo* by MRS or diffusion-weighted MRI may act as a surrogate marker of both necrotic and apoptotic cellular death. Similarly, the preservation of high-energy phosphates following neuroprotective interventions such as moderate hypothermia provides strong evidence that cell death can be inhibited.[37,38]

Conclusions

The use of noninvasive tools, especially magnetic resonance and near-infrared spectroscopy, has provided unique insights into the complex temporal sequence of energetic and hemodynamic disturbances that occur in the neonatal brain following a severe, transient episode of hypoxia-ischemia. It seems probable that acute and catastrophic interruption of fetal oxygen delivery during labor (e.g., as a result of uterine rupture or cord prolapse) will lead to the rapid development of primary energy failure in the human brain. It is currently impossible to perform MRS on the brain of the fetus during labor; hence, direct intrapartum assessment of cerebral energetics is impossible, and only indirect markers are available. On the basis of the current evidence, it seems that the most reliable early indicator of a preceding episode of cerebral energy failure is a marked suppression of background cortical electrical activity, which can be detected immediately after birth.

The precise time period of hypoxia-ischemia required for primary energy failure to occur depends on the balance between the degree of impairment of substrate delivery and the rate of ATP consumption. In animal experiments involving complete interruption of cerebral blood supply, energy failure occurs within 10–15 minutes; with partial or intermittent hypoxia-ischemia, 60 minutes to several hours duration may be required. In the assessment of encephalopathic infants, it might be possible, in theory, to deduce the severity and nature of the primary insult from the degree of secondary energy failure, but in practice, this has not yet proven feasible.

Studies of secondary cerebral energy failure in experimental models are likely to provide valuable information about fundamental mechanisms of cellular injury. Further work is required to relate the precise timing and nature of the primary insult to the severity and timing of the resultant secondary energy failure. The interaction between infective and ischemic processes in the initiation of cerebral energy failure is also of great interest and clinical importance.

In the future, noninvasive clinical assessment of cerebral energetics may enable both the severity and the spatial distribution of cellular injury to be determined in the first few days of life following an acute asphyxial insult. This will provide clinicians and parents with important prognostic information and guide novel therapeutic interventions.

Acknowledgments: The author gratefully acknowledges the major contribution of colleagues in the Departments of Paediatrics and Medical Physics and

Bioengineering, University College London, and the Department of Neonatal Medicine, Imperial College School of Medicine, United Kingdom.

References

1. Vannucci RC, Duffy TE: Cerebral metabolism in newborn dogs during reversible asphyxia. Ann Neurol 1977;1:528–534.
2. Yager JY, Brucklacher RM, Vannucci RC: Cerebral energy metabolism during hypoxia-ischemia and early recovery in immature rats. Am J Physiol 1992;262:H672–H677.
3. Yager JY, Brucklacher RM, Vannucci RC: Cerebral oxidative metabolism and redox state during hypoxia-ischemia and early recovery in immature rats. Am J Physiol 1992;261:H1102–H1188.
4. Hope PL, Costello AML, Cady EB, et al: Cerebral energy metabolism studied with phosphorus NMR spectroscopy in normal and birth-asphyxiated infants. Lancet 1984;ii:366–370.
5. Younkin DP, Delivoria-Papadopoulos M, Leonard JC, et al: Unique aspects of human newborn cerebral metabolism evaluated with phosphorus nuclear magnetic resonance spectroscopy. Ann Neurol 1984;16:581–586.
6. Azzopardi D, Wyatt JS, Cady EB, et al: Prognosis of newborn infants with hypoxic-ischemic brain injury assessed by phosphorus magnetic resonance spectroscopy. Pediatr Res 1989;25:445–451.
7. Laptook AR, Corbett RJ, Uauy R, et al: Use of ^{31}P magnetic resonance spectroscopy to characterize evolving brain damage after perinatal asphyxia. Neurology 1989;39:709–712.
8. Wyatt JS, Edwards AD, Azzopardi D, et al: Magnetic resonance and near infrared spectroscopy for the investigation of perinatal hypoxic-ischaemic brain injury. Arch Dis Child 1989;64:953–963.
9. Roth SC, Edwards AD, Cady EB, et al: Relation between cerebral oxidative metabolism following birth asphyxia and neurodevelopmental outcome at one year. Dev Med Child Neurol 1992;34:285–295.
10. Peden CJ, Rutherford MA, Sargentoni J, et al: Proton spectroscopy of the brain following hypoxic-ischaemic injury. Dev Med Child Neurol 1993;35:502–510.
11. Groenendaal F, Veenhoven RH, van der Grond J, et al: Cerebral lactate and N-acetyl-aspartate/choline ratios in asphyxiated full-term neonates demonstrated in vivo using proton magnetic resonance spectroscopy. Pediatr Res 1994;35:148–151.
12. Penrice J, Cady EB, Lorek A, et al: Proton magnetic resonance spectroscopy of the brain in normal preterm and term infants and early changes following perinatal hypoxia-ischemia. Pediatr Res 1996;40:6–14.
13. Hanrahan JD, Sargentoni J, Azzopardi D, et al: Cerebral metabolism within 18 hours of birth asphyxia: a proton magnetic resonance spectroscopy study. Pediatr Res 1996;39:584–590.
14. Corbett RJ, Laptook AR, Nunnally RL, et al: Intracellular pH, lactate, and energy metabolism in neonatal brain during partial ischemia measured in vivo by ^{31}P and ^{1}H nuclear magnetic resonance spectroscopy. J Neurochem 1988;51:1501–1509.
15. Martin E, Buchli R, Ritter S, et al: Diagnostic and prognostic value of cere-

bral ^{31}P magnetic resonance spectroscopy in neonates with perinatal asphyxia. Pediatr Res 1996;40:749–758.

16. Cady EB, Penrice J, Amess PN, et al: Lactate, N-acetyl aspartate, choline and creatine concentrations, and spin-spin relaxation in thalamic and occipito-parietal regions of developing human brain. Magn Res Med 1996;36:878–886.

17. Cady EB, Wylezinska M, Penrice J, et al: Quantitation of phosphorus metabolites in newborn brain using internal water as a reference standard. Magn Res Imaging 1996;14:293–304.

18. Robertson NJ, Cox IJ, Cowan FM, et al: Cerebral intracellular lactic alkalosis persisting months after neonatal encephalopathy measured by magnetic resonance spectroscopy. Pediatr Res 1999;46:287–296.

19. Roth SC, Baudin J, Cady EB, et al: Relation of deranged neonatal cerebral oxidative metabolism with neurodevelopmental outcome and head circumference at 4 years. Dev Med Child Neurol 1997;39:718–725.

20. Amess PN, Penrice J, Wylezinska M, et al: Early brain proton magnetic resonance spectroscopy and neonatal neurology related to neurodevelopmental outcome at 1 year in term infants after presumed hypoxic-ischaemic brain injury. Dev Med Child Neurol 1999;41:436–445.

21. Lorek A, Takei Y, Cady EB, et al: Delayed cerebral energy failure following acute hypoxia-ischemia in the newborn piglet: continuous 48-hour studies by phosphorus magnetic resonance spectroscopy. Pediatr Res 1994;36:699–706.

22. Penrice J, Lorek A, Cady EB, et al: Proton magnetic resonance spectroscopy of the brain during acute hypoxia-ischemia and delayed cerebral energy failure in the newborn piglet. Pediatr Res 1997;1:795–802.

23. Blumberg RM, Cady EB, Wigglesworth JS, et al: Relation between delayed impairment of cerebral energy metabolism and infarction following transient focal hypoxia-ischemia in the developing brain. Exp Brain Res 1997;13:130–137.

24. Busza AL, Allen KL, King MD, et al: Diffusion-weighted imaging studies of cerebral ischemia in gerbils: potential relevance to energy failure. Stroke 1992;23:1602–1612.

25. Campagne MVL, Thomas GR, Thibodeaux H, et al: Secondary reduction in the apparent diffusion coefficient of water, increase in cerebral blood volume and delayed neuronal death after middle cerebral artery occlusion and early reperfusion in the rat. J Cereb Blood Flow Metab 1999;19:1354–1364.

26. Thornton JS, Ordidge RJ, Penrice J, et al: Temporal and anatomical variations of brain water apparent diffusion coefficient in perinatal cerebral hypoxic-ischaemic injury: relationships to cerebral energy metabolism. Magn Reson Med 1998;39:920–927.

27. Thornton JS, Ordidge RJ, Penrice J, et al: Anisotropic water diffusion in white and grey matter of the neonatal piglet brain before and after transient hypoxia-ischemia. Magn Reson Imaging 1997;15:433–440.

28. Meek JH, Elwell CE, McCormick DC, et al: Abnormal cerebral hemodynamics in perinatally asphyxiated neonates related to outcome. Arch Dis Child Fetal Neonatal Ed 1999;81:F110–F115.

29. Quaresima V, Springett R, Cope M, et al: Oxidation and reduction of cytochrome oxidase in the neonatal brain observed by in vivo near infrared spectroscopy. Biochim Biophys Acta 1998;1366:291–300.

30. Tsuji M, Naruse H, Volpe J, et al: Reduction of cytochrome aa3 measured by near-infrared spectroscopy predicts cerebral energy loss in hypoxic piglets. Pediatr Res 1995;37:253–259.

31. Marks KA, Mallard EC, Roberts I, et al: Delayed vasodilatation and altered oxygenation after cerebral ischemia in fetal sheep. Pediatr Res 1996;39:48–54.

32. Brown GC, Cooper CE: Nanomolar concentrations of nitric oxide reversibly inhibit synaptosomal cytochrome oxidase respiration by competing with oxygen at cytochrome oxidase. FEBS Lett 1994;356:295–298.

33. Springett RJ, Penrice JM, Amess PN, et al: Non-invasive measurements of mitochondrial damage during neonatal hypoxia-ischemia: a role for nitric oxide? Biochem Soc Trans 1997;25:398.

34. Tan WKM, Williams CE, During MJ, et al: Accumulation of cytotoxins during the development of seizures and edema after hypoxic-ischemic injury in late-gestation fetal sheep. Pediatr Res 1996;39:791–797.

35. Marks KA, Mallard EC, Roberts I, et al: Nitric oxide synthase inhibition attenuates delayed vasodilatation and increases tissue injury following cerebral ischemia in fetal sheep. Pediatr Res 1996;40:185–191.

36. Mehmet H, Yue X, Penrice J, et al: Relation of impaired energy metabolism to apoptosis and necrosis following transient hypoxia-ischemia. Cell Death Differ 1998;5:321–329.

37. Thoresen M, Penrice J, Lorek A, et al: Mild hypothermia following severe transient hypoxia-ischemia ameliorates delayed cerebral energy failure in the newborn piglet. Pediatr Res 1995;37:667–670.

38. Amess PN, Penrice J, Cady EB, et al: Mild hypothermia after severe transient hypoxia-ischemia reduces the delayed rise in cerebral lactate in the newborn piglet. Pediatr Res 1997;41:803–808.

CHAPTER 7

Apoptosis and Necrosis in Perinatal Brain Injury

Huseyin Mehmet, A. David Edwards

Introduction

Delayed Injury After Cerebral Hypoxia-Ischemia

Studies with magnetic resonance spectroscopy (MRS) have demonstrated that term infants with clinical evidence of intrapartum hypoxia-ischemia show characteristic abnormalities in cerebral energy metabolism (see Chapter 6). These infants typically have normal cerebral energy metabolism soon after birth, but some hours later a progressive decline in cerebral high-energy phosphates occurs.[1] The magnitude of these delayed abnormalities in cerebral energy metabolism is related to the severity of later neurodevelopmental impairment.[2–5] These findings suggest that cerebral injury occurs not only during hypoxia-ischemia, but for a considerable time afterwards. Indeed, recent studies have shown that cerebral metabolism may be abnormal for many months following hypoxia-ischemia.[6] Mechanisms of cell death that explain such delayed and prolonged injury need to be elucidated. The demonstration that cells can die by apoptosis for a prolonged period after hypoxia-ischemia not only offers a suitable explanation for these findings, but also suggests that the previous view that hypoxia-ischemia induces cell death only by necrosis is incomplete.[7]

Recent research has begun to elucidate the complex relationship between apoptotic and necrotic cell death, although the majority of data have been acquired from experiments that have not involved perinatal brain cells. However, the mechanisms of apoptosis seem to be highly conserved, and it currently seems possible to construct a representation of events in the human newborn infant brain using data from a variety of paradigms. This chapter attempts to construct such a rep-

From Donn SM, Sinha SK, Chiswick ML (eds): *Birth Asphyxia and the Brain: Basic Science and Clinical Implications.* © 2002, Futura Publishing Co., Inc., Armonk, NY.

resentation, which must nevertheless be regarded as preliminary and in need of confirmation from specific studies of the developing brain.

Modes of Cell Death Following Oxidative Injury

Cell death can proceed by different routes, each with relatively characteristic morphologic criteria as endpoints. Death is conventionally classified as apoptotic or necrotic. In necrosis, cell death is triggered by an overwhelming external insult damaging cellular organelles, such as mitochondria, resulting in the loss of membrane integrity and the leaking of cytoplasmic contents into the extracellular matrix. In contrast, cells dying by apoptosis carry out a well-conserved and highly regulated genetic program of cell death. They do not immediately lose membrane integrity and the organelles remain largely intact. In the final stages, cell fragments are "shrink-wrapped" in the contracting plasma membrane and bud off as apoptotic bodies, which are subsequently phagocytosed by healthy neighboring cells. Since the apoptotic response to damage largely circumvents inflammatory responses, this mode of cell death would be particularly beneficial following injury to the brain, which has only a limited capacity for repair and regeneration.[8]

Apoptosis is a biochemically and genetically programmed cell death that requires time, energy and, in some cases, new gene transcription and translation. It can be triggered by a variety of stimuli, including ligand binding to specific cell surface receptors such as Fas or tumor necrosis factor-α (TNF-α), withdrawal of paracrine or autocrine survival factors, or damage to cell mechanisms or genetic material.[9] In many cells, apoptosis is a default pathway that is activated whenever survival signals, such as growth factors, are not available to the cell. The molecular mechanisms are becoming more clear, and important components of the death machinery, such as a specialized family of cysteine-aspartate proteases (caspases; Figure 1) have been described.[10] However, as discussed later, the distinction between apoptosis and necrosis is not always clear and, in many instances, these two modes of cell death can be regarded as a continuum of a single cell fate following injury.

Apoptosis and Necrosis Following Hypoxia-Ischemia

Both apoptotic and necrotic cells are found in tissue after hypoxia-ischemia. Necrosis can occur during hypoxia-ischemia or immediately

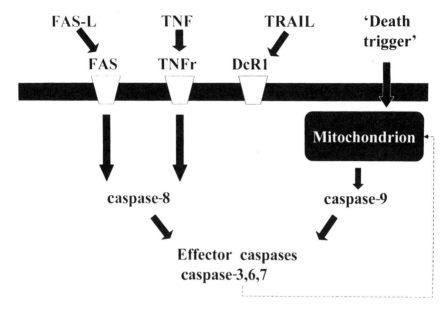

Figure 1. Examples of triggers of apoptosis and associated signal transduction pathways. The tumor necrosis factor receptor (TNFr) or the Fas receptor (FAS) bind TNF or FAS-L ligand, respectively, which triggers a cascade that activates caspase-8. In some cells, decoy receptors (DcR1) can bind and sequester death ligands (e.g., TRAIL), thus protecting the cell from apoptosis. Direct or indirect disruption of mitochondrial function can release apoptogenic factors which activate caspase-9. Both caspase-8 and caspase-9 activate the effector caspases-3, -6, and -7, which may feed back to induce opening of mitochondrial channels and release of further apoptogenic proteins. The effector caspases dismantle the cellular machinery and package the cell for phagocytosis.

following resuscitation, when blood flow is very low, and when an acute deficit in substrate delivery can result in a rapid reduction in cerebral energy production, membrane pump failure, and severe ionic imbalances that result in cell swelling. These acute early changes may be associated with an increase in excitotoxic amino acid levels and free radical production, the damaging effects of which can be blocked by specific receptor antagonists and scavengers (see Chapter 8).

Apoptotic cells are seen following hypoxic-ischemic injury in both the immature[11–13] and adult rat brain.[14,15] Administration of the anti-apoptotic survival factor insulin-like growth factor-1 (IGF-1) after the primary insult ameliorates delayed injury, while glutamate receptor blockade is only partially protective.[16] Apoptosis has been shown to be involved in human perinatal brain injury. Infants who die after intrauterine injury, either with or without evidence of hypoxia-ischemia, have a significant number of cells in the brain with the morphologic characteristics of apoptosis.[17,18]

The Relationship Between Apoptotic and Necrotic Death in Cerebral Injury

It might be convenient to consider immediate cell death following hypoxia-ischemia as necrotic, and delayed cell death as apoptotic. However, published data indicate that the relationship between these two modes of cell death is more complex. In experimental hypoxia-ischemia, apoptosis and necrosis can occur in adjacent populations of neurons and glial cells in the cingulate gyrus, while quantitative analysis of cell death showed that the numbers of apoptotic and necrotic cells were both linearly related to the severity of adenosine triphosphate (ATP) depletion during hypoxia-ischemia.[5,19] The cause of brain injury can also affect the mode of cell death. Thus, human infants who have suffered secondary energy failure have a preponderance of necrotic cells, while fetuses dying *in utero* show a higher proportion of apoptotic cells.[17]

These complexities may arise, in part, because some necrotic cells represent the secondary degradation of apoptotic cells. In this context, primary cell necrosis can be regarded as an acute response to severe injury and is the common pattern of change in cerebral infarcts. Secondary cell necrosis can occur in cells triggered to undergo apoptosis but unable to complete the program.[20] Oxygen-glucose deprivation may first induce apoptosis and then secondary necrosis in cerebellar granule cells.[21] Similarly, primary apoptosis precedes secondary necrosis following the injection of excitatory amino acid receptor agonists into the adult rat brain.[22] Cell necrosis should therefore be distinguished from tissue necrosis, in which a large number of cells undergo necrosis together, and may be primary, secondary, or both.

Molecular Evidence of Apoptosis Following Brain Injury

A number of molecular signals associated with apoptotic death are induced by impaired oxidative phosphorylation and oxidative injury. These signals are reviewed in the following sections.

Caspases and Poly(ADP-Ribose) Polymerase Cleavage

The nuclear enzyme, poly(ADP-ribose) polymerase (PARP), provides one of the most apparent links between oxidative stress, impaired energy metabolism, and cell damage. Free radicals such as nitric oxide and peroxynitrite can damage DNA, leading to activation of PARP, which catalyzes attachment of ADP-ribose units from nicotinamide adenine dinucleotide (NAD) to nuclear proteins. However, excessive activation of PARP can deplete NAD^+ and ATP (which is consumed in NAD regeneration), leading to an increase in the $NADH/NAD^+$ ratio, and eventually, cell death by energy depletion. PARP is induced by hypoxia-ischemia, and genetic disruption of PARP provides profound protection against both glutamate-mediated excitotoxic insults *in vitro* and major decreases in infarct volume after reversible middle cerebral artery occlusion.[23]

Although these results provide compelling evidence for a primary involvement of PARP activation in neuronal damage, the situation is complex. Genetic deletion of PARP or PARP inhibition by 3-aminobenzamide reduced infarct size after transient cerebral ischemia,[24] but did not reduce the density of apoptotic cells.[25] The susceptibility of primary neurons towards apoptosis is unaffected in PARP −/− mice, suggesting that PARP activation is not necessary for apoptosis.[26] Thus, in cerebral ischemia, PARP may contribute to cell death by NAD^+ depletion and primary energy failure without direct involvement in apoptotic responses.

PARP is involved in apoptosis in another way. Specific proteolytic cleavage of PARP by caspase-3 is an important event in at least one pathway to apoptosis,[27] possibly as a mechanism to maintain the ATP needed for successful completion of the apoptotic program. Caspases are the primary effectors of apoptotic death after a variety of death triggers.[10] Both caspase activity[28] and PARP cleavage[29] increase immediately following ischemic injury *in vivo,* followed several hours later by morphologic features of apoptosis.

Caspase inhibition can reduce neuronal loss following oxygen-glucose deprivation of cortical neurons[30] and following hypoxic-ischemic injury *in vivo.*[31,32] These results provide some of the most powerful evidence of the importance of apoptotic death in brain injury. However, some results suggest that while caspase inhibition may prevent the cellular manifestations of apoptosis, it does always not prevent cell death.[33] This complexity offers a further insight into the multiple pathways of apoptotic cell death.

Gene Expression and Activation

Neural apoptotic death is often preceded by the induction and activation of a considerable variety of genes, including immediate early genes,[34] β-amyloid precursor protein,[35] and nuclear factor-kappa B (NF-κB).[36] A number of these genes have been shown to possess either pro- or anti-apoptotic functions.[37] For example, the intermediate early gene product c-Jun, which is phosphorylated by stress-activated protein kinases (SAPKs), is strongly implicated in triggering neuronal apoptosis.[34]

In vivo studies of ischemia to neural cells have shown that SAPKs are activated by injury.[38] It remains to be determined whether these kinases are pro- or anti-apoptotic, but early activation of p38 SAPK has been shown to protect cells from apoptotic death following tumor necrosis factor (TNF) treatment.[39] Conversely, the specific SAPK inhibitor CEP-1347 is able to rescue motor neurons from apoptosis following the withdrawal of survival factors.[40]

Cytokines and Receptors

The activation of SAPKs as one of the earliest signals downstream of death receptor activation provides evidence that intercellular signaling may be involved in triggering cell death during tissue injury. Receptors for pro-apoptotic signals including Fas, TNF, and interleukin-1β (IL-1β), are expressed acutely in the injured brain and may contribute to the progression of neuronal damage following hypoxia-ischemia.[41-43] A recombinant human IL-1β receptor antagonist markedly protects against focal cerebral ischemia in the rat.[44] These observations demonstrate that the cerebral response to hypoxia-ischemia shares many components with the inflammatory response.

Further observations demonstrate the complexity of the endogenous inflammatory response after cerebral hypoxic-ischemic injury. Mice lacking NF-κB are more susceptible to TNF-induced damage.[45] On the other hand, TNF-null mice are more susceptible to hypoxic-ischemic injury,[46] while ventricular injection of recombinant IL-6 significantly reduces ischemic brain damage, suggesting that the large increases in TNF and IL-6 following cerebral ischemia are endogenous neuroprotective responses.[47] These data show that it may not be possible to immediately extrapolate from the systemic actions of inflammatory mediators to their role in the brain. (See Chapter 4.)

Factors Determining the Choice Between Apoptosis and Necrosis

A number of different factors influence whether a cell will undergo apoptosis or necrosis. These include the stage of development, the cell type, the severity of injury, and the availability of ATP.

Developmental Age, Differentiation, and Cell Type

A general principle of development in multicellular organisms is that excess numbers of cells are produced, and those superfluous to requirement are then selected to undergo programmed cell death by apoptosis during the maturation of functional organs.[48] In the developing nervous system, more than 50% of neurons are lost during development because of limiting trophic support from target tissues that they innervate.[49] Dividing progenitor cells are particularly sensitive to apoptotic stimuli, since the cell cycle machinery is intimately linked to apoptosis.[50] This capacity to undergo programmed cell death is diminished following maturation. Thus, following excitotoxic injury to the newborn rat striatum, neuronal death occurs by apoptosis, while in the adult rat the same insult produces rapid cytoplasmic disintegration, consistent with necrosis.[51]

Specific cell types may be particularly sensitized to either necrosis or apoptosis,[52] and the cellular stage of development may influence the choice between apoptosis and necrosis. For example, cerebellar Purkinje cells differentiate early in brain development. In the porcine model of hypoxic-ischemic injury, these cells are very sensitive indicators of injury but they only undergo necrosis, never apoptosis. In contrast, cerebellar granule cells (which continue to divide and migrate after birth) undergo apoptosis on a large scale following hypoxia-ischemia.[19]

Severity of Injury

The same cell type can be triggered to undergo apoptosis following mild injury, but necrosis if the damage is severe.[53] It is not always clear how the severity of injury dictates apoptosis or necrosis. One possibility is that the degree of damage to cell organelles influences the mode of cell death. Mitochondria are particularly sensitive to hypoxic injury and play a central role in both apoptosis and necrosis (Figure 2). For example, inhibitors of complex I trigger apoptosis at

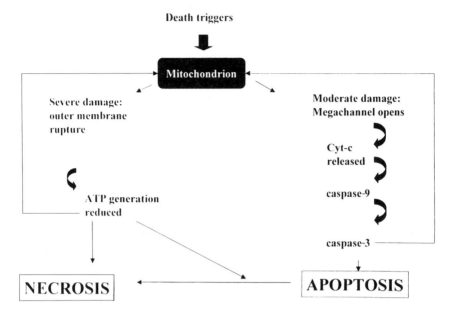

Figure 2. Postulated central role for mitochondria in both apoptotic and necrotic death. Cell injury can result in apoptosis or necrosis depending on the degree of mitochondrial damage. Severe damage results in disruption of the outer mitochondrial membrane, rapid depletion of adenosine triphosphate (ATP) stores, and necrotic cell death. Less severe damage can trigger cytochrome *c* release from mitochondria to the cytosol, where it participates in the activation of caspase-9, which in turn activates caspase-3, an effector caspase. ATP depletion may prevent the completion of the apoptotic pathway and drive a cell to necrotic death before apoptotic packaging of cellular contents is completed.

low concentrations, and necrosis at high concentrations, in neuronal cell lines in culture.[54] Indeed, Kroemer and colleagues have suggested that the severity of mitochondrial damage is the most important deciding factor between these two modes of cell death[55]; in this scenario, a small increase in mitochondrial membrane permeability can result in the controlled release of apoptogenic factors through the outer membrane, while severe mitochondrial damage releases a flood of Ca^{2+} and reactive oxygen species into the cytosol, leading to the disruption of plasma membrane integrity and cell necrosis.

Availability of Adenosine Triphosphate

Apoptosis requires energy,[56] while complete ATP depletion causes necrosis; thus, ATP availability is likely to be a significant determinant of apoptotic or necrotic death. When cells sustain a lethal insult, they will be able to execute the apoptotic program if ATP levels are sufficient, while in situations of limited ATP, the same degree of cellular injury can only result in necrosis. Consistent with this possibility, glutamate excitotoxicity has been shown to induce either necrosis or apoptosis depending on mitochondrial function. During and shortly after exposure to glutamate, neurons that died by necrosis had reduced mitochondrial membrane potential (mv/cm) and swollen nuclei. In contrast, neurons that recovered membrane potential and ATP levels subsequently underwent apoptosis.[53] Consumption of ATP by cell repair enzymes may thus also influence the mode of cell death; inhibition of PARP, therefore, preserves ATP levels and favors apoptosis in cells exposed to hydrogen peroxide.[57]

Preserving ATP levels can thus reduce the proportion of necrotic cells following hypoxic-ischemic injury and increase the relative amount of apoptosis. Gwag and colleagues demonstrated that, following severe ischemia, primary cell necrosis is reduced by the addition of the N-methyl-D-aspartate antagonist, MK-801. Residual neurons underwent a form of cell death with the hallmarks of apoptosis.[58] On the other hand, protection from apoptosis can condemn damaged cells to a necrotic death; cells treated with agents that reduce mitochondrial permeability alone underwent apoptosis, whereas those kept in identical conditions in the presence of the caspase inhibitor, Z-VADfmk, died from necrosis.[59]

Oxidative Stress

The newborn infant, particularly the preterm infant, is thought to be particularly prone to tissue damage from oxidative stress because of reduced total antioxidant capacity, and several studies have investigated the possibility of reducing morbidity by ameliorating the effects of oxidative stress in the newborn.[60] Oxidative stress is considered to be a major mediator of apoptosis in several cellular systems including neurons. Stimuli that cause oxidative stress, including culture in high oxygen,[61] exposure to β-amyloid,[62] or nitric oxide species[63] trigger apoptosis. Oxidative signals for apoptosis can originate both extracellularly and intracellularly, and can also be generated by reduced concentrations of antioxidants. A number of cerebroprotective strategies are directed specifically at reducing oxidative stress. For example, glutathione depletion in immature embryonic cortical neurons leads to death by apoptosis. This can be prevented by the administration of antioxidants.[64]

The Role of Mitochondria in Apopotosis and Necrosis

While mitochondrial failure and falling ATP levels might be either the trigger or the consequence of death, it has been understood for many years that mitochondrial failure can cause necrosis, while direct inhibition of mitochondrial metabolism can also trigger apoptosis[54,65] (Figure 3). The precise mechanisms are now beginning to be elucidated and much current interest is focused upon the mitochondrial membrane permeability transition, which some suggest may be a common element in several different pathways to apoptotic death.[55]

The Mitochondrial Permeability Transition Pore

One of the possible effects of free radical damage on mitochondria was first hypothesized by Skulachev,[66] and confirmed later by direct experimentation. The hypothesis suggested that the mitochondrial megachannel or permeability transition pore is involved in preventing free radical accumulation. High concentrations of free radicals in the mitochondria would trigger opening of the pore, allowing release of radicals into the cytosol. The resulting decrease in mitochondrial free radicals would subsequently allow pore closure. Conversely, persistent free

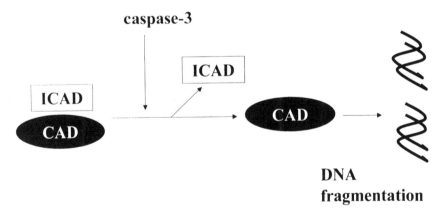

Figure 3. Apoptotic endonuclease activation. Caspase-activated deoxyribonuclease (CAD) is bound to its inhibitor (ICAD) in healthy cells. Following commitment to apoptosis, activated caspase-3 cleaves ICAD and inactivates its CAD-inhibitory effect. This activation of CAD downstream of the caspase cascade is responsible for internucleosomal DNA degradation during apoptosis.

radical accumulation in mitochondria would prevent pore closure and eventually lead to the release of the apoptosis-inducing proteins such as Apaf-1 and cytochrome *c* into the cytosol.[67] In this way, cells producing excess amounts of free radicals would be eliminated by apoptosis. In favor of this hypothesis, it is clear that the mitochondrial permeability transition pore is activated by accumulation of reactive oxygen sepcies.[68] The opening of the megachannel can also be triggered independently, although the result in all cases is a sudden increase in the permeability of the inner mitochondrial membrane to small molecules[69] (Figure 4).

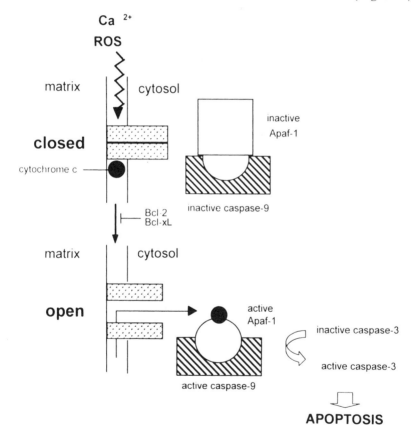

Figure 4. The mitochondrial permeability transition pore opens in response to various stimuli such as excess reactive oxygen species (ROS) or intramitochondrial calcium (Ca²⁺), and may allow release of apoptogenic proteins such as cytochrome *c*. This activates the Apaf-1/caspase-9 complex, which cleaves pro-caspase-3 (inactive) to the active form and leads to apoptotic execution. The apoptotic process is inhibited by anti-apoptotic members of the Bcl-2 family, such as Bcl-2 and Bcl-xL.

Although the exact composition of the permeability transition pore is currently under debate, experiments using specific inhibitors of mitochondrial protein function have identified key components. For example, bongkrekic acid, a ligand of the mitochondrial adenine nucleotide translocator, abolishes mitochondrial permeability transition and inhibits p53-dependent thymocyte apoptosis induced by DNA damage.[70] Similarly, the anti-apoptotic effects of cyclosporin A implicate cyclophilin D as a key component of the permeability transition pore. Other members include cytosolic hexokinase, porin (the voltage-dependent anion channel), creatine kinase, and at least one member of the Bcl-2 family of proteins.[55]

Mitochondrial Permeability Transition and Cell Death

In intact cells, the mitochondrial permeability transition leads to a reduction in mitochondrial membrane potential,[71] and a disruption of outer membrane integrity leads to the release of proteins that are involved in apoptotic execution.[72] Much of the information regarding the identity of mitochondrial factors released in apoptosis has been obtained from cell-free systems established to reproduce the apoptotic program *in vitro*.[73] In one such model, apoptosis could be initiated by addition of deoxyadenosine triphosphate (dATP) but also required cytochrome *c*. Intact cells undergoing apoptosis show a translocation of cytochrome *c* (normally, an electron carrier in the respiratory chain) from mitochondria to the cytosol,[74] which in turn results in the activation of specific caspases.[75] Among these enzymes, caspase-3 is thought to be pivotal in apoptotic execution, since cells that lack detectable levels of this enzyme fail to undergo cytochrome *c*-dependent apoptosis.[76] While caspase inhibitors substantially reduce mitochondrial membrane potential and cell death, they do not prevent the passage of cytochrome *c* from mitochondria to the cytosol, which must occur upstream of caspase activation in some cases.

Along with cytochrome *c* and dATP, Apaf-1 has been identified as an important protein that participates in the activation of caspase-3.[77] Apaf-1 shares significant homology with Caenorhabditis elegans CED-4, a protein that is required for apoptosis in the nematode. A third protein factor, Apaf-3, is also required for caspase-3 activation *in vitro*. Apaf-3 was identified as a member of the caspase family, caspase-9.[78] Genetic studies suggest that caspase-9 is one of the most upstream members of the apoptotic protease cascade and the formation of an

Apaf-1/caspase-9 complex activates caspase-3 in a cytochrome *c*- and dATP-dependent manner.

The effects of cytochrome *c* translocation to the cytosol are paradoxical. While ATP is required for apoptotic execution, the mitochondrial cytochrome *c* deficit will eventually result in shutdown of the respiratory chain, and consequently, ATP synthesis will cease. Thus, Fas-driven apoptosis in Jurkat cells results in the inactivation of cytochrome *c* with cessation of oxygen consumption.[79] However, the converse is not always true; it was found that apoptosis induced by branched chain amino acids is preceded by a fall in oxygen consumption without cytochrome *c* release.[80] Other reports have confirmed that apoptosis can proceed in the absence of cytosolic translocation of cytochrome *c*.[81]

Nevertheless, the release of pro-apoptotic factors from mitochondria is an important link between mitochondria and apoptosis in at least some systems, and it emphasizes the important role of mitochondria in regulating the cell death pathway. The fact that mitochondrial dysfunction can also cause necrotic death through depletion of ATP demonstrates the critical importance of mitochondrial biology in the elucidation of hypoxic-ischemic cerebral injury.

Bcl-2 Family Members and Mitochondria

Bcl-2 is a mitochondrial outer membrane protein that blocks the apoptotic death of many cell types.[82] The precise mechanism of Bcl-2 protection is unclear. There is some evidence that Bcl-2 regulates an antioxidant pathway at sites of free radical generation.[83] However, new data indicating that Bcl-2 family members prevent the mitochondrial permeability transition[84] suggest that the inhibition of free radical generation may be a secondary effect. Consistent with this role, release of apoptosis-initiating proteins such as cytochrome *c* or Apaf-1 from mitochondria can be initiated by the pro-apoptotic protein Bax.[85] On the other hand, in some cell types Bcl-2 cannot prevent or delay the decrease of the cellular ATP level subsequent to metabolic inhibition, suggesting that it blocks apoptosis at a point downstream of the collapse of cellular-energy homeostasis.[86]

Whatever the precise mechanism of Bcl-2 action, it has been shown to protect neurons from apoptosis following cerebral ischemia. Specifically, overexpression of the human Bcl-2 protein under the control of neuron-specific promoters reduced neuronal loss following permanent middle cerebral artery occlusion.[87]

Conclusions

Both apoptotic and necrotic cell death are important components of neuronal loss, and our present understanding suggests a central role for the mitochondria in both modes of death. However, the distinction between apoptosis and necrosis is becoming less clear. The mode of cell death is determined by a number of cellular factors including developmental status, the severity of injury, and mitochondrial function. The complexity of the events involved in oxidative damage to the brain underlines the need for therapeutic approaches that will combat multiple mechanisms of injury, and interrupt both apoptotic and necrotic processes.

References

1. Hamilton PA, Hope PL, Cady EB, et al: Impaired energy metabolism in brains of newborn infants with increased cerebral echodensities. Lancet 1986;1:1242–1246.
2. Hope PL, Costello AM, Cady EB, et al: Cerebral energy metabolism studied with phosphorus NMR spectroscopy in normal and birth-asphyxiated infants. Lancet 1984;2:366–370.
3. Roth SC, Edwards AD, Cady EB, et al: Relation between cerebral oxidative metabolism following birth asphyxia and neurodevelopmental outcome and brain growth at one year. Dev Med Child Neurol 1992;34:285–295.
4. Roth SC, Baudin J, Cady E, et al: Relation of deranged neonatal cerebral oxidative metabolism with neurodevelopmental outcome and head circumference at 4 years. Dev Med Child Neurol 1997;39:718–725.
5. Yue X, Mehmet H, Penrice J, et al: Apoptosis and necrosis in the newborn piglet brain following transient cerebral hypoxia-ischemia. Neuropathol Appl Neurobiol 1997;23:16–25.
6. Hanrahan D, Cox IJ, Edwards AD, et al: Persistent increases in cerebral lactate concentration after birth asphyxia. Pediatr Res 1998;44:304–311.
7. Du C, Hu R, Csernansky CA, et al: Very delayed infarction after mild focal cerebral ischemia: a role for apoptosis? J Cereb Blood Flow Metab 1996; 16:195–201.
8. Dobkin BH: Experimental brain injury and repair. Curr Opin Neurol 1997; 10:493–497.
9. Nagata S, Golstein P: The Fas death factor. Science 1995;267:1449–1456.
10. Thornberry NA, Lazebnik Y: Caspases, enemy within. Science 1998;281: 1312–1316.
11. Beilharz EJ, Bassett NS, Sirimanne ES, et al: Insulin-like growth factor II is induced during wound repair following hypoxic-ischemic injury in the developing rat brain. Brain Res Mol Brain Res 1995;29:81–91.
12. Ferrer I, Tortosa A, Macaya A, et al: Evidence of nuclear DNA fragmentation following hypoxia-ischemia in the infant rat brain, and transient forebrain ischemia in the adult gerbil. Brain Pathol 1994;4:115–122.
13. Mehmet H, Yue X, Squier MV, et al: Increased apoptosis in the cingulate

sulcus of newborn piglets following transient hypoxia-ischemia is related to the degree of high energy phosphate depletion during the insult. Neurosci Lett 1994;181:121–125.

14. Linnik MD, Zorbrist RH, Hatfield MD: Evidence supporting a role for programmed cell death in focal cerebral ischemia in rats. Stroke 1993;24: 2002–2008.

15. MacManus JP, Buchan AM, Hill IE, et al: Global ischemia can cause DNA fragmentation indicative of apoptosis in rat brain. Neurosci Lett 1993; 164:89–92.

16. Gluckman PD, Klempt N, Guan J, et al: A role for IGF-1 in the rescue of CNS neurons following hypoxic-ischemic injury. Biochem Biophys Res Commun 1992;182:593–599.

17. Edwards AD, Yue X, Cox P, et al: Apoptosis in the brains of infants suffering intrauterine cerebral injury. Pediatr Res 1997;42:684–689.

18. Scott RJ, Hegyi L: Cell death in perinatal hypoxic-ischemic brain injury. Neuropathol Appl Neurobiol 1997;23:307–314.

19. Mehmet H, Yue X, Penrice J, et al: Relation of impaired energy metabolism to apoptosis and necrosis following transient cerebral hypoxia-ischemia. Cell Death Diff 1998;5:321–329.

20. Majno G, Joris I: Apoptosis, oncosis, and necrosis: an overview of cell death. Am J Pathol 1995;146:3–15.

21. Kalda A, Eriste E, Vassiljev V, Zharkovsky A: Medium transitory oxygen-glucose deprivation induced both apoptosis and necrosis in cerebellar granule cells. Neurosci Lett 1998;240:21–24.

22. Ferrer I, Martin F, Serrano T, et al: Both apoptosis and necrosis occur following intrastriatal administration of excitotoxins. Acta Neuropathol Berl 1995;90:504–510.

23. Eliasson MJ, Sampei K, Mandir AS, et al: Poly(ADP-ribose) polymerase gene disruption renders mice resistant to cerebral ischemia. Nat Med 1997;3:1089–1095.

24. Takahashi K, Greenberg JH, Jackson P, et al: Neuroprotective effects of inhibiting poly(ADP-ribose) synthetase on focal cerebral ischemia in rats. J Cereb Blood Flow Metab 1997;17:1137–1142.

25. Endres M, Wang ZQ, Namura S, et al: Ischemic brain injury is mediated by the activation of poly(ADP-ribose) polymerase. J Cereb Blood Flow Metab 1997;17:1143–1151.

26. Leist M, Single B, Kunstle G, et al: Apoptosis in the absence of poly-(ADP-ribose) polymerase. Biochem Biophys Res Commun 1997;233:518–522.

27. Lazebnik YA, Kaufmann SH, Desnoyers S, et al: Cleavage of poly(ADP-ribose) polymerase by a proteinase with properties like ICE. Nature 1994; 371:346–347.

28. Namura S, Zhu J, Fink K, et al: Activation and cleavage of caspase-3 in apoptosis induced by experimental cerebral ischemia. J Neurosci 1998; 18:3659–3668.

29. Joashi UC, Greenwood K, Taylor DL, et al: Poly(ADP ribose) polymerase cleavage precedes neuronal death in the hippocampus and cerebellum following injury to the developing rat forebrain. Eur J Neurosci 1999;11: 91–100.

30. Gottron FJ, Ying HS, Choi DW: Caspase inhibition selectively reduces the apoptotic component of oxygen-glucose deprivation-induced cortical neuronal cell death. Mol Cell Neurosci 1997;9:159–169.

31. Endres M, Namura S, Shimizu-Sasamata M, et al: Attenuation of delayed neuronal death after mild focal ischemia in mice by inhibition of the caspase family. J Cereb Blood Flow Metab 1998;18:238–247.
32. Loddick SA, MacKenzie A, Rothwell NJ: An ICE inhibitor, z-VAD-DCB attenuates ischemic brain damage in the rat. Neuroreport 1996; 7:1465–1468.
33. McCarthy NJ, Whyte MK, Gilbert CS, Evan GI: Inhibition of Ced-3/ICE-related proteases does not prevent cell death induced by oncogenes, DNA damage, or the Bcl-2 homologue Bak. J Cell Biol 1997;136:215–227.
34. Dragunow M, Preston K: The role of inducible transcription factors in apoptotic nerve cell death. Brain Res Rev 1995;21:1–28.
35. Baiden-Amissah K, Cox PM, Joashi U: Induction of beta-amyloid precursor protein (β-APP) expression after neonatal hypoxic ischemic cerebral injury (HII). J Pathol 1997;182:A49.
36. Clemens JA, Stephenson DT, Dixon EP: Global cerebral ischemia activates nuclear factor-kappa B prior to evidence of DNA fragmentation. Brain Res Mol Brain Res 1997;48:187–196.
37. MacManus JP, Linnik MD: Gene expression induced by cerebral ischemia: an apoptotic perspective. J Cereb Blood Flow Metab 1997;17:815–832.
38. Walton KM, DiRocco R, Bartlett BA, et al: Activation of p38(MAPK) in microglia after ischemia. J Neurochem 1998;70:1764–1767.
39. Roulston A, Reinhard C, Amiri P, Williams LT: Early activation of c-Jun N-terminal kinase and p38 kinase regulate cell survival in response to tumor necrosis factor α. J Biol Chem 1998;273:10232–10239.
40. Maroney AC, Glicksman MA, Basma AN, et al: Motoneuron apoptosis is blocked by CEP-1347 (KT 7515), a novel inhibitor of the JNK signaling pathway. J Neurosci 1998;18:104–111.
41. Botchkina GI, Meistrell ME 3rd, Botchkina IL, Tracey KJ: Expression of TNF and TNF receptors (p55 and p75) in the rat brain after focal cerebral ischemia. Mol Med 1997;3:765–781.
42. Silverstein F, Barks J, Hagan P, et al: Cytokines and perinatal brain injury. Neurochem Int 1997;30:375–383.
43. Felderhoff-Muser U, Taylor DL, Greenwood K, et al: Fas/CD95/APO-1 can function as a death receptor in neural cells in vitro and in vivo and is upregulated following cerebral hypoxia-ischemia to the developing brain. Brain Pathol 2000;10:17–24.
44. Loddick SA, Rothwell NJ: Neuroprotective effects of human recombinant interleukin-1 receptor antagonist in focal cerebral ischemia in the rat. J Cereb Blood Flow Metab 1996;16:932–940.
45. Beg AA, Baltimore D: An essential role for NF-kappaB in preventing TNF-α-induced cell death. Science 1996;274:782–784.
46. Bruce AJ, Boling W, Kindy MS, et al: Altered neuronal and microglial responses to excitotoxic and ischemic brain injury in mice lacking TNF receptors. Nat Med 1996;2:788–794.
47. Loddick SA, Turnbull AV, Rothwell NJ: Cerebral interleukin-6 is neuroprotective during permanent focal cerebral ischemia in the rat. J Cereb Blood Flow Metab 1998;18:176–179.
48. Jacobson MD, Weil M, Raff MC: Programmed cell death in animal development. Cell 1997;88:347–354.
49. Oppenheim RW: Cell death during development of the nervous system. Ann Rev Neurosci 1991;14:453–501.

50. Ross ME: Cell division and the nervous system: regulating the cycle from neural differentiation to death. Trends Neurosci 1996;19:62–68.

51. Portera-Cailliau C, Price DL, Martin LJ: Non-NMDA and NMDA receptor-mediated excitotoxic neuronal deaths in adult brain are morphologically distinct: further evidence for an apoptosis-necrosis continuum. J Comp Neurol 1997;378:88–104.

52. Sloviter RS, Dean E, Sollas AL, Goodman JH: Apoptosis and necrosis induced in different hippocampal neuron populations by repetitive perforant path stimulation in the rat. J Comp Neurol 1996;366:516–533.

53. Ankarcrona M, Dypbukt JM, Bonfoco E, et al: Glutamate-induced neuronal death: a succession of necrosis or apoptosis depending on mitochondrial function. Neuron 1995;15:961–973.

54. Hartley A, Stone JM, Heron C, et al: Complex I inhibitors induce dose-dependent apoptosis in PC12 cells: relevance to Parkinson's disease. J Neurochem 1994;63:1987–1990.

55. Kroemer G, Dallaporta B, Resche-Rigon M: The mitochondrial death/life regulator in apoptosis and necrosis. Annu Rev Physiol 1998;60:619–642.

56. Kass GE, Eriksson JE, Weis M, et al: Chromatin condensation during apoptosis requires ATP. Biochem J 1996;318:749–752.

57. Watson AJ, Askew JN, Benson RS: Poly(adenosine diphosphate ribose) polymerase inhibition prevents necrosis induced by H_2O_2 but not apoptosis. Gastroenterology 1995;109:472–482.

58. Gwag BJ, Lobner D, Koh JY, et al: Blockade of glutamate receptors unmasks neuronal apoptosis after oxygen-glucose deprivation in vitro. Neuroscience 1995;68:615–619.

59. Hirsch T, Susin SA, Marzo I, et al: Mitochondrial permeability transition in apoptosis and necrosis. Cell Biol Toxicol 1998;14:141–145.

60. Saugstad OD: Mechanisms of tissue injury by oxygen radicals: implications for neonatal disease. Acta Paediatr 1996;85:1–4.

61. Enokido Y, Hatanaka H: Apoptotic cell death occurs in hippocampal neurons cultured in a high oxygen atmosphere. Neuroscience 1993;57:965–972.

62. Behl C, Davis JB, Lesley R, Schubert D: Hydrogen peroxide mediates amyloid beta protein toxicity. Cell 1994;77:817–827.

63. Khan S, Kayahara M, Joashi U, et al: Differential induction of apoptosis in Swiss 3T3 cells by nitric oxide and the nitrosonium cation. J Cell Sci 1997;110:2315–2322.

64. Ratan RR, Murphy TH, Baraban JM: Oxidative stress induces apoptosis in embryonic cortical neurons. J Neurochem 1994;62:376–379.

65. Wolvetang EJ, Johnson KL, Krauer K, et al: Mitochondrial respiratory chain inhibitors induce apoptosis, FEBS Lett 1994;339:40–44.

66. Skulachev VP: Why are mitochondria involved in apoptosis? Permeability transition pores and apoptosis as selective mechanisms to eliminate superoxide-producing mitochondria and cell. FEBS Lett 1996;397:7–10.

67. Scarlett JL, Murphy MP: Release of apoptogenic proteins from the mitochondrial intermembrane space during the mitochondrial permeability transition. FEBS Lett 1997;418:282–286.

68. Chernyak BV: Redox regulation of the mitochondrial permeability transition pore. Biosci Rep 1997;17:293–302.

69. Kroemer G, Zamzami N, Susin SA: Mitochondrial control of apoptosis. Immunol Today 1997;18:44–51.

70. Marchetti P, Castedo M, Susin SA, et al: Mitochondrial permeability tran-

sition is a central coordinating event of apoptosis. J Exp Med 1996;184: 1155–1160.

71. Petit PX, Susin SA, Zamzami N, et al: Mitochondria and programmed cell death: back to the future. FEBS Lett 1996;396:7–13.

72. Petit PX, Goubern M, Diolez P, et al: Disruption of the outer mitochondrial membrane as a result of large amplitude swelling: the impact of irreversible permeability transition. FEBS Lett 1998;426:111–116.

73. Ellerby HM, Martin SJ, Ellerby LM, et al: Establishment of a cell-free system of neuronal apoptosis: comparison of premitochondrial, mitochondrial, and postmitochondrial phases. J Neurosci 1997;17:6165–6178.

74. Liu X, Kim CN, Yang J, et al: Induction of apoptotic program in cell-free extracts: requirement for dATP and cytochrome c. Cell 1996;86:147–157.

75. Bossy-Wetzel E, Newmeyer DD, Green DR: Mitochondrial cytochrome c release in apoptosis occurs upstream of DEVD-specific caspase activation and independently of mitochondrial transmembrane depolarization. EMBO J 1998;17:37–49.

76. Li F, Srinivasan A, Wang Y, et al: Cell-specific induction of apoptosis by microinjection of cytochrome c: Bcl-xL has activity independent of cytochrome c release. J Biol Chem 1997;272:30299–30305.

77. Zou H, Henzel WJ, Liu X, et al: Apaf-1, a human protein homologous to C. elegans CED-4, participates in cytochrome c-dependent activation of caspase-3. Cell 1997;90:405–413.

78. Li P, Nijhawan D, Budihardjo I, et al: Cytochrome c and dATP-dependent formation of Apaf-1/caspase-9 complex initiates an apoptotic protease cascade. Cell 1997;91:479–489.

79. Adachi S, Cross AR, Babior BM, Gottlieb RA: Bcl-2 and the outer mitochondrial membrane in the inactivation of cytochrome c during Fas-mediated apoptosis. J Biol Chem 1997;272:21878–21882.

80. Jouvet P, Rustin P, Felderhoff U, et al: Maple syrup urine disease metabolites induce apoptosis in neural cells without cytochrome c release or changes in mitochondrial membrane potential. Biochem Soc Trans 1998; 26:S341.

81. Chauhan D, Pandey P, Ogata A, et al: Cytochrome c-dependent and -independent induction of apoptosis in multiple myeloma cells. J Biol Chem 1997;272:29995–29997.

82. Hockenbery D, Nunez G, Milliman C, et al: Bcl-2 is an inner mitochondrial membrane protein that blocks programmed cell death. Nature 1990; 348:334–336.

83. Hockenbery DM, Oltvai ZN, Yin XM, et al: Bcl-2 functions in an antioxidant pathway to prevent apoptosis. Cell 1993;75:241–251.

84. Vander Heiden MG, Chandel NS, Williamson EK, et al: Bcl-xL regulates the membrane potential and volume homeostasis of mitochondria. Cell 1997;91:627–637.

85. Jurgensmeier JM, Xie Z, Deveraux Q, et al: Bax directly induces release of cytochrome c from isolated mitochondria. Proc Natl Acad Sci USA 1998; 95:4997–5002.

86. Marton A, Mihalik R, Bratincsak A, et al: Apoptotic cell death induced by inhibitors of energy conservation: Bcl-2 inhibits apoptosis downstream of a fall of ATP level. Eur J Biochem 1997;50:467–475.

87. Martinou JC, Dubois-Dauphin M, Staple JK, et al: Overexpression of Bcl-2 in transgenic mice protects neurons from naturally occurring cell death and experimental ischemia. Neuron 1994;13:1017–1030.

Effects of Nitric Oxide on Neuronal and Cerebrovascular Function

Donna M. Ferriero, Stephen Ashwal

Introduction

Other than congenital anomalies and genetic malformations, many types of brain injuries in the newborn, especially hypoxic-ischemic damage, may result from a neurotoxic biochemical cascade of events that includes the generation of free radicals and excitatory amino acid receptor overactivation.[1] One of the factors in the injury cascade, nitric oxide (NO), will be examined in this chapter. Over the past 10 years, the role of NO as a signaling molecule has become elucidated.[2] Its importance in the regulation of certain developmental processes in the brain, as well as its toxicity to the nervous system, have been recognized. The focus of this chapter is on how NO is synthesized, its developmental expression in the brain, and some of its known physiologic roles. The effects of nitric oxide on both neuronal and cerebrovascular function will be considered, and the role of reactive oxygen metabolites and nitric oxide synthase (NOS) in the pathophysiology of neonatal hypoxic-ischemic injury will be addressed.

Nitric Oxide Synthase Enzyme and Nitric Oxide Synthesis

Nitric oxide synthase (EC 1.14.23) is the enzyme that produces NO during the conversion of arginine to citrulline. NO, a free radical that acts as a neural messenger molecule, mediates several biologic actions in higher mammals, including relaxation of blood vessels, macrophage-mediated cytotoxicity, and the formation of cyclic guanine monophosphate (cGMP). NOS has at least three isoforms (Table 1): the

From Donn SM, Sinha SK, Chiswick ML (eds): *Birth Asphyxia and the Brain: Basic Science and Clinical Implications.* © 2002, Futura Publishing Co., Inc., Armonk, NY.

Table 1

Nitric Oxide Synthase Isoforms

Isoform	Primary Sites	Constitutive	Inducible	Calcium-Dependent
NOS 1 (neuronal, nNOS)	neurons, skeletal muscle	+	+	+
NOS 2 (inducible, iNOS)	macrophages, microglia	−	+	−
NOS 3 (endothelial, eNOS)	endothelial cells	+	+	+/−

NOS = nitric oxide synthase.

endothelial isoform (type 3 NOS or eNOS), which is membrane-associated and found in endothelial cells; the inducible isoform (type 2 NOS or iNOS), found in macrophages and microglia; and the neuronal isoform (type 1 NOS or nNOS), found predominantly in neurons of the central and peripheral nervous systems and in skeletal muscle. These NOS isoforms are encoded by three distinct genes that are 50–60% homologous. Although the eNOS isoform was named because of its localization to vascular endothelial cells, this isoform is found co-localized in a wide range of neurons throughout the brain, and is selectively enriched, occurring independently of nNOS, in pyramidal cells of the hippocampus.[3] Initially, the iNOS form of the enzyme was thought to be the only inducible form. However, it is clear from a number of studies that the constitutive isoforms, eNOS and nNOS, as well as iNOS, are inducible. Following neuronal damage, for example, nNOS levels increase markedly in discrete populations of cells.[4] Although iNOS is found predominantly in macrophages, it has been cloned from hepatocytes and chondrocytes, cells unrelated to macrophages or microglia,[5,6] and has been induced in reactive astrocytes after transient global ischemia.[7] Data now exist showing that a mitochondrial NOS isoform exists, which is similar to iNOS.[8]

The NOS enzyme is composed of an N-terminal oxygenase domain and a C-terminal reductase domain with a short amino acid recognition sequence for calcium calmodulin (CaM) located between the two domains (Figure 1) (for a review, see reference 9). The N-terminal leader sequence contains PIN and PDZ domains that function to target the enzyme in cells. This leader sequence is more extensive in nNOS than in eNOS. The oxygenase domain forms the active catalytic site containing a beta-hairpin loop, a core region that binds heme,

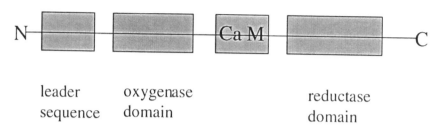

Figure 1. Structure of the nitric oxide synthase (NOS) enzyme. The NOS enzyme is composed of an oxygenase domain located near the N-terminus and reductase domain located near the C-terminus. There is a short amino acid recognition sequence for calcium calmodulin (CaM) between the two domains.

tetrahydrobiopterin, and arginine. A caveolin-binding sequence is also located in this domain. Caveolins are structural scaffolding proteins present in membrane caveoli. It appears that the caveolins inhibit NO synthesis, a process that can be reversed by CaM.[10] The reductase domain contains the CaM inhibitory loop in the nNOS and eNOS isoforms, as well as the important binding sites for flavin mononucleotide (FMN), flavin adenine dinucleotide (FAD), and nicotinamide adenine dinucleotide phosphate (NADPH). During NO synthesis, the reductase flavins acquire electrons from NADPH and transfer them to the heme iron, which permits it to bind and activate oxygen.

Tetrahydrobiopterin (BH4) appears to be a critical cofactor in the regulation of NOS. BH4 is needed for iNOS to dimerize and it couples heme iron reduction to NO synthesis. It works in an anticooperative manner such that the first BH4 binding lowers the enzyme's affinity for the binding of the second. This is biologically important because nNOS can produce superoxide in the absence of BH4.[11] Likewise, CaM also plays a critical role in activating NOS, since its binding causes electron transfer to the heme.[9]

NO mechanisms are probably related to the numerous NO-derived species that exist. There are NO-derived N-oxides with oxidation numbers from +1 (nitroxyl anion) to +6 (peroxynitrite [$ONOO^-$ and NO_3^-]).[12] The availability of the different cofactors dictates which reactive nitrogen species is generated. Regulation is then provided by the steric properties, chemistries, and partition coefficients of the various NO species. Targets of NO-related species in brain include guanylate cyclase, the N-methyl-D-aspartate (NMDA) receptor, synaptosomal associated protein of 25 kDa (SNAP-25), syntaxin 1a, n-sec1, neurogranin, H-adenosine triphosphatase (ATPase), cyclic nucleotide-gated channel, Ca^{2+} channel in rods, Na^+/K^+-ATPase, and adenosine diphosphate (ADP) ribosyltransferase.[13]

Regional and Cellular Location of Neuronal Nitric Oxide Synthase

Specific antibodies and oligonucleotide probes have localized brain NOS to the neuronal population in the rat and primate brain which coincides with NADPH-diaphorase histochemical staining.[14] nNOS is concentrated at synaptic junctions in brain and motor endplates in skeletal muscle. The N-terminus of nNOS, which contains the PDZ protein motif, interacts with similar motifs in post-synaptic density-proteins (PSD-95, PSD-93).[15] The synaptic actions of NO are enabled by the subcellular targeting of nNOS to these specialized membrane structures. This structural coupling of nNOS to the NMDA receptor allows for nNOS activity to be markedly enhanced in response to NMDA receptor stimulation.

The localization of NOS mRNA and immunoreactivity in rat brain to distinct *neuronal* populations and the finding that nNOS co-localizes with NADPH-diaphorase staining suggest a role for NO in modulating glutamate neurotoxicity. Recently, it has been shown that the anatomic pattern of nNOS expression during development in the rat brain correlates well with areas that are susceptible to hypoxic-ischemic injury.[16] For example, there is no nNOS expression in the basal ganglia prior to birth, but during the first postnatal week, when the basal ganglia become selectively vulnerable to hypoxic-ischemic and excitotoxic injury, nNOS mRNA and protein become abundant. Further evidence of the link between excitotoxicity and nNOS expression comes from data co-localizing the NMDA-R1 subunit of the glutamate receptor with nNOS in both pre- and post-synaptic sites in the cerebral cortex of rat brain.[17] By immunoelectron microscopy, it was shown that nNOS is most frequently located at synapses and particularly within spines, where it is clustered directly over post-synaptic densities. NMDA-R1 is present at post-synaptic sites exhibiting nNOS immunoreactivity, but this presence is not obligatory, and nNOS can appear independent of the NMDA receptor as well.

Development of Neuronal Nitric Oxide Synthase

In the developing rat brain, the expression of nNOS by *in situ* hybridization and immunohistochemisty could be detected as early as embryonic day 10. From embryonic day 14 to 18, the highest level of expression was in the cortical plate, where the majority of neurons were positive. This expression diminished with time, with only a few nNOS positive neurons remaining in the adult cortex. nNOS could be detected in the hippocampus at embryonic day 16, remaining constant with regional localization in layers CA1 and CA3 in the adult. In the developing cerebellum, nNOS expression was observed only after birth with positive cells limited to the molecular cell layer. As the cerebellum matured, nNOS expression could be detected in the inner granular layer and by postnatal day 21, the adult distribution was observed.

In another study in rat brain, although the transcripts for all three major NOS isoforms were present permanently from embryonic day 10 onward, the respective protein isoforms varied over time and in different regions. These data suggest that the isoform expression is controlled post-transcriptionally.[18]

In the guinea pig brain, NOS *activity* was not detected until midgestation, reaching adult levels before birth and peaking at 140% of adult activity in the forebrain and 250% in the cerebellum 1 week after birth. This rise in activity could be blunted by treatment with tamoxifen, suggesting that estrogens play a role in determination of NOS activity.[19]

In mouse, nNOS immunoreactivity appeared at embryonic day 14 in the spinal cord near the central canal, and then in the thalamus and striatum.[20] The first cortical region to show NOS reactivity was the parietal cortex at embryonic days 18 to 20. The immunoreactivity increased in all cortical areas, reaching a plateau at postnatal day 4. The neuronal packing density declined until adulthood, with a brief but transient increase at puberty.

In human brain, nNOS immunoreactive cells are seen as early as 18 gestational weeks in the subcortical plate and white matter.[21] After 26 weeks gestation, neurons are seen in cortical layers II-IV. Immunoreactive neurons are seen in the basal ganglia as early as 13 weeks gestation, with a peak at 23–24 weeks in putamen and 33–36 weeks in caudate. The cerebellum exhibited immunoreactivity within Purkinje cells after 23 weeks gestation and in basket cells after 31 weeks. The central gray matter of the brainstem had immunoreactive neurons with peaks at term for the pontine nucleus and 23–24 weeks gestation in the inferior olivary nucleus. Another study in human brain compared second trimester brain with adult and found nNOS neurons concentrated in the subplate zone, striatum, and restricted brainstem nuclei, with sparse distribution in the hippocampus and no cells in the cerebellum.[22] In the adult brain, the highest density of nNOS neurons was found in striatum followed by the neocortex. In all of the studies, the regional specificity suggests a role of NO in developmental processes.

Physiologic Roles of Nitric Oxide

Recognition that NO has physiologic roles in mammalian cells came when it was discovered that the endothelial-derived relaxing factor (EDRF) was indeed NO.[23] It had been known that EDRF served as a regulator of blood vessel relaxation and thus as a principal mediator of blood flow and pressure. Following this discovery, NO became implicated in the ability of activated macrophages to kill tumor cells and bacteria.[24] A role for NO in mediating the ability of glutamate to act via the NMDA receptor to stimulate cGMP formation in brain formed the basis for understanding the role of NO in glutamate neurotoxicity.[25,26] Numerous experiments have implicated NO in a number of physiologic roles in the central nervous system (CNS) such as vision, memory, feeding, nociception, and olfaction.[27] In the peripheral nervous system, NO may participate in: sensory transmission; development of penile erections; nonadrenergic, noncholinergic vasodilation; and relaxation of trachea, gastrointestinal tract, and bladder.

NO inhibits platelet aggregation and adhesion, in part through a cGMP mechanism (see reference 27). Platelets also liberate NO, thereby forming a feedback mechanism to inhibit platelet activation. NO can inhibit leukocyte activation and proliferation of smooth muscle cells, thus participating in vasomotor control at a number of levels.

The presence of a distinct isoform of NOS occurring in mitochondria has implications in energy metabolism and mitochondrial respiration. NO inhibits mitochondrial aconitase and complexes I, II, and IV of the electron transport chain in various cell types. NO binds to metalloproteins, particularly hemoproteins in both ferrous and ferric states, explaining its predilection for the cytochrome c enzymatic functions in mitochondria.[12]

The Role of Nitric Oxide in Disease States

Free radicals (see Chapter 9), compounds carrying one or more unpaired electrons, exist only transiently within cells.[28] Examples of free radicals in living tissues include superoxide (O_2^-), hydroxyl (^-OH), and nitric oxide (NO). These free radicals and other reactive oxygen species, including hydrogen peroxide and peroxynitrite, are products of normal cellular metabolism and are injurious to cellular components such as membrane lipids, proteins, and DNA.[28] Under normal conditions, most free radicals and other reactive oxygen species are neutralized ("scavenged") before they inflict damage, and the damage they cause is rapidly repaired. The cellular antioxidant defense system consists of superoxide dismutase (SOD) which exists as a cytoplasmic copper- and zinc- containing SOD (SOD1) and a mitochondrial manganese-containing SOD (SOD2). These enzymes reduce the superoxide anion to hydrogen peroxide that is then detoxified by catalase (CAT) and glutathione peroxidase (GSH-Px). The latter enzyme consumes reducing equivalents of glutathione (GSH), a major source of nonprotein thiol in tissue, converting reduced GSH to the oxidized form (GSSG). This compound is reduced back to GSH by glutathione reductase (GSH-Rd) using reducing equivalents of NADPH.

Effects of Nitric Oxide on Neuronal and Cerebrovascular Function

Nitric Oxide and Cerebral Blood Flow Regulation

The role of NO in cerebrovascular regulation is now well established and based on several earlier observations involving the systemic circulation including: (1) recognition in 1980 that an intact endothelium was required for acetylcholine-induced vasodilation; (2) determination in 1987 that this "endothelial-derived relaxing factor" was NO; and (3) demonstration in 1989 that infusion of an NOS inhibitor into the brachial artery of humans caused a marked reduction in cerebral blood flow (CBF).[29] NO-induced vasodilation is mediated by cGMP activation which inhibits contractile mechanisms of the vascular smooth muscle. Several reviews of NO in the adult cerebrovascular circulation have been published.[30–34] Little information concerning its regulatory role early in development is available.

Sources of Nitric Oxide Affecting Cerebral Blood Vessels

Several sources of NO derived from all three NOS isoforms affect the cerebral circulation[30,32,35] (Figure 2). NOS 1 (calcium-dependent, constitutive) is present in a relatively small number of neurons in the brain, some of which contain processes in close association with cerebral microvessels.[36] NOS 1 is also present in perivascular nerves that originate from several cranial autonomic ganglia (primarily the pterygopalatine ganglion).[37–39] Although there is no apparent relation between the number of NOS 1 neurons and the effects of NOS inhibitors on CBF or regional NOS activity,[40,41] selective NOS 1 inhibitors such as 7-nitroindazole (7-NI) that do not appear to alter eNOS have been shown to reduce resting CBF between 20% in the hippocampus and 58% in the substantia nigra.[42]

NOS 2 (calcium-independent, inducible) is not normally present in substantial concentrations in brain but is present within the endothelium and vascular smooth muscle cells.[43] Previous studies using aminoguanidine (AMG), an inhibitor of NOS 2, reported no effect on

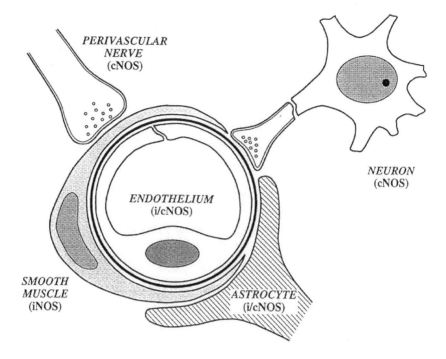

Figure 2. Illustration of the cellular localization of the different NOS isoforms at the microvascular level. Endothelial NOS (NOS 3 or eNOS) regulates resting cerebral blood flow and also is released during ischemia and reperfusion. Neuronally derived NOS (NOS 1 or nNOS) can also be released from perivascular nerves and brain parenchyma and may preferentially improve collateral flow during ischemia. Inducible NOS (NOS 2 or iNOS; calcium-independent) is not normally present in substantial concentrations in brain but is present within the endothelium and vascular smooth muscle cells. nNOS can affect the vascular tone of cerebral arteries stimulated with lipopolysaccharide, but it is unlikely that it contributes to any significant degree of cerebrovascular regulation during global or focal ischemia. cNOS = constitutive NOS (either nNOS or eNOS). From Iadecola et al, with permission.[30]

resting CBF or the cerebrovascular vasodilation elicited by hypercapnia.[44] The majority of NOS 2 is derived from migrating neutrophils that enter the brain as part of a post-ischemic inflammatory response and are typically found at the periphery of an infarct.[45] Based on studies in carotid arteries isolated from NOS 2 deficient mice, it appears that NOS 2 mediates impairment of vascular contraction after treatment with lipopolysaccharide.[46] After intraventricular administration of lipopolysaccharide, induction of NOS 2 expression resulting in increased CBF has been reported.[47] However, it is unclear whether NOS 2 activation was from neutrophils or vascular smooth muscle. Although there are substantial data that inhibition of NOS 2 reduces infarct volume,[48] the role of NOS 2 in the regulation of CBF during focal ischemia and reperfusion has yet to be defined, as differences in its effects depend on the type of model of ischemia used (i.e., permanent versus temporary middle cerebral artery occlusion [MCAO]). In models of temporary ischemia, NOS 2 is predominantly localized in vascular cells rather than in neutrophils and is maximally expressed in the postischemic brain at 12 hours.[49] In studies using AMG, changes in CBF were not observed although reduction in infarct volume occurred.[44]

NOS 3 (constitutive) is found primarily within the endothelium and serves as the principal source of NO that acts as a vasodilator. NOS 3 (and NOS 2) isoforms are contained within astrocytes,[50] but their role in vascular regulation remains uncertain. NOS 3 immunoreactivity has been demonstrated in vessels of the human brain at different developmental stages. NOS 3-positive endothelial cells are present in vessels of the leptomeninges and deep white matter by 10–13 weeks gestation, in the cortex at 18–21 weeks, and in the subcortical white matter at 23–26 weeks.[51] Such regional developmental differences might account for the topographical predilection for hemorrhagic or hypoxic-ischemic lesions.

Resting Cerebral Blood Flow

Several lines of evidence have shown that NO participates in the regulation of basal CBF.[30] Studies in isolated blood vessels have demonstrated that topical application of the NOS inhibitor monoethyl L-arginine (L-NMMA) can constrict the rat basilar artery. This effect is reversed by L-arginine, the amino acid substrate converted by NOS to NO and citrulline.[52] Also, using a craniotomy window technique, topical administration of L-arginine dilates pial arterioles in several species in a dose-dependent manner.[53,54] In addition, systemic administration of L-NMMA (30 mg/kg) reduced resting CBF by 20–30% in rats.[55] In humans, administration of L-arginine (16.7 mg/kg/min) has been shown to increase resting CBF by 9.5%, suggesting that basal CBF in humans is likely to be NO-dependent.[56] Because NOS inhibitors have not been found to affect resting cerebral glucose utilization or oxygen consumption, their effect on CBF is considered to result from the direct impact of NO on the cerebral vasculature rather than to reduced cerebral energy metabolism.[30,57,58] It is also recognized that the contribution of NO to basal CBF is region- and species-specific.[59] For example, using dynamic susceptibility contrast magnetic resonance imaging (MRI) in nonischemic spontaneously hypertensive rats,it has been shown that L-arginine administration (300 mg/kg) increased cortical CBF without significantly increasing striatal CBF.[60]

Nitric oxide contributes to control of resting CBF in the fetal and newborn circulation. Studies in the near-term fetal lamb (using microspheres) found that total CBF decreased (129 to 89 mL/100 g/min) and cerebrovascular resistance increased (0.46 to 0.80 mmHg/mL/100 g/min) after infusion of N[omega]-nitro-L-arginine (L-NNLA),[61] although other investigators using the same NOS inhibitor found no effect on resting CBF.[62] Other studies in the fetal lamb have found that the fourfold increase in regional cortical NOS activity between 92 and 135 days gestation was associated with twofold increases in CBF and oxygen consumption and that inhibition of NOS with NG-nitro-L-arginine methyl ester ([L-NAME] 60 mg/kg) resulted in 27% and 25% reductions in CBF at 93 and 133 days gestation, respectively.[63] These findings suggest that the emergence of NOS activity participated in the establishment of mature patterns of CBF regulation parallel the development of synaptic and electrical activity. Inhalation of NO (up to 60 ppm) in fetal lambs has been shown to lower pulmonary artery pressure without directly affecting CBF and electrocortical activity, but CBF can indirectly be influenced by NO-mediated changes in Pco_2.[64]

In vitro studies using newborn piglet arteries have shown endothelium-dependent vasodilation elicited by bradykinin that was enhanced with L-arginine and decreased by L-NAME.[65] Also in newborn piglets, administration of the nonselective NOS inhibitor L-NAME (10 and 20 mg/kg) reduced CBF as detected by measuring changes in total cerebral hemoglobin content using near-infrared spectroscopy.[66] In addition, administration of the NO donor sodium nitroprusside ([SNP] 1.5 mg/kg) increased CBF. Other studies in piglets using L-NG-mono-methyl-L-arginine ([L-NMMA] 100 mg) found that forebrain CBF decreased to 81% of control values, whereas neurohypophyseal flow decreased to 56% with no effect on cerebral oxygen consumption.[67]

Physiologic Control of Cerebral Blood Flow

Numerous reports have examined the role of NO under varying physiologic conditions, including changes in: (1) autoregulation; (2) carbon dioxide tension; (3) oxygen tension; and (4) glucose concentration. These varying conditions are reviewed briefly in the following sections.

Autoregulation

Cerebrovascular autoregulation refers to the ability of the cerebral arteries to adjust their level of resistance (by dilating or constricting) as systemic blood pressure fluctuates to maintain CBF within an established range.[68] Several studies have suggested that NO does not mediate this response in the adult cerebrovascular circulation,[30] although more recent evidence suggests that NO exerts a role in maintaining the lower limit of autoregulation.[69–73] However, not all investigators agree.[74] It has also been suggested that even though NO does not participate in regulatory control during hypertension, it may contribute to the loss of autoregulatory control when increases in CBF occur above the upper limits of blood pressure regulation.[75]

Few investigators have examined autoregulation in the newborn. Studies in 2- to 14-day-old piglets, have shown that NO may mediate vasodilation that occurs in response to reduction in transmural flow and pressure.[76]

Carbon Dioxide

Studies using NOS inhibitors in several species have demonstrated somewhat contradictory results,[77] but the overall impression is that they attenuate the increase in CBF seen with hypercapnia.[30,78–82] The magnitude of this attenuation ranges from 36% to 94%, can be reversed by co-administration of L-arginine, and depends on the amount and nature of the specific inhibitor used and the time interval between inhibitor administration and the hypercapnic challenge. The effect of NOS inhibition is maximal when the P_{CO_2} ranges between 50 and 60 mmHg; P_{CO_2} levels greater than 100 mmHg do not show the same response.[83] The mechanism of the NO response is uncertain but may be related to further decreasing perivascular pH, one of the principal mechanisms responsible for hypercapnic vasodilation.[84] It is also clear that other mechanisms, aside from those related to NO, regulate the cerebrovascular response to changes in P_{CO_2} particularly at high P_{CO_2} tensions. The effect of NO on this hypercapnic response may also be augmented by the release of prostaglandins.[85]

The source of NO during hypercapnia is also uncertain. As reviewed by Iadecola and colleagues, evidence against NO originating from endothelial cells, perivascular nerves, and neurons has been reported.[30] Of interest is that NOS 1 knockout mice have preservation of cerebrovascular responses – including hypercapnia – to the same degree as wild-type mice, a finding that supports the concept that NOS 1 does not mediate hypercapnic vasodilation.[86] It also has been suggested that mechanisms may be different at varying levels of cerebrovascular resistance (i.e., large versus small arteries) and that the vasodilator response to changes in PCO_2 could be propagated from more distant vessels. In humans, data both supporting[87] and arguing against[88] a role for NO in hypercapnia-induced vasodilation have been published.

Data from two studies in newborn piglets have suggested that NO is not an important mediator of CBF-PCO_2 reactivity. In one study, cerebrovascular resistance was measured using near-infrared spectroscopy in response to changes in PCO_2 before and after L-NAME or SNP administration.[66] Neither agent affected changes in vascular resistance as PCO_2 was varied. In a second study using 133-xenon in mechanically ventilated piglets less than 24 hours postnatal age, CBF-PCO_2 reactivity was 18.4% before and 15.2% per kPa after administration of L-NAME.[89] This difference in PCO_2 reactivity was not considered statistically different.

Oxygen

Studies using NOS inhibitors during hypoxia have also demonstrated conflicting results.[90] The overall consensus suggests that the contribution of NO to cerebral hypoxic vasodilation is relatively minor.[30] In several studies, no attenuation of the response to decreasing PO_2 has been reported[91-93] even when NOS activity was reduced.[94] Other studies, however, have found a moderate attenuation of the response to hypoxemia after intravenous administration of L-NMMA in the rat[95] and L-NAME administration in the awake dog.[96] More recently, it has been suggested that NO plays a role in hypoxemic vasodilation but not during hemodilution,[97] and also that NOS 1 may mediate the vasodilator effect at the capillary (rather than arterial) level.[98]

Studies in fetal lambs have suggested that NO mediates the cerebral vasodilatory response to hypoxia.[62] In one study, the increase in CBF (129 to 187 mL/100 g/min) secondary to hypoxemia could be blocked by administration of the NOS inhibitor L-NNLA with resultant CBF values of 143 mL/100 g/min, an effect that could be reversed with L-arginine.[61] Other studies by the same group of investigators indicated no modulating role of NO when fetal arterial oxygen content was increased above normal.[99]

Glucose

Studies examining the influence of NO on post-hypoglycemic increases in CBF have shown different results. In adult models, L-NAME attenuated the hypoglycemic-induced hyperemic response in goats,[100] whereas no effect was noted in rats.[101] In 1- to 2-week-old piglets rendered hypoglycemic with insulin (200 U/kg IV), L-NAME (40 mg/kg IV) attenuated cortical and cerebellar increases in CBF.[102] Differences in these observations may be species- or method-related and indicate that further studies are needed before any conclusions can be drawn concerning the role of NO on CBF during hypoglycemia.

Nitric Oxide and Cerebrovascular Disease

A better understanding of the relative neurotoxic versus neuroprotective effects of NO during ischemia and reperfusion is slowly emerging.[103–106] The cerebroprotective role of NO has been attributed to its role as a cerebral vasodilator (enhancing collateral circulation) and as an inhibitor of platelet aggregation and leukocyte adhesion (preventing microvascular plugging by platelets and leukocytes).[105] An oversimplification between the competing roles of NO describes a sequence of events that includes: (1) early cerebral protection from increased CBF as a consequence of vascular NO release; (2) neurotoxicity from neuronally derived NO; and (3) delayed neurotoxicity from post-ischemic inflammatory responses, which causes inducible NO synthesis and release.[107]

The overall effect of NO derived from different isoforms remains complex, as many factors contribute to its role, including the nature (focal versus global) and duration of the ischemic insult, the degree of post-ischemic reperfusion, the vulnerability of different brain regions, and whether the injury leads to necrotic or apoptotic cell death. In addition, few studies of the role of NO during focal or global ischemia have involved direct measurements of CBF. Several experimental observations have suggested that NO increases CBF. These include: (1) administration of high-dose nonselective NOS inhibitors increased infarct volume, presumably by inhibiting NOS 3 and reducing CBF; and (2) administration of L-arginine before, or soon after, ischemia reduced infarct volume by preferentially affecting vascular NO production.[31,34] The following sections review available experimental data (in adult models and then in newborns) for focal and global cerebral ischemia based on the method by which NO was manipulated, or by measurement of changes in NOS 3 activity or expression as follows: (1) L-arginine infusion; (2) infusion of NO donors; (3) use of NOS inhibitors; (4) use of NOS knockout models; and (5) NOS activity and mRNA expression.

Focal Cerebral Ischemia

Numerous studies on the relation between NO and CBF during focal cerebral ischemia in adult models of MCAO have been reported.

Few studies are available concerning newborns and almost all of these have used the Rice-Vannucci model of unilateral carotid artery occlusion with 8% hypoxia. Several reviews have examined the validity and results obtained with different models of focal ischemia in the newborn.[108–111]

L-arginine Infusion

Initial studies by Morikawa and colleagues used L-arginine (30 mg/kg IV) administered 5 minutes after unilateral common carotid/ MCAO and demonstrated an increase in regional CBF within the dorsolateral ischemic cortex in spontaneously hypertensive rats.[112,113] Higher doses of L-arginine (300 mg/kg) increased CBF from 22% to 33% of baseline as measured by laser-Doppler flowmetry; this effect was reversible with topical L-NAME (1 μM), as measured by decreased pial arteriole caliber from 115% to 106% of baseline. Subsequent studies from the same group of investigators showed that L-arginine (300 mg/kg IV) given immediately after the onset of MCAO elevated regional CBF by 20% in the dorsolateral cortex of Sprague-Dawley rats; 30 mg/kg of L-arginine increased blood flow distal to the MCAO (i.e., the ischemic penumbra) by 50%.[114] These findings were associated with a 35% reduction in infarct volume.

Administration of L-arginine during reperfusion also increases CBF, but this is dependent on the duration of ischemia. Five minutes of ischemia does not impair the vasodilatory effect of L-arginine, but 20 minutes of ischemia does reduce this effect.[115] Restoration of the L-arginine effect after pretreatment with L-NAME suggests that cytotoxic substances such as NO and related compounds might mediate this vascular response.

The effects of L-arginine are most likely on endothelial NO production, as the effects of L-arginine-induced pial artery dilation can be blocked by topical application of L-NAME without reducing brain NOS activity.[113] Other studies have found that CBF increases to L-arginine precede penumbral changes in the electroencephalogram (EEG) and this has been interpreted as indicating that the vascular response is not based on increased neuronal activity.[116]

Infusion of Nitric Oxide Donors

Administration of the NO donors, sodium nitroprusside (SNP) or 3-morpholino sydnonimine (SIN-1), increases CBF in the ischemic area, improves EEG recovery, and reduces focal ischemic injury.[117,118]

Initially, it was suggested that the protective effect by NO donors was unrelated to its inhibition of platelet aggregation,[118] and that the primary reason that NO enabled cerebral protection was related to its ability to increase CBF.[30] However, several recent studies have found that SNP and SIN-1 possess potent antithrombotic activities.[119]

Use of Nitric Oxide Synthase Inhibitors

Much confusion has been generated by the varying results that examined the magnitude of infarct volume reduction after using non-selective or selective NOS inhibitors at different concentrations and routes of administration.[30,31,33,34] Interestingly, few studies have compared changes in CBF, infarct volume reduction, and changes in NOS activity under identical circumstances using the same inhibitors.

In cats, L-NAME administered before MCAO, at a dose that completely inhibited cortical NOS activity (10 mg/kg), reduced caudate nucleus injury volume (80% to 52%) without affecting local CBF.[120] However, no differences in ipsilateral cerebral hemispheric injury between control and L-NAME-treated cats were observed.

In rats, L-NAME (1.5 mg/kg/min) infused 15 minutes after MCAO reduced ischemic blood flow by 36%.[121] These investigators also showed that, despite a decrease in CBF, NOS inhibition mildly improved the oxygen supply and consumption balance in the ischemic cortex.

Other investigators have shown that L-NAME (0.1 mg/kg bolus, 0.01 mg/kg/min IV) reduced CBF in the area of infarction at 30 minutes by 36%. After 180 minutes, it reduced CBF by 33%, and 15 minutes into reperfusion, L-NAME increased CBF in the area of infarction by 69% compared with controls.[122] Infarct volume reduction was similar irrespective of when L-NAME was given, and this suggested that the major neurotoxic role of NO occurs early during reperfusion rather than during ischemia. These findings may be related to recent observations that neuronal NO production appears to play an important role in regulating vascular tone and CBF to collateral-dependent tissue after MCAO.[123] Thus, inhibition of NOS during hypotension and MCAO increases arterial pressure, decreases blood flow to normal cerebrum, and increases blood flow to collateral-dependent cortical brain regions.[124]

Additional studies also lend support to earlier observations that NO may inhibit platelet aggregation based on studies using NO donors.[119] In a model of focal ischemia, L-NAME-treated rats had significant increases in total platelets in the ischemic hemisphere encompassing the anterior and posterior border zone areas, as well as widespread reductions (25%) in CBF.[125]

Use of Nitric Oxide Synthase Knockout Models

Use of genetically altered mice has also contributed to our understanding of CBF regulation and NO. NOS 1 knockout mice, deficient in nNOS, demonstrate reduced infarct volumes and neurologic deficits after MCAO that did not correlate with changes in CBF or differences in the vascular anatomy compared with control mice.[126] However, when nitro-L-arginine was given to nonselectively inhibit NOS 3, infarct volumes increased, suggesting that NOS 3 conferred some degree of cerebral protection. In subsequent studies, Huang and co-investigators, using NOS 3 knockout mice in which eNOS was reduced, demonstrated that regional CBF values recorded in the MCA territory by laser-Doppler flowmetry were more severely reduced after occlusion. In addition, the CBF values were disproportionately reduced during controlled hemorrhagic hypotension in autoregulation experiments.[127] These mice also had infarct volumes after filament MCAO that were increased by 21% compared with wild-type mice. These findings again suggested that NO production within endothelium could protect brain tissue by hemodynamic mechanisms. Additional studies by the same investigators using the NOS 3 knockout MCAO model and functional computed tomographic scanning techniques found that hemodynamic deficits were more severe in mutant mice than in the wild type.[128] The calculated relative perfusion index within the hemodynamic penumbra was significantly lower in the NOS 3 gene deletion group (35.6%) compared to 43.0% in the wild-type mice.

Nitric Oxide Synthase Activity and mRNA Expression

Studies in a rat filament model of MCAO have shown that NOS 3 is upregulated within 1 hour throughout the ischemic core and progressively increases up to 24 hours after ischemia.[129] In penumbral regions, a delayed (24-hour) upregulation of NOS 3 remained constant throughout the duration of ischemia. These findings of a rapid and intense differential expression of NOS 3 in core and penumbral areas support a role for NOS 3 in mediating changes in CBF.

Taken together, five separate approaches examining the role of NO and CBF during focal ischemia provide convincing data that release of vascular NO is important. The relative distribution of sources of NO, the magnitude and time course of its release, and the effect of NO on vascular cGMP-induced vasodilation require further investigation. Such studies will allow a better understanding of the overall cerebral protective effect of NO, a determination of when this effect occurs, and whether it can be enhanced.

Newborns

Studies have not yet examined the role of NO in CBF regulation in models of newborn stroke. However, in the newborn lamb, after intrastriatal injection of NMDA produced a histopathologic lesion, it was found that co-administration of L-NAME did not effect lesion size or post-NMDA hyperemia.[130] Interpretation of these data suggested that NO does not play a major part in NMDA-induced neonatal neuronal injury and might be only partially responsible for regional hyperemia during NMDA injection.

Global Ischemia

Although the role of NO during global ischemia is less well established than in focal ischemia, several studies have suggested its overall neurotoxic effect.[131] Few studies have examined changes in CBF during global ischemia and reperfusion, whether vascular release of NO occurs, and how this may be protective.

L-arginine Infusion

L-arginine (300 mg/kg IV), in a model of bilateral carotid artery occlusion for 30 minutes followed by 60 minutes recirculation in spontaneously hypertensive rats, increased post-ischemic CBF by 171% of resting CBF values compared to 126% in saline-treated controls.[132] During ischemia, CBF had significantly decreased to below 8% of resting values in all groups. Markers of tissue injury (reduced levels of adenosine triphosphate [ATP] and glucose; presence of lactate) were reduced in the L-arginine-treated animals. These findings suggested that enhanced post-ischemic hyperemia is beneficial to the ischemic brain and administration of L-arginine might be useful.

Infusion of Nitric Oxide Donors

Studies have not examined the influence of NO donors on CBF during global ischemia. However, the influence of acute ischemia on the ability of cerebral blood vessels to subsequently relax upon exposure to

NO donors has been evaluated. In goats, 20 minutes of global ischemia reduced the ability of several NO donors (including SNP) to relax middle cerebral artery rings 1 week after insult.[133]

Use of Nitric Oxide Synthase Inhibitors

Several studies using NOS inhibitors in rat models of global ischemia (bilateral carotid occlusion with/without cauterization of the vertebral arteries) have shown reduction in CBF during ischemia and reperfusion.[134] In one study, decreased CBF during ischemia was observed after L-NMMA administration without definite evidence of improvement in the severity of neuronal injury.[135] During reperfusion, L-NAME (30 mg/kg) prevented the return to baseline CBF,[136] and in other studies pretreatment with L-NAME (2, 10, and 50 mg/kg), produced dose-related depression of post-ischemic hyperemia.[137] These findings suggest that NO is instrumental in development of post-ischemic cerebral hyperemia. Similar findings of reduced hyperemia during reperfusion after L-NAME administration have also been reported in cats.[138]

Use of Nitric Oxide Synthase Knockout Models

Studies using NOS 1 or NOS 3 knockout mice during global ischemia that examined CBF have not been reported.

Nitric Oxide Synthase Activity and mRNA Expression

Although studies have demonstrated increased NOS 3 activity during reperfusion in a rat model of global ischemia (75% in parietal cortex; 40% in hippocampus),[139] the effects on CBF have not been examined.

Newborns

Studies in newborns have also endorsed a role for NO and its relation to CBF during global asphyxia. In infant piglets, L-NAME (3 mg/kg) administered before cardiac arrest increased arterial pressure and cardiac output, and decreased CBF by 18% compared to placebo.[140] L-NAME also attenuated post-resuscitation hyperemia in several brain regions including the cerebellum, diencephalon, and watershed regions supplied by the anterior and middle cerebral arteries. Other piglet studies have also shown blunting of the post-ischemic hyperemic response with L-NAME but without significant changes in cerebrovascular resistance.[141] In newborn lambs subjected to asphyxia, no differences in carotid artery blood flow were observed during reperfusion between L-NNLA-treated animals and controls.[142] However, the L-NNLA-treated group had preservation of the cerebral metabolic rate of oxygen and electrocortical brain activity in the NLA groups.

In rats, developmental age may be a critical factor in the response to hypoxia. Regional CBF decreased to 93% of baseline during hypoxia and increased to 124% of baseline during reoxygenation in 7-day-old rats, whereas CBF increased during hypoxia (125%) and reoxygenation (168%) in 14-day-old rats.[143] Although L-NAME attenuated the hyperemic response at both ages, it appeared that the 7-day-old rats had less capacity to activate NO production. Other studies in newborn rats (delivered by cesarean section and placed into a water bath) have shown little changes in NOS 1 activity 20 minutes after asphyxia despite fourfold increases in CBF.[144]

Reactive Oxygen Metabolites, Nitric Oxide Synthase, and Hypoxia-Ischemia

There is a growing body of evidence that reactive oxygen metabolites (see Chapter 9) play a significant role in the generation of injury to the brain after ischemia and reperfusion[145] (Figure 3). In adult rat brain following forebrain ischemia, brain superoxide dismutase (CuZn-SOD, EC 1.15.1.1) activity increases regionally in areas of brain associated with increased lipid peroxidation.[146] NOS can reduce molecular oxygen by one electron to O_2^-.[147] The generation of O_2^- and the reaction of the superoxide anion with NO lead to formation of another reactive metabolite, peroxynitrite.[148] Free radicals cause enzyme inactivation, DNA degradation, lipid peroxidation, and proteolysis, leading to disintegration of cell membrane integrity. In rat forebrain neuronal cultures, SOD blocked hypoxia-induced glutamate release, and NOS inhibitors and hemoglobin protected the cells from glutamate or hypoxic-induced cell death.[149] These data are consistent with the hypothesis that *glutamate release and free radical formation* can lead to NOS activation, which in turn yields a cooperative toxicity between O_2^- and NO. However, when sodium nitroprusside was injected into the hippocampus or striatum at postnatal day 7, little damage was seen suggesting that the neonatal

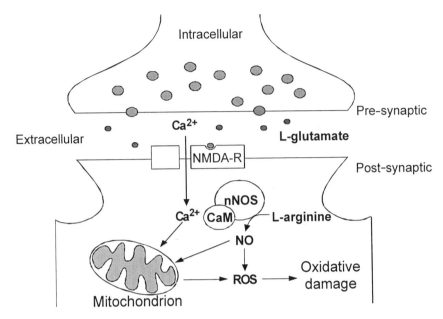

Figure 3. Hypothetical schema of the mechanisms involved in neuronal injury after hypoxic-ischemic injury. During ischemia, decreased glutamate uptake leads to post-synaptic activation of NMDA receptors and influx of Ca^{2+}, which in turn specifically activates nNOS. Both Ca^{2+} influx and formation of NO leads to mitochondrial dysfunction, formation of ROS, oxidative damage, and ultimately cell death. In this schema, oxidative damage can result even when nNOS activity is inhibited pharmacologically. NMDA-R = N-methyl-D-aspartate receptor; nNOS = neuronal nitric oxide synthase; CaM = calcium calmodulin; NO = nitric oxide; ROS = reactive oxygen species. Adapted from Bredt,[186] with permission.

brain is not sensitive to increased NO concentrations locally without other stress to neurons like excess glutamate production after hypoxic-ischemic injury.[150]

A recent developmental study of neuronal and glial cell-enriched fractions of rat brain showed that the cerebral cortex of rat brain contains higher concentrations of SOD early in development (postnatal day 15) and that SOD activity decreases with age. In addition, the authors showed that the neuronal activity of SOD is always less than glial SOD at all ages.[151] These data might help to explain the differential susceptibility of the developing CNS to hypoxic-ischemic injury. Selectively vulnerable populations of neurons exist in different regions at different stages of development.[152] Therefore, the premature brain may show a predilection for damage to the periventricular white matter zones because of the regional changes in NOS and SOD activity in these areas.

In primary cerebral cortical cell culture, glutamate neurotoxicity can be prevented by nitro-L-arginine, an NOS inhibitor; and hemoglobin, which complexes NO and prevents the neurotoxic effects of NMDA.[153] In coronal slices of mature rat brain incubated with NMDA, pre-incubation with nitro-L-arginine attenuates the toxicity of NMDA.[154] Therefore, the neurotoxicity associated with cerebral ischemia appears to involve glutamatergic stimulation of NOS via NMDA receptors. NMDA stimulates NO formation in NOS neurons, but these neurons are selectively resistant to NMDA neurotoxicity. It is unclear why the neurons that generate NO are not susceptible to its destructive effects. Recent evidence suggests that, in the setting of hypoxia-ischemia, NOS is induced in neurons by increased intracellular calcium after it binds to calmodulin.[153] The increased NOS activity results in large amounts of NO diffusing out of the neuron into the extracellular space where it can combine with superoxide anion to form peroxynitrite. The generation of this neurotoxic species results in lipid peroxidation and cytotoxicity to nearby cells.[148]

Early studies of the NADPH-diaphorase neurons in rats showed them to be resistant to systemic administration of other toxins such as carbon monoxide, sulfanilamide, 3-acetyl-pyridine, tetrachloromethane, and thalidomide.[155] The physiologic function of NADPH diphorase is not completely understood, although its recent identification as NOS has yielded important information.[156]

Although these NOS neurons are selectively resistant to NMDA, they are more susceptible than other neurons to kainate or quisqualate toxicity.[157] In fact, low concentrations of quisqualate will kill NADPH-diaphorase-containing neurons without producing generalized neuronal injury in murine cortical neuronal culture. This differential susceptibility is not absolute, since high doses of any glutamate agonist will produce nonselective neuronal injury. The demonstration that the NADPH-diaphorase-positive neurons have a differential susceptibility to glutamate agonists provides a basis for explaining the developmental patterns of neuronal cell loss that change over time in NMDA-mediated toxicity. Conflicting data do exist, however, for the response of the developing CNS to NO inhibition during excitotoxicity. For example, NO mediates quinolinate neurotoxicity in the rat pup brain and a nonspecific inhibitor of NO synthesis is neuroprotective after focal stroke.[158] In another study, when the same inhibitor was given prior to *or* after the hypoxic-ischemic injury, damage was prevented only when the animal was pretreated.[159] These results may represent a problem with nonselective inhibition of NOS activity that leads to unpredictable results in a given setting.

Although NO appears to be a critical mediator in the pathogenesis of hypoxic-ischemic injury in the newborn and adult, other negative studies have shown that neither pharmacologic inhibition of enzymatic activity nor scavenging of metabolites provides protection when administered after the insult. These results are in keeping with previous findings that enzymatic inhibition of NADPH diaphorase using cysteamine could be accomplished without significant protection of neonatal forebrain after a hypoxic-ischemic insult.[160] These findings are surprising given that elimination of NOS activity, either by selective destruction of the neurons or targeted disruption of the neuronal nNOS gene, results in protection from hypoxia-ischemia in the neonatal brain.[161,162]

Enzymatic inhibition has been more successful, but not robustly, in the mature nervous system. Using the NOS inhibitor, 7-NI, infarct volume was reduced by 25% after proximal MCAO in the rat and this effect was blocked by co-administration of L-arginine.[163] In an MCAO/reperfusion model, low-dose L-NAME given from the beginning of the insult through the reperfusion period reduced infarct volume from 40% to 27%.[164] In the neonatal rat, NG-nitro-L-arginine (L-NO-Arg) proved efficacious if the drug was administered prior to the insult, but not afterward.[159] Similar results were obtained with documented inhibition of NOS with L-NO-Arg 15 hours prior to the onset of a hypoxic-ischemic insult, which provided almost complete protection against neuronal damage.[158]

In perfused respiring brain slices taken from 7-day-old rat pups, pretreatment with 7-NI and L-NAME (but not L-NO-Arg) protected tissue from hypoxia-induced energy loss of ATP.[165] In addition, there was no production of nitrotyrosine (a marker for peroxynitrite) in inhibited slices. These studies illustrate that the inhibition of nNOS must occur prior to the onset of the insult in order for energy loss and subsequent tissue destruction to be prevented. In 7-day-old Wistar rat pups with permanent left MCAO, nitrotyrosine immunoreactivity was seen in blood vessels close to the cortical infarct and in white blood cells. The appearance of the nitrotyrosine paralleled an increase in iNOS production by these cells as well as by glia.[166]

In a post-treatment study in fetal sheep, a continuous infusion of L-NNA at a dose of 50 mg/hr instituted 2 hours after a 30-minute *in utero* ischemic insult delayed the increase in cerebral blood volume, but did not decrease the extent of cerebral injury.[167] Some of the negative effects of these drugs can be explained by nonselectivity of the inhibition. That is, if the endothelial isoform of NOS is also inhibited, then compensatory changes in blood flow that might be protective would be blocked, thus contributing to the damage caused by the initial insult. This effect was well documented in animals lacking the nNOS transgene. When the NOS inhibitor, L-NAME, was administered after MCAO to inhibit eNOS activity in the mutant, the protective effect of knocking down nNOS was lost, and infarct volume was similar in both transgenic and wild-type animals.[126] In one study (Sheldon and Ferriero, unpublished observation), both the wild-type and nNOS knockout animals given L-NAME after the hypoxic-ischemic insult had markedly increased mortality, potentially indicating the important role of CBF during hypoxia and recovery in the newborn. Supporting this idea is a recent study in newborn piglets, in which nonselective inhibition with n-nitro-L-arginine given before cerebral hypoxic-ischemic injury tended to compromise cerebral energy status during and after hypoxia-ischemia, as measured by ^{1}H- and ^{31}P-magnetic resonance spectroscopy (MRS).[168] In another study investigating the role of NOS in post-ischemic energy failure, 14-day-old Wistar rat pups subjected to hypoxic-ischemic injury and treated with L-NAME exhibited a decrease in nNOS activity in the infarcted region with an increase in iNOS activity. L-NAME did not prevent delayed impairment of cerebral energy metabolism as measured by ^{31}P-MRS, nor did it ameliorate infarct size.[169]

In conditions of energy failure, NOS produces NO and the reaction between superoxide and NO forms the powerful oxidant, peroxynitrite, which further contributes to cytotoxicity.[170] Together these compounds cause single strand breaks in DNA. The damaged DNA then activates poly(ADP-ribose) polymerase (PARP) in the nucleus, to assist in the repair of the DNA. Activated PARP transfers ADP-ribose moieties from the oxidized form of NAD (NAD$^+$) to nuclear proteins. The NAD$^+$ resynthesis depletes ATP, leading to a major cellular energy deficit in a futile cycle.[171] Therefore, another method of downstream modulation of NO toxicity would be to eliminate the excessive peroxynitrite formed when nNOS is activated in the setting of superoxide leakage from mitochondria. Recently, phenylbutylnitrone, used for the detection of reactive oxygen intermediates in various experimental systems, has been shown to provide protection from oxidative injury in the CNS without toxicity associated with other drugs causing mortality from changes in CBF and mean blood pressure.[172,173]

Potential protective mechanisms associated with the generation of NO have been proposed and the timing of this NO generation may be critical in determining whether this reactive oxygen species will be protective or cytotoxic. The most valuable effect of NO in most cerebrovascular systems has been its effect on facilitating blood flow through vasodilation, an effect attributed to the activation of soluble guanylate cyclase with resultant increased cGMP.[174] Nitrosylation of K^+ channel protein might also contribute to a calcium-dependent relaxation of blood vessels.[175] NO may improve microvascular flow through the inhibition of platelet aggregation and leukocyte adhesion through activation of guanylate cyclase and inhibition of 12-lipoxygenase.[176] Another complex and controversial protective effect of NO is the inhibition of the NMDA receptor via a redox modulatory site that would inhibit calcium flux through the channel.[177] NO has been reported to lessen the direct cytotoxicity produced by hydrogen peroxide,[178] has been implicated as an OH^- scavenger, and can prevent radical propagation reactions by reacting with alkoxyl and peroxyl radicals.[105] These latter mechanisms may be operative in the developing nervous system after hypoxic-ischemic stress, since the neonatal brain does produce excess hydrogen peroxide after the insult.[179]

The net result of these cytotoxic and neuroprotective effects of NO is determined by the amount of NO produced in temporal and spatial relationship to the injury. In the 7-day-old rat model of hypoxia-ischemia, NO metabolites were measured by a NO analyzer in the lesion during the hypoxia and reoxygenation periods, and were seen to increase in the lesioned areas. Pretreatment with 7-NI, the nNOS inhibitor, blunted the rise during both of these time periods, while pretreatment with aminoguanidine, an iNOS inhibitor, blocked only the reoxygenation rise.[180] These data provide strong support for the role of all forms of NOS in the pathogenesis of neonatal hypoxia-ischemia. In an investigation of intrauterine hypoxia-ischemia in rat brain, nNOS activity was increased for 2 days after birth, but then declined through postnatal day 14. Expression of iNOS mRNA was increased immediately after the insult and nNOS was reduced through postnatal day 14.[181] These data illustrate that NOS expression can change for prolonged periods after the insult.

The chemical biology of NO is very complex. Its effects depend on either a direct interaction with biological molecules, or an indirect reaction with oxygen species to form reactive nitrogen oxide species. Direct effects occur at concentrations less than 1 μM. The constitutive NOS isoforms (nNOS and eNOS) generate these low fluxes of NO, whereas the inducible isoform is largely responsible for greater production of NO and thus indirect biological effects such as nitrosation, nitration, and oxidation.[182] In the setting of neonatal hypoxia-ischemia, it may be that the direct effects of NO are blocked by the inhibitors and scavengers used in these studies, but that the larger NO production is not blocked.

In one study using the iNOS inhibitor, aminoguanidine, focal cerebral ischemic damage was reduced after MCAO in the adult rat.[48] There is an influx of microglia expressing NOS immunoreactivity after an insult,[57,183,184] and it may be that this second phase of insult contributed by the release of NO from iNOS in microglia is not adequately blocked by inhibiting the neuronal and endothelial isoforms of NOS. In a neonatal rat model of hypoxic preconditioning, in which a prior hypoxic insult protected the brain from a more severe hypoxic-ischemic insult 24 hours later, NO production and activity was critical to the induction of tolerance.[185] However, the effect of NO was mediated by the eNOS isoform, rather than iNOS or nNOS.

References

1. Volpe JJ: *Neurology of the Newborn.* W.B. Saunders, Philadelphia, 1995.
2. Brenman JE, Bredt DS: Synaptic signaling by nitric oxide. Curr Opin Neurobiol 1997;7:374–378.
3. Dinerman JL, Dawson TM, Schell MJ, et al: Endothelial nitric oxide synthase localized to hippocampal pyramidal cells: implications for synaptic plasticity. Proc Natl Acad Sci USA 1994;91:4214–4218.
4. Verge VM, Xu Z, Xu XJ, et al: Marked increase in nitric oxide synthase mRNA in rat dorsal root ganglia after peripheral axotomy: in situ hybridization and functional studies. Proc Natl Acad Sci USA 1992;89: 11617–11621.
5. Geller DA, Lowenstein CJ, Shapiro RA, et al: Molecular cloning and expression of inducible nitric oxide synthase from human hepatocytes. Proc Natl Acad Sci USA 1993;90:3491–3495.
6. Charles IG, Palmer RM, Hickery MS, et al: Cloning, characterization, and expression of a cDNA encoding an inducible nitric oxide synthase from the human chondrocyte. Proc Natl Acad Sci USA 1993;90:11419–11423.
7. Endoh M, Maiese K, Wagner J: Expression of the inducible form of nitric oxide synthase by reactive astrocytes after transient global ischemia. Brain Res 1994;651:92–100.
8. Tatoyan A, Giulivi C: Purification and characterization of a nitric-oxide synthase from rat liver mitochondria. J Biol Chem 1998;273:11044–11048.
9. Stuehr DJ: Mammalian nitric oxide synthases. Biochim Biophys Acta 1999;1411:217–230.
10. Venema VJ, Ju H, Zou R, et al: Interaction of neuronal nitric-oxide synthase with caveolin-3 in skeletal muscle: identification of a novel caveolin scaffolding/inhibitory domain. J Biol Chem 1997;272:28187–28190.
11. Mayer B, John M, Heinzel B, et al: Brain nitric oxide synthase is a biopterin- and flavin-containing multi-functional oxido-reductase. FEBS Lett 1991;288:187–191.
12. Henry Y, Guissani A: Interactions of nitric oxide with hemoproteins: roles of nitric oxide in mitochondria. Cell Mol Life Sci 1999;55:1003–1014.
13. Stamler JS, Toone EJ, Lipton SA, et al: (S)NO signals: translocation, regulation, and a consensus motif. Neuron 1997;18:691–696.

14. Bredt DS, Glatt CE, Hwang PM, et al: Nitric oxide synthase protein and mRNA are discretely localized in neuronal populations of the mammalian CNS together with NADPH diaphorase. Neuron 1991;7:615–624.

15. Brenman JE, Chao DS, Gee SH, et al: Interaction of nitric oxide synthase with the postsynaptic density protein PSD-95 and alpha1-syntrophin mediated by PDZ domains. Cell 1996;84:757–767.

16. Black SM, Bedolli MA, Martinez S, et al: Expression of neuronal nitric oxide synthase corresponds to regions of selective vulnerability to hypoxia-ischaemia in the developing rat brain. Neurobiol Dis 1995;2:145–155.

17. Aoki C, Rhee J, Lubin M, et al: NMDA-R1 subunit of the cerebral cortex co-localizes with neuronal nitric oxide synthase at pre- and postsynaptic sites and in spines. Brain Res 1997;750:25–40.

18. Keilhoff G, Seidel B, Noack H, et al: Patterns of nitric oxide synthase at the messenger RNA and protein levels during early rat brain development. Neuroscience 1996;75:1193–1201.

19. Lizasoain I, Weiner CP, Knowles RG, et al: The ontogeny of cerebral and cerebellar nitric oxide synthase in the guinea pig and rat. Pediatr Res 1996;39:779–783.

20. Oermann E, Bidmon HJ, Mayer B, et al: Differential maturational patterns of nitric oxide synthase-I and NADPH diaphorase in functionally distinct cortical areas of the mouse cerebral cortex. Anat Embryol (Berl) 1999;200:27–41.

21. Ohyu J, Takashima S: Developmental characteristics of neuronal nitric oxide synthase (nNOS) immunoreactive neurons in fetal to adolescent human brains. Brain Res Dev Brain Res 1998;110:193–202.

22. Downen M, Zhao ML, Lee P, et al: Neuronal nitric oxide synthase expression in developing and adult human CNS. J Neuropathol Exp Neurol 1999;58:12–21.

23. Ignarro LJ, Buga GM, Wood KS, et al: Endothelium-derived relaxing factor produced and released from artery and vein is nitric oxide. Proc Natl Acad Sci USA 1987;84:9265–9269.

24. Stuehr DJ, Nathan CF: Nitric oxide. A macrophage product responsible for cytostasis and respiratory inhibition in tumor target cells. J Exp Med 1989;169:1543–1555.

25. Bredt DS, Snyder SH: Nitric oxide mediates glutamate-linked enhancement of cGMP levels in the cerebellum. Proc Natl Acad Sci USA 1989;86:9030–9033.

26. Garthwaite J, Garthwaite G, Palmer RM, et al: NMDA receptor activation induces nitric oxide synthesis from arginine in rat brain slices. Eur J Pharmacol 1989;172:413–416.

27. Moncada S, Higgs A: The L-arginine-nitric oxide pathway. N Engl J Med 1993;329:2002–2012.

28. Halliwell B, Gutteridge JMC: *Free Radicals in Biology and Medicine.* Clarendon Press, Oxford, 1989, pp 237–245.

29. Billiar TR: Nitric oxide: novel biology with clinical relevance. Ann Surg 1995;221:339–349.

30. Iadecola C, Pelligrino DA, Moskowitz MA, et al: Nitric oxide synthase inhibition and cerebrovascular regulation. J Cereb Blood Flow Metab 1994;14:175–192.

31. Nagafuji T, Sugiyama M, Matsui T, et al: Nitric oxide synthase in cerebral ischemia: possible contribution of nitric oxide synthase activation in brain

microvessels to cerebral ischemic injury. Mol Chem Neuropathol 1995;26:107–157.

32. Toda N: Nitric oxide and the regulation of cerebral arterial tone. In Vincent SR (ed): *Nitric Oxide in the Nervous System*. Vol 26. Academic Press, San Diego, 1995, pp 207–225.

33. Dawson DA: Nitric oxide and focal cerebral ischemia: multiplicity of actions and diverse outcome. Cerebrovasc Brain Metab Rev 1994;6:299–324.

34. Watkins LD: Nitric oxide and cerebral blood flow: an update. Cerebrovasc Brain Metab Rev 1995;7:324–337.

35. Faraci FM, Brian JE Jr: Nitric oxide and the cerebral circulation. Stroke 1994;25:692–703.

36. Regidor J, Edvinsson L, Divac I: NOS neurones lie near branchings of cortical arteriolae. Neuroreport 1993;4:112–114.

37. Nozaki K, Moskowitz MA, Maynard KI, et al: Possible origins and distribution of immunoreactive nitric oxide synthase-containing nerve fibers in cerebral arteries. J Cereb Blood Flow Metab 1993;13:70–79.

38. Rand MJ, Li CG: Nitric oxide in the autonomic and enteric nervous system. In Vincent SR (ed): *Nitric Oxide in the Nervous System*. Academic Press, San Diego, 1995, pp 227–279.

39. Toda N, Okamura T: Neurogenic nitric oxide (NO) in the regulation of cerebroarterial tone. J Chem Neuroanat 1996;10:259–265.

40. Bredt DS, Hwang PM, Snyder SH: Localization of nitric oxide synthase indicating a neural role for nitric oxide. Nature 1990;347:768–770.

41. Kovách AG, Szabó C, Benyó Z, et al: Effects of NG-nitro-L-arginine and L-arginine on regional cerebral blood flow in the cat. J Physiol (Lond) 1992;449:183–196.

42. Kelly PA, Ritchie IM, Arbuthnott GW: Inhibition of neuronal nitric oxide synthase by 7-nitroindazole: effects upon local cerebral blood flow and glucose use in the rat. J Cereb Blood Flow Metab 1995;15:766–773.

43. Licinio J, Prolo P, McCann SM, et al: Brain iNOS: current understanding and clinical implications. Mol Med Today 1999;5:225–232.

44. Iadecola C, Zhang F, Xu X: Inhibition of inducible nitric oxide synthase ameliorates cerebral ischemic damage. Am J Physiol 1995;268:R286–R292.

45. Nogawa S, Forster C, Zhang F, et al: Interaction between inducible nitric oxide synthase and cyclooxygenase-2 after cerebral ischemia. Proc Natl Acad Sci USA 1998;95:10966–10971.

46. Gunnett CA, Chu Y, Heistad DD, et al: Vascular effects of LPS in mice deficient in expression of the gene for inducible nitric oxide synthase. Am J Physiol 1998;275:H416–H421.

47. Okamoto H, Ito O, Roman RJ, et al: Role of inducible nitric oxide synthase and cyclooxygenase-2 in endotoxin-induced cerebral hyperemia. Stroke 1998;29:1209–1218.

48. Zhang F, Casey RM, Ross ME, et al: Aminoguanidine ameliorates and L-arginine worsens brain damage from intraluminal middle cerebral artery occlusion. Stroke 1996;27:317–323.

49. Iadecola C, Zhang F, Casey R, et al: Inducible nitric oxide synthase gene expression in vascular cells after transient focal cerebral ischemia. Stroke 1996;27:1373–1380.

50. Murphy S, Simmons ML, Agullo L, et al: Synthesis of nitric oxide in CNS glial cells. Trends Neurosci 1993;16:323–328.

51. Miyawaki T, Sohma O, Mizuguchi M, et al: Development of endothelial

nitric oxide synthase in endothelial cells in the human cerebrum. Brain Res Dev Brain Res 1995;89:161–166.

52. Faraci FM: Role of nitric oxide in regulation of basilar artery tone in vivo. Am J Physiol 1990;259:H1216–H1221.

53. Rosenblum WI, Nishimura H, Nelson GH: Endothelium-dependent L-arg- and L-NMMA-sensitive mechanisms regulate tone of brain microvessels. Am J Physiol 1990;259:H1396–H1401.

54. Busija DW, Leffler CW, Wagerle LC: Mono-L-arginine-containing compounds dilate piglet pial arterioles via an endothelium-derived relaxing factor-like substance. Circ Res 1990;67:1374–1380.

55. Tanaka K, Gotoh F, Gomi S, et al: Inhibition of nitric oxide synthesis induces a significant reduction in local cerebral blood flow in the rat. Neurosci Lett 1991;127:129–132.

56. Reutens DC, McHugh MD, Toussaint PJ, et al: L-arginine infusion increases basal but not activated cerebral blood flow in humans. J Cereb Blood Flow Metab 1997;17:309–315.

57. Macrae IM, Dawson DA, Norrie JD, et al: Inhibition of nitric oxide synthesis: effects on cerebral blood flow and glucose utilisation in the rat. J Cereb Blood Flow Metab 1993;13:985–992.

58. Cholet N, Seylaz J, Lacombe P, et al: Local uncoupling of the cerebrovascular and metabolic responses to somatosensory stimulation after neuronal nitric oxide synthase inhibition. J Cereb Blood Flow Metab 1997;17:1191–1201.

59. Kajita Y, Takayasu M, Suzuki Y, et al: Regional differences in cerebral vasomotor control by nitric oxide. Brain Res Bull 1995;38:365–369.

60. Caramia F, Yoshida T, Hamberg LM, et al: Measurement of changes in cerebral blood volume in spontaneously hypertensive rats following L-arginine infusion using dynamic susceptibility contrast MRI. Magn Reson Med 1998;39:160–163.

61. van Bel F, Sola A, Roman C, et al: Role of nitric oxide in the regulation of the cerebral circulation in the lamb fetus during normoxemia and hypoxemia. Biol Neonate 1995;68:200–210.

62. McCrabb GJ, Harding R: Role of nitric oxide in the regulation of cerebral blood flow in the ovine foetus. Clin Exp Pharmacol Physiol 1996;23:855–860.

63. Northington FJ, Tobin JR, Harris AP, et al: Developmental and regional differences in nitric oxide synthase activity and blood flow in the sheep brain. J Cereb Blood Flow Metab 1997;17:109–115.

64. Lopes Cardozo RH, de Beaufort AJ, Gesink BJ, et al: Inhalation of nitric oxide: effect on cerebral hemodynamics and activity, and antioxidant status in the newborn lamb. Biol Neonate 1996;69:284–292.

65. Martínez-Orgado J, Salaices M, Rodríguez-Martínez MA, et al: Role of nitric oxide on the endothelium-dependent vasodilation in newborn piglet cerebral arteries. Gen Pharmacol 1994;25:899–902.

66. Takei Y, Edwards AD, Lorek A, et al: Effects of N-omega-nitro-L-arginine methyl ester on the cerebral circulation of newborn piglets quantified in vivo by near-infrared spectroscopy. Pediatr Res 1993;34:354–359.

67. Greenberg RS, Helfaer MA, Kirsch JR, et al: Nitric oxide synthase inhibition with NG-mono-methyl-L-arginine reversibly decreases cerebral blood flow in piglets. Crit Care Med 1994;22:384–392.

68. Paulson OB, Strandgaard S, Edvinsson L: Cerebral autoregulation. Cerebrovasc Brain Metab Rev 1990;2:161–192.

69. Preckel MP, Leftheriotis G, Ferber C, et al: Effect of nitric oxide blockade on the lower limit of the cortical cerebral autoregulation in pentobarbital-anaesthetized rats. Int J Microcirc Clin Exp 1996;16:277–283.

70. Rise IR, Kirkeby OJ: Effect of reduced cerebral perfusion pressure on cerebral blood flow following inhibition of nitric oxide synthesis. J Neurosurg 1998;89:448–453.

71. Kajita Y, Takayasu M, Dietrich HH, et al: Possible role of nitric oxide in autoregulatory response in rat intracerebral arterioles. Neurosurgery 1998;42:834–841.

72. Tanaka K, Fukuuchi Y, Gomi S, et al: Inhibition of nitric oxide synthesis impairs autoregulation of local cerebral blood flow in the rat. Neuroreport 1993;4:267–270.

73. Kobari M, Fukuuchi Y, Tomita M, et al: Role of nitric oxide in regulation of cerebral microvascular tone and autoregulation of cerebral blood flow in cats. Brain Res 1994;667:255–262.

74. Takahashi S, Cook M, Jehle J, et al: Preservation of autoregulatory cerebral vasodilator responses to hypotension after inhibition of nitric oxide synthesis. Brain Res 1995;678:21–28.

75. Talman WT, Dragon DN: Inhibition of nitric oxide synthesis extends cerebrovascular autoregulation during hypertension. Brain Res 1995; 672:48–54.

76. Shimoda LA, Norins NA, Jeutter DC, et al: Flow-induced responses in piglet isolated cerebral arteries. Pediatr Res 1996;39:574–583.

77. Fabricius M, Rubin I, Bundgaard M, et al: NOS activity in brain and endothelium: relation to hypercapnic rise of cerebral blood flow in rats. Am J Physiol 1996;271:H2035–H2044.

78. Iadecola C, Zhang F, Xu X: SIN-1 reverses attenuation of hypercapnic cerebrovasodilation by nitric oxide synthase inhibitors. Am J Physiol 1994;267:R228–R235.

79. Smith JJ, Lee JG, Hudetz AG, et al: The role of nitric oxide in the cerebrovascular response to hypercapnia. Anesth Analg 1997;84:363–369.

80. Horvath I, Sandor NT, Ruttner Z, et al: Role of nitric oxide in regulating cerebrocortical oxygen consumption and blood flow during hypercapnia. J Cereb Blood Flow Metab 1994;14:503–509.

81. Okamoto H, Hudetz AG, Roman RJ, et al: Neuronal NOS-derived NO plays permissive role in cerebral blood flow response to hypercapnia. Am J Physiol 1997;272:H559–H566.

82. Sandor P, Komjati K, Reivich M, et al: Major role of nitric oxide in the mediation of regional CO_2 responsiveness of the cerebral and spinal cord vessels of the cat. J Cereb Blood Flow Metab 1994;14:49–58.

83. Iadecola C, Zhang F: Nitric oxide-dependent and -independent components of cerebrovasodilation elicited by hypercapnia. Am J Physiol 1994; 266:R546–R552.

84. Niwa K, Lindauer U, Villringer A, et al: Blockade of nitric oxide synthesis in rats strongly attenuates the CBF response to extracellular acidosis. J Cereb Blood Flow Metab 1993;13:535–539.

85. Heinert G, Nye PC, Paterson DJ: Nitric oxide and prostaglandin pathways interact in the regulation of hypercapnic cerebral vasodilatation. Acta Physiol Scand 1999;166:183–193.

86. Irikura K, Huang PL, Ma J, et al: Cerebrovascular alterations in mice lacking neuronal nitric oxide synthase gene expression. Proc Natl Acad Sci USA 1995;92:6823–6827.

87. Schmetterer L, Findl O, Strenn K, et al: Role of NO in the O_2 and CO_2 responsiveness of cerebral and ocular circulation in humans. Am J Physiol 1997;273:R2005–R2012.

88. White RP, Deane C, Vallance P, et al: Nitric oxide synthase inhibition in humans reduces cerebral blood flow but not the hyperemic response to hypercapnia. Stroke 1998;29:467–472.

89. Patel J, Pryds O, Roberts I, et al: Limited role for nitric oxide in mediating cerebrovascular control of newborn piglets. Arch Dis Child Fetal Neonatal Ed 1996;75:F82–F86.

90. Berger C, von Kummer R: Does NO regulate the cerebral blood flow response in hypoxia? Acta Neurol Scand 1998;97:118–125.

91. Kozniewska E, Oseka M, Stys T: Effects of endothelium-derived nitric oxide on cerebral circulation during normoxia and hypoxia in the rat. J Cereb Blood Flow Metab 1992;12:311–317.

92. Pelligrino DA, Koenig HM, Albrecht RF: Nitric oxide synthesis and regional cerebral blood flow responses to hypercapnia and hypoxia in the rat. J Cereb Blood Flow Metab 1993;13:80–87.

93. Buchanan JE, Phillis JW: The role of nitric oxide in the regulation of cerebral blood flow. Brain Res 1993;610:248–255.

94. McPherson RW, Koehler RC, Traystman RJ: Hypoxia, alpha 2-adrenergic, and nitric oxide-dependent interactions on canine cerebral blood flow. Am J Physiol 1994;266:H476–H482.

95. Berger C, von Kummer R, Gerlach L, et al. Role of nitric oxide in local cerebral blood flow under hypoxic conditions. International Symposium on Cerebral Blood Flow Vessels '93. Zao, Japan, 1993.

96. Audibert G, Saunier CG, Siat J, et al: Effect of the inhibitor of nitric oxide synthase, NG-nitro-L-arginine methyl ester, on cerebral and myocardial blood flows during hypoxia in the awake dog. Anesth Analg 1995;81: 945–951.

97. Todd MM, Farrell S, Wu B: Cerebral blood flow during hypoxemia and hemodilution in rabbits: different roles for nitric oxide? J Cereb Blood Flow Metab 1997;17:1319–1325.

98. Hudetz AG, Shen H, Kampine JP: Nitric oxide from neuronal NOS plays critical role in cerebral capillary flow response to hypoxia. Am J Physiol 1998;274:H982–H989.

99. van Bel F, Sola A, Roman C, et al: Perinatal regulation of the cerebral circulation: role of nitric oxide and prostaglandins. Pediatr Res 1997;42: 299–304.

100. Diéguez G, Fernández N, García JL, et al: Role of nitric oxide in the effects of hypoglycemia on the cerebral circulation in awake goats. Eur J Pharmacol 1997;330:185–193.

101. Horinaka N, Artz N, Jehle J, et al: Examination of potential mechanisms in the enhancement of cerebral blood flow by hypoglycemia and pharmacological doses of deoxyglucose. J Cereb Blood Flow Metab 1997;17:54–63.

102. Ichord RN, Helfaer MA, Kirsch JR, et al: Nitric oxide synthase inhibition attenuates hypoglycemic cerebral hyperemia in piglets. Am J Physiol 1994;266:H1062–H1068.

103. Dalkara T, Moskowitz MA: The complex role of nitric oxide in the pathophysiology of focal cerebral ischemia. Brain Pathol 1994;4:49–57.

104. Dalkara T, Moskowitz MA: Neurotoxic and neuroprotective roles of nitric oxide in cerebral ischaemia. Int Rev Neurobiol 1997;40:319–336.

105. Iadecola C: Bright and dark sides of nitric oxide in ischemic brain injury. Trends Neurosci 1997;20:132–139.
106. Samdani AF, Dawson TM, Dawson VL: Nitric oxide synthase in models of focal ischemia. Stroke 1997;28:1283–1288.
107. Love S: Oxidative stress in brain ischemia. Brain Pathol 1999;9:119–131.
108. Vannucci RC, Vannucci SJ: A model of perinatal hypoxic-ischemic brain damage. Ann NY Acad Sci 1997;835:234–249.
109. Hagberg H, Bona E, Gilland E, et al: Hypoxia-ischaemia model in the 7-day-old rat: possibilities and shortcomings. Acta Paediatr Suppl 1997; 422:85–88.
110. Romijn HJ, Hofman MA, Gramsbergen A: At what age is the developing cerebral cortex of the rat comparable to that of the full-term newborn human baby? Early Hum Dev 1991;26:61–67.
111. Roohey T, Raju TN, Moustogiannis AN: Animal models for the study of perinatal hypoxic-ischemic encephalopathy: a critical analysis. Early Hum Dev 1997;47:115–146.
112. Morikawa E, Huang Z, Moskowitz MA: L-arginine decreases infarct size caused by middle cerebral arterial occlusion in SHR. Am J Physiol 1992; 263:H1632–H1635.
113. Morikawa E, Rosenblatt S, Moskowitz MA: L-arginine dilates rat pial arterioles by nitric oxide-dependent mechanisms and increases blood flow during focal cerebral ischaemia. Br J Pharmacol 1992;107:905–907.
114. Morikawa E, Moskowitz MA, Huang Z, et al: L-arginine infusion promotes nitric oxide-dependent vasodilation, increases regional cerebral blood flow, and reduces infarction volume in the rat. Stroke 1994;25:429–435.
115. Sporer B, Martens KH, Koedel U, et al: L-arginine-induced regional cerebral blood flow increase is abolished after transient focal cerebral ischemia in the rat. J Cereb Blood Flow Metab 1997;17:1074–1080.
116. Dalkara T, Yoshida T, Irikura K, et al: Dual role of nitric oxide in focal cerebral ischemia. Neuropharmacology 1994;33:1447–1452.
117. Zhang F, Iadecola C: Nitroprusside improves blood flow and reduces brain damage after focal ischemia. Neuroreport 1993;4:559–562.
118. Zhang F, White JG, Iadecola C: Nitric oxide donors increase blood flow and reduce brain damage in focal ischemia: evidence that nitric oxide is beneficial in the early stages of cerebral ischemia. J Cereb Blood Flow Metab 1994;14:217–226.
119. Sasaki Y, Seki J, Giddings JC, et al: Effects of NO-donors on thrombus formation and microcirculation in cerebral vessels of the rat. Thromb Haemost 1996;76:111–117.
120. Nishikawa T, Kirsch JR, Koehler RC, et al: Effect of nitric oxide synthase inhibition on cerebral blood flow and injury volume during focal ischemia in cats. Stroke 1993;24:1717–1724.
121. Wei HM, Chi OZ, Liu X, et al: Nitric oxide synthase inhibition alters cerebral blood flow and oxygen balance in focal cerebral ischemia in rats. Stroke 1994;25:445–449.
122. Ashwal S, Cole DJ, Osborne TN, et al: Dual effects of L-NAME during transient focal cerebral ischemia in spontaneously hypertensive rats. Am J Physiol 1994;267:H276–H284.
123. Robertson SC, Loftus CM: Effect of N-methyl-D-aspartate and inhibition of neuronal nitric oxide on collateral cerebral blood flow after middle cerebral artery occlusion. Neurosurgery 1998;42:117–123;discussion 123–114.

124. Muhonen MG, Heistad DD, Faraci FM, et al: Augmentation of blood flow through cerebral collaterals by inhibition of nitric oxide synthase. J Cereb Blood Flow Metab 1994;14:704–714.

125. Stagliano NE, Zhao W, Prado R, et al: The effect of nitric oxide synthase inhibition on acute platelet accumulation and hemodynamic depression in a rat model of thromboembolic stroke. J Cereb Blood Flow Metab 1997;17:1182–1190.

126. Huang Z, Huang PL, Panahian N, et al: Effects of cerebral ischemia in mice deficient in neuronal nitric oxide synthase. Science 1994;265:1883–1885.

127. Huang Z, Huang PL, Ma J, et al: Enlarged infarcts in endothelial nitric oxide synthase knockout mice are attenuated by nitro-L-arginine. J Cereb Blood Flow Metab 1996;16:981–987.

128. Lo EH, Hara H, Rogowska J, et al: Temporal correlation mapping analysis of the hemodynamic penumbra in mutant mice deficient in endothelial nitric oxide synthase gene expression. Stroke 1996;27:1381–1385.

129. Zhang ZG, Chopp M, Zaloga C, et al: Cerebral endothelial nitric oxide synthase expression after focal cerebral ischemia in rats. Stroke 1993;24:2016–2021.

130. Taylor GA, Trescher WH, Johnston MV, et al: Experimental neuronal injury in the newborn lamb: a comparison of N-methyl-D-aspartic acid receptor blockade and nitric oxide synthesis inhibition on lesion size and cerebral hyperemia. Pediatr Res 1995;38:644–651.

131. O'Neill MJ, Hicks C, Ward M, et al: Neuroprotective effects of the antioxidant LY231617 and NO synthase inhibitors in global cerebral ischaemia. Brain Res 1997;760:170–178.

132. Sadoshima S, Nagao T, Okada Y, et al: L-arginine ameliorates recirculation and metabolic derangement in brain ischemia in hypertensive rats. Brain Res 1997;744:246–252.

133. Salom JB, Barberá MD, Centeno JM, et al: Relaxant effects of sodium nitroprusside and NONOates in goat middle cerebral artery: delayed impairment by global ischemia-reperfusion. Nitric Oxide 1999;3:85–93.

134. Strasser A, Yasuma Y, McCarron RM, et al: Effect of nitro-L-arginine on cerebral blood flow and monoamine metabolism during ischemia/reperfusion in the mongolian gerbil. Brain Res 1994;664:197–201.

135. Sakashita N, Ando Y, Yonehara T, et al: Role of superoxide dismutase and nitric oxide on the interaction between brain and systemic circulation during brain ischemia. Biochim Biophys Acta 1994;1227:67–73.

136. Prado R, Watson BD, Wester P: Effects of nitric oxide synthase inhibition on cerebral blood flow following bilateral carotid artery occlusion and recirculation in the rat. J Cereb Blood Flow Metab 1993;13:720–723.

137. Humphreys SA, Koss MC: Role of nitric oxide in post-ischemic cerebral hyperemia in anesthetized rats. Eur J Pharmacol 1998;347:223–229.

138. Clavier N, Kirsch JR, Hurn PD, et al: Cerebral blood flow is reduced by N-omega-nitro-L-arginine methyl ester during delayed hypoperfusion in cats. Am J Physiol 1994;267:H174–H181.

139. Beasley TC, Bari F, Thore C, et al: Cerebral ischemia/reperfusion increases endothelial nitric oxide synthase levels by an indomethacin-sensitive mechanism. J Cereb Blood Flow Metab 1998;18:88–96.

140. Schleien CL, Kuluz JW, Gelman B: Hemodynamic effects of nitric oxide synthase inhibition before and after cardiac arrest in infant piglets. Am J Physiol 1998;274:H1378–H1385.

141. Greenberg RS, Helfaer MA, Kirsch JR, et al: Effect of nitric oxide synthase inhibition on postischemic cerebral hyperemia. Am J Physiol 1995; 269:H341–H347.

142. Dorrepaal CA, Shadid M, Steendijk P, et al: Effect of post-hypoxic-ischemic inhibition of nitric oxide synthesis on cerebral blood flow, metabolism and electrocortical brain activity in newborn lambs. Biol Neonate 1997;72: 216–226.

143. Ioroi T, Yonetani M, Nakamura H: Effects of hypoxia and reoxygenation on nitric oxide production and cerebral blood flow in developing rat striatum. Pediatr Res 1998;43:733–737.

144. Lubec B, Kozlov AV, Krapfenbauer K, et al: Nitric oxide and nitric oxide synthase in the early phase of perinatal asphyxia of the rat. Neuroscience 1999;93:1017–1023.

145. Chan PH: Role of oxidants in ischemic brain damage. Stroke 1996;27: 1124–1129.

146. Sutherland G, Bose R, Louw D, et al: Global elevation of brain superoxide dismutase activity following forebrain ischemia in rat. Neurosci Lett 1991;128:169–172.

147. Pou S, Pou WS, Bredt DS, et al: Generation of superoxide by purified brain nitric oxide synthase. J Biol Chem 1992;267:24173–24176.

148. Beckman JS: The double-edged role of nitric oxide in brain function and superoxide-mediated injury. J Dev Physiol 1991;15:53–59.

149. Cazevieille C, Muller A, Meynier F, et al: Superoxide and nitric oxide cooperation in hypoxia/reoxygenation-induced neuron injury. Free Radic Biol Med 1993;14:389–395.

150. Maragos WF, Silverstein FS: Resistance to nitroprusside neurotoxicity in perinatal rat brain. Neurosci Lett 1994;172:80–84.

151. Geremia E, Baratta D, Zafarana S, et al: Antioxidant enzymatic systems in neuronal and glial cell-enriched fractions of rat brain during aging. Neurochem Res 1990;15:719–723.

152. Ferriero DM, Arcavi LJ, Sagar SM, et al: Selective sparing of NADPH-diaphorase neurons in neonatal hypoxia-ischemia. Ann Neurol 1988;24: 670–676.

153. Dawson VL, Dawson TM, London ED, et al: Nitric oxide mediates glutamate neurotoxicity in primary cortical cultures. Proc Natl Acad Sci USA 1991;88:6368–6371.

154. Kollegger H, McBean GJ, Tipton KF: Reduction of striatal N-methyl-D-aspartate toxicity by inhibition of nitric oxide synthase. Biochem Pharmacol 1993;45:260–264.

155. Thomas E, Pearse AGE: The solitary active cells histochemical demonstration of damage-resistant nerve cells with a TPN-diaphorase reaction. ACTA Neuropathologica 1964;3:238–249.

156. Bredt DS, Snyder SH: Transient nitric oxide synthase neurons in embryonic cerebral cortical plate, sensory ganglia, and olfactory epithelium. Neuron 1994;13:301–313.

157. Koh JY, Choi DW: Vulnerability of cultured cortical neurons to damage by excitotoxins: differential susceptibility of neurons containing NADPH-diaphorase. J Neurosci 1988;8:2153–2163.

158. Trifiletti RR: Neuroprotective effects of NG-nitro-L-arginine in focal stroke in the 7-day old rat. Eur J Pharmacol 1992;218:197–198.

159. Hamada Y, Hayakawa T, Hattori H, et al: Inhibitor of nitric oxide syn-

thesis reduces hypoxic-ischemic brain damage in the neonatal rat. Pediatr Res 1994;35:10–14.

160. Spanggord H, Sheldon RA, Ferriero DM: Cysteamine eliminates nitric oxide synthase activity but is not protective to the hypoxic-ischemic neonatal rat brain. Neurosci Lett 1996;213:41–44.

161. Ferriero DM, Sheldon RA, Black SM, et al: Selective destruction of nitric oxide synthase neurons with quisqualate reduces damage after hypoxia-ischemia in the neonatal rat. Pediatr Res 1995;38:912–918.

162. Ferriero DM, Holtzman DM, Black SM, et al: Neonatal mice lacking neuronal nitric oxide synthase are less vulnerable to hypoxic-ischemic injury. Neurobiol Dis 1996;3:64–71.

163. Yoshida T, Limmroth V, Irikura K, et al: The NOS inhibitor, 7-nitroindazole, decreases focal infarct volume but not the response to topical acetylcholine in pial vessels. J Cereb Blood Flow Metab 1994;14:924–929.

164. Ashwal S, Cole DJ, Osborne TN, et al: Low dose L-NAME reduces infarct volume in the rat MCAO/reperfusion model. J Neurosurg Anesthesiol 1993;5:241–249.

165. Litt L, Espanol MT, Hasegawa K, et al: NOS inhibitors decrease hypoxia-induced ATP reductions in respiring cerebrocortical slices. Anesthesiology 1999;90:1392–1401.

166. Coeroli L, Renolleau S, Arnaud S, et al: Nitric oxide production and perivascular tyrosine nitration following focal ischemia in neonatal rat. J Neurochem 1998;70:2516–2525.

167. Marks KA, Mallard CE, Roberts I, et al: Nitric oxide synthase inhibition attenuates delayed vasodilation and increases injury after cerebral ischemia in fetal sheep. Pediatr Res 1996;40:185–191.

168. Groenendaal F, de Graaf RA, van Vliet G, et al: Effects of hypoxia-ischemia and inhibition of nitric oxide synthase on cerebral energy metabolism in newborn piglets. Pediatr Res 1999;45:827–833.

169. Blumberg RM, Taylor DL, Yue X, et al: Increased nitric oxide synthesis is not involved in delayed cerebral energy failure following focal hypoxic-ischemic injury to the developing brain. Pediatr Res 1999;46:224–231.

170. Huie RE, Padmaja S: The reaction of no with superoxide. Free Radic Res Commun 1993;18:195–199.

171. Murphy MP: Nitric oxide and cell death. Biochim Biophys Acta 1999; 1411:401–414.

172. Cao X, Phillis JW: alpha-Phenyl-tert-butyl-nitrone reduces cortical infarct and edema in rats subjected to focal ischemia. Brain Res 1994;644:267–272.

173. Zhao Q, Pahlmark K, Smith ML, et al: Delayed treatment with the spin trap alpha-phenyl-N-tert-butyl nitrone (PBN) reduces infarct size following transient middle cerebral artery occlusion in rats. Acta Physiol Scand 1994;152:349–350.

174. Iadecola C: Regulation of the cerebral microcirculation during neural activity: is nitric oxide the missing link? Trends Neurosci 1993;16:206–214.

175. Bolotina VM, Najibi S, Palacino JJ, et al: Nitric oxide directly activates calcium-dependent potassium channels in vascular smooth muscle. Nature 1994;368:850–853.

176. Kubes P: Nitric oxide affects microvascular permeability in the intact and inflamed vasculature. Microcirculation 1995;2:235–244.

177. Lei SZ, Pan ZH, Aggarwal SK, et al: Effect of nitric oxide production on

the redox modulatory site of the NMDA receptor-channel complex. Neuron 1992;8:1087–1099.

178. Wink DA, Hanbauer I, Krishna MC, et al: Nitric oxide protects against cellular damage and cytotoxicity from reactive oxygen species. Proc Natl Acad Sci USA 1993;90:9813–9817.

179. Fullerton HJ, Ditelberg JS, Chen SF, et al: Copper/zinc superoxide dismutase transgenic brain accumulates hydrogen peroxide after perinatal hypoxia ischemia. Ann Neurol 1998;44:357–364.

180. Higuchi Y, Hattori H, Kume T, et al: Increase in nitric oxide in the hypoxic-ischemic neonatal rat brain and suppression by 7-nitroindazole and aminoguanidine. Eur J Pharmacol 1998;342:47–49.

181. Cai Z, Hutchins JB, Rhodes PG: Intrauterine hypoxia-ischemia alters nitric oxide synthase expression and activity in fetal and neonatal rat brains. Brain Res Dev Brain Res 1998;109:265–269.

182. Wink DA, Mitchell JB: Chemical biology of nitric oxide: insights into regulatory, cytotoxic, and cytoprotective mechanisms of nitric oxide. Free Radic Biol Med 1998;25:434–456.

183. Ivacko JA, Sun R, Silverstein FS: Hypoxic-ischemic brain injury induces an acute microglial reaction in perinatal rats. Pediatr Res 1996;39:39–47.

184. Ditelberg JS, Sheldon RA, Epstein CJ, et al: Brain injury after perinatal hypoxia-ischemia is exacerbated in copper/zinc superoxide dismutase transgenic mice. Pediatr Res 1996;39:204–208.

185. Gidday JM, Shah AR, Maceren RG, et al: Nitric oxide mediates cerebral ischemic tolerance in a neonatal rat model of hypoxic preconditioning. J Cereb Blood Flow Metab 1999;19:331–340.

186. Bredt DS: NO NMDA receptor activity. Nat Biotechnol 1996;14:944.

CHAPTER 9

Free Radical-Mediated Processes

Ola Didrik Saugstad

Introduction

The Oxygen Paradox

Tissue injury may be aggravated when oxygen is administered following a significant period of hypoxia. This phenomenon is known as the "oxygen paradox," a term introduced by Ruff and Strughold in 1939 (according to Latham, 1951[1]). In 1954, Gerschman and co-workers proposed that oxygen is toxic because it generates oxygen free radicals.[2] This so-called oxygen radical hypothesis was an immense leap forward and paved the way for a more thorough understanding of the mechanisms involved in the oxygen paradox.

In 1968, McCord and Fridovich described superoxide dismutase, an important enzyme to detoxify superoxide radicals.[3] They also studied the free radical-generating system xanthine-xanthine oxidase, and showed that the amount of oxygen radicals produced in this system is dependent on both the oxygen and xanthine concentration present.[4] Since the 1960s, other studies have shown that hypoxanthine, the precursor of xanthine, accumulates during experimentally induced hypoxia[5–9] and following clinical intrauterine asphyxia.[10] A significant increase in the concentration of this metabolite during reperfusion in a canine *E. coli* sepsis model has also been reported.[11] Subsequently, it was suggested that one explanation of the "oxygen paradox" might be that, during reoxygenation, accumulated hypoxanthine was oxidized to uric acid with a simultaneous burst in oxygen radical production.[12] Other investigators quickly grasped this point and developed the hypothesis further.[13–15]

A number of metabolites in addition to hypoxanthine may play a

This work was supported by the Norwegian Council for Research, The Laerdal Foundation for Acute Medicine, The Norwegian Council on Cardiovascular Research, The Norwegian Women's Public Health Association, The Anders Jahres Research Foundation, and The Norwegian SIDS Society.

From Donn SM, Sinha SK, Chiswick ML (eds): *Birth Asphyxia and the Brain: Basic Science and Clinical Implications.* © 2002, Futura Publishing Co., Inc., Armonk, NY.

pivotal role in hypoxia-reoxygenation injury, or in ischemia-reperfusion injury. Accumulation of activated phagocytes in such a process contributes to free radical production as well. Recent interest has focused on the role of nitric oxide (NO) under such conditions, as well as its interrelationship between excitatory amino acids and production of toxic peroxynitrite radicals. There seems to be a close but complex relationship between free radicals, activated phagocytes, adhesion molecules, and activation of microglial cells in the brain. In addition, free radicals appear to be important regulators for growth and development as second messengers and for signal transduction.

Generation of Free Radicals

Free radicals are molecules or atoms of independent existence that contain one or more unpaired electrons in the outer electron shell. These are sometimes highly reactive with an extremely short half-life, interacting with other compounds and thus initiating chain reactions. Radicals can be formed by the loss of a single electron or by the gain of a single electron from a nonradical.[16] Although a number of free radicals exist, much interest has been focused on the oxygen radical species. Oxygen itself is essentially nonreactive; however, during normal metabolism aerobic cells produce a variety of very reactive O_2 intermediate by-products of metabolism, especially via the mitochondrial respiratory chain of enzymes and the P-450 system. These reactive oxygen species are potentially extremely cytotoxic because they have the ability to interact with and alter the principal components of the cells, including proteins, lipids, carbohydrates, and even DNA.

The major reactive oxygen species that can produce these cytotoxic effects include superoxide radical, hydrogen peroxide (which, strictly speaking, is not a free radical), hydroxyl radical, and singlet oxygen. Mitochondrial respiration is the major physiologic source for generation of reactive oxygen species. For every four electrons fed into the cytochrome oxidase complex, a molecule of oxygen is reduced to two molecules of water. Cytochrome oxidase itself releases no detectable oxygen radicals into free solutions, but several partially reduced oxygen intermediates have been identified bound to the cytochrome oxidase complex. Components other than cytochrome oxidase leak a few electrons onto oxygen before passing them to the next component in the respiratory chain. A small part of the oxygen consumed in the mitochondria is therefore partially reduced by electrons, which leak from electron carriers in the respiratory chain of healthy, intact mitochondria. Two distinct sites of leakage have been identified: ubisemiquinone, and nicotinamide adenine dinucleotide phosphate (NADPH) dehydrogenase. Because of such electron leakage, instead of accepting four electrons (e^-) simultaneously, oxygen is reduced stepwise by accepting one electron at a time. Reactive oxygen species are formed as intermediates:

$$O_2 + e^- \rightarrow O_2^- \text{ (superoxide radical)} \tag{1}$$
$$O_2^- + e^- \rightarrow H_2O_2 \text{ (hydrogen peroxide)} \tag{2}$$
$$H_2O_2 + e^- \rightarrow OH^- \text{ (hydroxyl radical)} \tag{3}$$
$$OH^- + e^- \rightarrow H_2O \text{ (water)} \tag{4}$$

In a reduced state, as in hypoxia-ischemia when the adenine nucleotide pool is partially degraded, the percentage of electron leakage is increased. Therefore, during reoxygenation relatively more oxygen radicals are produced compared with the normal resting situation. In addition, more superoxide dismutase is lost.[17]

Free Radicals, Iron, and Other Transition Metals

Transition metals such as iron, copper, chromium, molybdenum, cobalt, manganese, nickel, and vanadium contain unpaired electrons and, therefore, fulfill criteria for free radicals. Copper, however, does not strictly qualify as a free radical, but by forming Cu^{2+} it loses two electrons, leaving an unpaired electron.

Iron is the most abundant transition metal in humans. It catalyzes the reaction between superoxide anion and hydrogen peroxide so that the toxic hydroxyl radical is formed. In 1884, Fenton (according to Simic and Taylor[18]) oxidized organic molecules by ferrous-hydrogen peroxide mixtures. In 1932, Haber and Weiss provided an explanation of the process, which is another source of an intermediate reactive oxygen species:

$$H_2O_2 + Fe^{2+} \rightarrow OH^- + OH^- + Fe^{3+} \tag{5}$$

This is the so-called Haber-Weiss reaction; the mixture of H_2O_2 and divalent iron is the Fenton reagent. This entire hydroxyl radical-generating process is known as the Fenton-Haber-Weiss process. Ferric ion (Fe^{3+}) is rapidly reduced by ascorbate producing ferrous ion and ascorbate radical. The latter has a low redox potential and can reduce a number of oxidants. This might be of special interest during birth, since ascorbic acid (vitamin C) concentrations are high at birth and decline rapidly thereafter.[19,20] The recycling to ferrous ion (Fe^{2+}) by ascorbate has been of interest because even low levels of ferrous ion may perpetuate the process of free radical formation. Free iron has been detected in birth asphyxia, especially in preterm deliveries (see below).[21,22] These two components, vitamin C and free iron, might substantially add to the oxidative stress during birth asphyxia.

The plasma proteins apotransferrin and ceruloplasmin have strong antioxidant activities. The antioxidative activity of apotransferrin depends on its ability to bind two ferric ions, and ceruloplasmin is a potent antioxidant by facilitating binding of iron to transferrin. The antioxidant capacity of these two proteins in brain homogenate is 200–300-fold that of α-tocopherol (vitamin E).[23,24] Nonprotein-bound iron is not normally present in plasma because any free ferrous present is oxidized to ferric ion by the ferroxidase activity of ceruloplasmin and rigorously bound to transferrin. Low levels of these proteins in newborns, especially premature infants, decrease their transferrin iron-binding and ferroxidase antioxidant capacities, and nonprotein-bound iron can be detected in plasma, i.e., after asphyxia.[21,22] The superoxide radical produced by both activated leukocytes and xanthine oxidase, especially during aerobic conditions *per se,* releases iron from ferritin.[25,26] Thus, a vicious cycle might be established with increased lipid peroxidation. Hydroxyl radicals produced by the release of iron during oxidative stress damage erythrocyte membranes. This mechanism is thought to play a key role in red cell aging.[27]

Other Free Radical-Generating Systems

Oxygen free radicals are also produced by enzymatic systems such as (hypo) xanthine-xanthine oxidase, as well as the P-450 system, oxidation of arachidonic acid and catecholamines, together with a number of other systems. Nitric oxide (NO) is a free radical that may react with superoxide radical (O_2^-) to form the toxic peroxynitrite radical ($ONOO^-$).

$$NO + O_2^- \rightarrow ONOO^- \tag{6}$$

Activated phagocytes also produce oxygen free radicals during the respiratory burst as an important part of the defense against microorganisms.[28] In fact, *in vivo* activated neutrophils are important inducers of the Fenton reaction. Phagocytic cells mediate their antimicrobial functions by the release of mediators such as lysozymes, peroxidases, and proteases, in addition to oxygen radicals and NO.

$$NADPH + 2O_2 \rightarrow H^+ + 2O_2^- \tag{7}$$

In human neutrophils and monocytes, hydroxyl radical formation is iron dependent, since it decreases in iron deficiency and increases during iron supplementation.[29]

Hypochlorous acid is a strong oxidant and is generated during the respiratory burst by the reaction of hydrogen peroxide with myeloperoxidase. By reacting with ferrocyanide hydroxyl, radicals are generated three orders of magnitude faster than the Fenton reaction involving hydrogen peroxide.[30,31] There is reason to suggest that hypochlorous acid generated by activated phagocytes may be a source of hydroxyl radicals. Hypochlorous acid (HOCl) might also react with hydrogen peroxide to form singlet oxygen (O_2^*).

$$HOCl + H_2O_2 \rightarrow O_2^* + H^+ + H_2O + Cl^- \tag{8}$$

Defense Against Free Radicals

Mammalian organisms have developed a series of different systems to defend themselves against oxygen toxicity. When the oxygen concentration in the atmosphere increased some 2 billion years ago, blue-green algae developed superoxide dismutase-like enzymes as protection against superoxide radicals. This represents one of the most important leaps in the evolutionary process enabling living organisms to exist in an oxygen-enriched atmosphere. In the plant kingdom, there was an absolute need for efficient protection against oxidative stress because of the fact that chlorophyll is in close contact with oxygen. Therefore, a rich variety of antioxidants has been developed in fruit and vegetables.

There are different mechanisms of biochemical protection against free radicals, including: scavengers (mannitol or DMSO); repair agents; reduced glutathione; antioxidants (vitamin C or uric acid); and antioxidant enzymes (glutathione peroxidase, catalase, and superoxide dismutases). Table 1 provides some examples of protective mechanisms. There are both intracellular and extracellular antioxidative defense systems.

Intracellular Defenses

Antioxidant enzymes such as superoxide dismutases, catalases, and glutathione peroxidases, together with glutathione constitute important parts of the intracellular defense. Superoxide radical, which induces

Table 1

Protection Against Free Radicals

Scavengers (S)	$S + OH^- \rightarrow S^- + H_2O$
Repair agents	$GSH + {}^-CH_3 \rightarrow GS^- + CH_4$
Antioxyenzymes	
Catalase	$2 H_2O_2 \rightarrow O_2 + H_2O$
Glutathione peroxidase	$ROOH + 2GSH \rightarrow ROH + H_2O + GSSG$
Superoxide dismutase	$2O_2^- + 2H^+ \rightarrow H_2O_2$
Antioxidants (A)	$ROO^- + A\text{-}OH \rightarrow ROOH + AR\text{-}O^-$

lipid peroxidation of unsaturated fatty acids in cell membranes, is transformed to hydrogen peroxide and molecular oxygen by superoxide dismutase. Hydrogen peroxide oxidizes proteins and is inactivated by catalase and glutathione peroxidase. Peroxyl radicals, also inactivated by glutathione peroxidase, may depolymerize polysaccharides. Singlet oxygen, which may attack nucleic acids by base hydroxylation, DNA strand scission and cross-linkage, is scavenged by β-carotene.

Glutathione is a substrate for glutathione peroxidase, which removes hydrogen peroxide and scavenges hydroxyl radicals and singlet oxygen. Its reduced form, GSH, is oxidized to GSSG, which results in the reduction of hydrogen peroxide to water. Glutathione reductase catalyzes the reductions of GSSG to GSH, leading to the oxidation of NADPH to NADP$^+$. The ratio of GSH/GSSG in normal cells is kept high and declines in oxidative stress. This ratio is a good indicator for oxidative stress *in vivo*.

Development of the Intracellular Defense Systems

In utero, the fetus is essentially protected from possible toxic effects of oxygen, although oxidative stress probably is present in several conditions (e.g., inflammation). However, immediately after birth the newborn will encounter a more oxygen-enriched atmosphere with a four- to fivefold increase in Pao$_2$. To meet this challenge, a maturation of the antioxidative defense systems in the lungs occurs. In different species (e.g., rabbit, guinea pig, rat, hamster, and sheep), an increase of 300–700% in the activities of superoxide dismutase, catalase, and glutathione peroxidase was found during the latter 15–20% of the gestational period. There are accumulating data showing that a similar maturation also occurs in humans, and that the maturational process occurs during approximately the latter 40% of gestation.[32]

This implies that preterm infants are born with a lowered antioxidant defense compared to term infants. Further, term animals are better able to effect increased activities of antioxidative enzymes of the lung after 48 hours of exposure to hyperoxia. Studies in rat pups have shown that prenatal administration of glucocorticoids accelerates the normal maturational pattern not only of the surfactant system, but also of antioxidant enzymes in the lung. By contrast, prenatal treatment with either thyroid hormone or thyroid-releasing hormone depresses the normal maturation of these systems despite their maturational effects on the surfactant system.[32] Preterm infants have a lower concentration, and also a lowered synthesis, of glutathione compared to term infants.[33,34]

Extracellular Defenses

In contrast to the intracellular defense system, the capacity of the extracellular antioxidant defense system seems to be similar in preterm and term infants. At birth, the oxidative defense in extracellular fluids is the same as in adults, but gradually decreases over 6 weeks. Total antioxidant capacity of extracellular fluid has been measured at 900 μmol/L in the newborn, decreasing to 600 μmol/L at 2 weeks. At 6 weeks, breast-fed infants have higher levels of antioxidants than formula-fed infants. The importance of the various components does, however, vary with postnatal age.

At birth, uric acid and vitamin C constitute most of the extracellular capacity, approximately 50% and 25%, respectively. At a postnatal age of 2 weeks, uric acid represents 30%, and vitamin C only 5%, of the capacity. Bilirubin now seems to be the most important extracellular antioxidant, constituting more than 30% of the total capacity, up from 6% at birth. Vitamin C, which is the most effective aqueous phase antioxidant *in vitro,* is higher in umbilical cord blood than in maternal blood but falls dramatically in the first 3 days of life and then gradually rises over the next 6 weeks.[19] Other important extracellular antioxidants are sulfhydryl groups. Glutathione does not seem to play an important role in plasma; however, in alveolar and tracheal lining fluid it is an important antioxidant with 100-fold higher concentration than in plasma.[35,36] It might be tempting to supplement infants exposed to increased oxidative stress with extracellular antioxidants. However, care should be exercised, since some antioxidants such as vitamin C may also act as a pro-oxidant in combination with iron.[37]

Thus, intracellular defense against free radicals is lower in fetal life, and as such is lower in the preterm compared to the term infant.

In contrast, the extracellular defenses of the preterm and term infant seem to be similar. The net consequence, however, is that oxidative stress, defined as an imbalance between oxidative and antioxidative forces, is elevated in the preterm infant.

Action of Free Radicals

It is well known that free radicals act on a number of cellular components: peroxidation of polyunsaturated fatty acids, resulting in disruption of the cellular membrane; protein oxidation, leading to inactivation of enzymes and other proteins; and depolymerization of carbohydrates. Free radicals also act on DNA by cross linkage and scission of DNA strands. Lubec recently summarized actions of oxygen radicals and specifically the hydroxyl radical.[38]

Lipid-Based Radicals

Lipid-based free radicals are formed when oxygen radicals attack polyunsaturated fatty acids in lipid components of the cell. Fatty acid molecules become less resistant to oxidative attack as the number of double bonds increases. Unsaturated fatty acids as linoleate, linolenate, and arachidonic acid produce free radicals by auto-oxidation. If oxygen reacts at either end position of these radicals a mixture of hydroperoxides is produced.[39]

Superoxide itself is insufficiently reactive to abstract hydrogen from lipids. Because of its charge, it is not expected to enter the interior of membranes, which are hydrophobic. The lipid peroxidation sequence of polyunsaturated fatty acids positioned in the cell membrane may, however, be initiated by an attack of a hydroxyl radical. A hydrogen atom is consequently abstracted from a methylene group ($^-CH_2^-$):

$$^-CH_2^- + OH^- \rightarrow \ ^-CH^- + H_2O \tag{9}$$

Extraction of a hydrogen atom leaves behind an unpaired electron on the methylene group. This carbon radical seems to stabilize by molecular rearrangements to form conjugated dienes. By combining with oxygen (oxygen is a hydrophobic molecule that concentrates into the interior of membranes), peroxyl radicals (CHO_2^-) are formed:

$$^-CH^- + O_2 \rightarrow CHO_2^- \tag{10}$$

Peroxyl radicals are capable of abstracting hydrogen atoms from other lipid molecules. When reacting with oxygen they form other peroxyl radicals, and thus a chain reaction of lipid peroxidation can continue. Generation of alkoxy radicals from hydroperoxides is similar to the Haber-Weiss reaction:

$$ROOH + Fe^{2+} \rightarrow RO^- + OH^- + Fe^{3+} \qquad (11)$$

In the presence of transition metals, lipid peroxidation is accelerated.

Vitamin E, which is fat-soluble, tends to concentrate in the interior of cell membranes and plays an important role by inhibiting this chain reaction; it is therefore designated as a chain breaker. This occurs by reacting with lipid radicals, and donating a hydrogen atom to them. Simultaneously, a stable and nonreactive tocopherol radical is generated, and the chain reaction is terminated. Vitamin C reduces the tocopherol radical to tocopherol. Vitamin E also quenches and reacts with singlet oxygen.[40]

Protein and DNA Damage

Protein damage induced by oxygen radicals as singlet oxygen or the hydroxyl radical results in a conformational change that also renders the proteins more susceptible to proteolysis by proteolytic enzymes, such as elastase. Hydroxyl radicals may also attack the proteins at specific sites, leading to specific protein fragments and oxidation products. Protein carbonylation is typically generated by the Fenton reaction with the presence of hydrogen peroxide and transition metal.[41]

The formation of 8-hydroxydesoxyguanosine reflects nonenzymatic hydroxyl radical attack on DNA. Hydroxyl radical-induced DNA damage causes selective base substitution, since the four bases have different susceptibility to hydroxyl radical-induced mutations. Oncogene activation may therefore be one potential mechanism by which hydroxyl radicals contribute to carcinogenesis.[42]

Role of Nitric Oxide as a Free Radical

Nitric oxide is a free radical which, in combination with superoxide radical, forms the toxic peroxynitrite molecule.[43,44] It therefore is interesting that N-nitro-L-arginine methyl ester (L-NAME), an inhibitor of NO synthesis, increases lipid peroxidation in rat liver following ischemia-reperfusion.[45]

In hypoxia and reoxygenation, excitatory amino acids (i.e., glutamate) are released from the pre-synaptic membrane, activating the N-methyl-D-aspartate (NMDA) receptors in the post-synaptic membrane of the neurons. The increased influx of calcium into the neurons induces a number of enzymes such as NO synthetase, leading to increased NO production in the reoxygenation period, with a simultaneous formation of superoxide radicals. If these come into contact with NO, toxic peroxynitrite might be formed.[43,44] Peroxynitrite, which is a powerful oxidant, is stable in alkaline solutions. Although peroxynitrite is not truly a free radical, Beckman et al have shown that in physiologic conditions peroxynitrite (ONOO$^-$) initiates many reactions, which implies production of toxic hydroxyl radicals and nitrogen dioxide (NO$_2$).[43]

$$ONOO^- + H^+ \rightarrow OH^- + NO_2^- \qquad (12)$$

Peroxynitrite is far more toxic and can diffuse 10,000 times further than the hydroxyl radical.[46]

Free Radicals and Apoptosis

Free radicals also play an important role in apoptosis and necrosis (see Chapter 7).[47–49] Following hypoxia, both apoptopic and necrotic cells are found in the brain. Human infants who have suffered secondary energy failure have a preponderance of necrotic cells, while those dying *in utero* show a high proportion of apoptopic cells.[50] Further, apoptotic cells are found in brains following hypoxia-ischemia in newborn piglets and immature rats.[51,52] Necrosis can occur during hypoxia-reoxygenation or during ischemia. The acute oxygen deficiency may lead to a rapid reduction in mitochondrial energy production, and consequently, necrotic cell death. These acute changes may be associated with an increase in both free radical production and an increase in excitotoxic amino acids. In contrast, apoptosis requires time as well as energy, and does not involve an inflammatory reaction. This mode of cell death is therefore particularly beneficial in the brain, which has only limited capacity for repair.[53]

Whether a cell dies of apoptosis or necrosis following hypoxia-reoxygenation is probably dependent on a number of factors, such as the duration and degree of the hypoxic insult and the maturational level of the cells involved. It is clear that apoptosis can be induced by reactive oxygen species.[49,53,54] Decreased superoxide dismutase activity in neuronal cells induces, and antioxidants inhibit, apoptosis. Bcl-2 is a mitochondrial membrane protein that blocks apoptosis. One effect of Bcl-2 is to inhibit free radical formation.[47] Overexpression of Bcl-xL, a key regulator of apoptosis with similarities to Bcl-2, protects astrocytes from oxidative injury.[55]

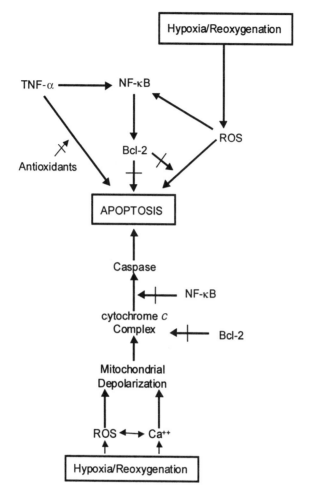

Figure 1. Hypoxia-reoxygenation and apoptosis. Hypoxia-reoxygenation or ischemia-reperfusion may induce both necrosis and apoptosis. Reactive oxygen species (ROS) are produced in the reoxygenation period. Simultaneously, excitatory amino acids are released pre-synaptically, activating NMDA and metabotropic post-synaptic receptors and inducing influx as well as intracellular release of calcium. Both ROS and calcium depolarize the mitochondria, inducing release of cytochrome *c* complex. This activates caspase-9, which activates caspase-3. Tumor necrosis factor-α (TNF-α) may activate caspase-8, which also activates caspase-3. Caspase-3 activation infers DNA fragmentation and apoptosis. ROS as well as TNF-α may induce apoptosis directly. This latter substance also may have an antiapoptotic action by inducing nuclear factor-κB (NF-κB), which induces Bcl-2. Bcl-2 is a powerful anti-apoptotic agent as well as an antioxidant. Antioxidants may block apoptosis at a number of levels indicating novel potential strategies to prevent apoptosis.

There is a complex interrelation between hypoxia-reoxygenation, oxygen radicals, neuronal excitatory processes, inflammation, and apoptosis. For example, NO may induce apoptosis through excessive stimulation of neurotransmitter release by activation of NMDA receptors, and also via activation of caspases.[56] Antioxidants may prevent apoptosis by inhibition at a number of levels, and other new potential therapeutic strategies are possible in hypoxia-reoxygenation, such as inhibition of caspase activation (Figure 1).

Reactive Oxygen Species and Physiologic Processes

Oxygen radicals are not only toxic but also play a role in regulating physiologic processes. It is well known that oxygen radical-generating systems have profound vasoactive effects.[57,58] Oxygen radical-generating systems such as hypoxanthine-xanthine oxidase induce both vasoconstriction and vasodilation, probably depending on the organ and the dose used. For instance, this system potently dilates isolated fetal lamb ductal rings via synthesis of prostaglandin E_2,[59] and constricts the intact pulmonary circulation of pigs.[60,61] For this reason, it is suggested that reactive oxygen species play a role in regulating the perinatal circulation.

Free Radicals as Second Messengers and in Signal Transduction

It has recently become clear that redox-dependent reactions have proven to be important in regulating numerous processes that determine the physiologic and pathophysiologic function of cells and tissues.[62] Oxygen radicals, as well as reactive species derived from NO, serve as intracellular messengers that drive signal transduction. It is also well established that the free radical NO acts as a second messenger for biologic processes such as smooth muscle relaxation, neurotransmission, platelet inhibition, and immune regulation. A number of ligand receptor interactions produce reactive oxygen species, which in turn elicit signaling by targeting some signal transduction component molecules. It has been hypothesised that oxidants serve as physiologic messengers for receptor-mediated cell signaling.

Among ligands utilizing reactive oxygen species as second messengers are tumor necrosis factor-α (TNF-α), interleukin-1β (IL-1β), transforming growth factor-β1 (TGF-1β), platelet-derived factor, insulin, angiotensin II, vitamin D_3, and parathyroid hormone. TNF-α and other cytokines may produce an oxidative stress response. TNF-α activates both AP-1 (controls expression of cell growth mediators) and nuclear factor-κB ([NF-κB] activated by several cytokines and prevents neuronal apoptosis; controls cytokines, chemokines, and cell adhesion molecules). The ability of TNF-α to kill tumor cells has been inhibited by antioxidants. Bcl-2 protects cells from TNF-α-induced apoptosis (Figure 1). Reactive oxygen species also have the ability to modulate the activity of transcription factors such as AP-1 and NF-κB. Induction of AP-1-binding activity is regulated by intracellular glutathione levels, and is associated with hydroxyl radical generation.[63–65]

Antioxidants also induce various biologic processes, such as gene expression, by stimulating signal transduction and protein phosphorylation. Reactive oxygen species such as superoxide anion, hydrogen peroxide, hydroxyl radical, and lipid hydroperoxides play a role in signal transduction, stimulating Ca^{2+} signaling by increasing cytosolic Ca^{2+} concentration. The oxygen radical-generating system hypoxanthine-xanthine oxidase enhances release of inositol triphosphate from sarcoplasmic reticulum of different cell types. Also, linoleic acid hydroperoxide has a similar effect on aortic endothelial cells. Phospholipase A_2 (PLA_2) is activated by oxidants and acts as a rate-determining step in eicosanoid synthesis. The products of PLA_2 are mediators of inflammatory processes and immune responses, and NADPH oxidase activation.

In addition to the stimulation of signal transduction, it is postulated that reactive oxygen species may be second messengers for transcription factor activation, apoptosis, bone resorption, cell growth, and chemotaxis. The hydroxyl radical also plays a role in viral replication, since scavengers of this oxygen free radical inhibited HIV-1 replication in monocyte-derived phagocytes.[66] Oxidative stress may therefore influence growth and development in ways not yet completely understood.[62]

Inflammation and Oxidative Stress

There is a close relationship between inflammation and oxidative stress (see Chapter 4). Hypoxia-ischemia followed by reoxygenation induces inflammatory responses by activating pro-inflammatory cytokines such as IL-1β and TNF-α, as well as a number of inflammatory proteins. This is followed by invasion of neutrophils. It is well known that neutrophils become activated during ischemia-reperfusion. This leads to increased adhesiveness to the endothelium and release of reactive oxygen species and proteases. Inflammatory mediators can stimulate endothelium to produce the adhesion molecule E-selectin, which is a slow process over approximately an hour, or P-selectin, which is a fast process within minutes. Simultaneously activated neutrophils express L-selectin. The interaction between E-selectin with L- and P-selectin results in rolling and initial binding of the neutrophil to the endothelial surface. Interaction of neutrophil CD18 molecules with endothelial intracellular adhesion molecule-1 (ICAM-1) is responsible for the firm attachment of the neutrophil to the endothelium, eventually leading to transendothelial migration.[67-70] Hydrogen peroxide promotes endothelial adhesion via induction of adhesion molecule ICAM-1 gene expression,[71] a process which might involve inducible NO synthase.[72]

Toxic oxygen metabolites and proteases produced in neutrophils are released into a microenvironment, which is protected from naturally occurring antioxidants and antiproteases in plasma; thus, the antioxidant defense in this compartment is low. Activated mononuclear cells produce IL-1 and TNF-α, increasing the permeability of the blood-brain barrier and facilitating the passage of cytokines into the brain. IL-1 and TNF-α production is also induced by excitotoxins. TNF-α is capable of inducing oligodendrocyte damage; this is the cell responsible for deposition of myelin.[73] Microglia are also stimulated and activate proliferation of astroglia.

Generation of Oxygen Free Radicals During Hypoxia-Reoxygenation and Ischemia-Reperfusion

One important advance in the understanding of the relationship between free radicals and hypoxia was the observation that hypoxanthine accumulated during hypoxemia,[5-8,11] coupled with McCord and Fridovich's observation that xanthine/xanthine oxidase (XO) produced oxygen free radicals.[3,4] It was obvious that a burst of free radicals could be produced during reoxygenation.

$$\text{Hypoxanthine} + O_2 \xrightarrow{\text{XO}} \text{uric acid} + O_2^- \qquad (13)$$

The existence of a positive relationship between the hypoxanthine and oxygen concentration, and oxygen free radical production, was a logical assumption.[12] This had in fact been shown in *in vitro* studies.[4] This hypothesis became very popular and it was tested not only in intrapartum asphyxia, but also in conditions such as cardiac arrest, myocardial ischemia, and organ transplantation. One critical prerequisite for this hypothesis is the presence of xanthine oxidase in tissues. Much confusion arose, however, because several investigators were unaware of the vast difference in xanthine oxidase distribution between organs and more importantly between species. Xanthine oxidase in humans is restricted to a few organs such as the liver and intestine. It was postulated that xanthine oxidase is released during hypoxemia and reoxygenation and circulated in a way that several organs could be attacked simultaneously.[10,74] It has now been established that this is indeed the case[75-78] and that xanthine oxidase is limited to a few tissues in man.[79] Increased levels of xanthine oxidase have been observed in the blood of sick premature infants.[80]

Zweier et al showed that xanthine oxidase is present in human aortic endothelial cells in culture. When these cells are subjected to anoxia and reoxygenation, electron paramagnetic resonance measurements, using a spin trap agent, show free radical generation. Accumulated hypoxanthine and xanthine oxidase is the primary source for this production. The oxygen radical production can be completely inhibited by superoxide dismutase, as well as with the iron chelator, deferoxamine.[81] Bågenholm et al found a twofold increase in the production of free radicals within 10–20 minutes of reperfusion following ischemia of the fetal sheep brain.[82] In 7-day-old rats, a combination of left carotid artery ligation and exposure to 8% oxygen for 70 minutes produced severe brain injury assessed by brain weight. Elevated lipid peroxidation products were found in the left hemisphere in the first 60 minutes after reoxygenation.[83]

It has also been shown that superoxide radicals are generated in the cerebral cortex in newborn pigs during asphyxia and re-ventilation.[84] In a further study in 1- to 5-day-old piglets, the same authors observed that the superoxide radical production occurred mainly during re-ventilation rather than during asphyxia. Both indomethacin and allopurinol prevented superoxide anion formation.[85]

Dorrepaal et al measured nonprotein-bound and lipid peroxidation by iron and thiobarbituric acid reactive species in asphyxiated and nonasphyxiated newborn infants. Nonprotein-bound iron was present in severe asphyxia and was the most significant variable for neurodevelopmental outcome at 1 year of age. There was also increased oxidative lipid damage in asphyxiated infants.[21] Buonocore et al recently showed that free iron in erythrocytes correlated very well with the degree of asphyxia assessed by plasma hypoxanthine levels. Thus, post-asphyxial oxygen radical production results from both activation of the hypoxanthine-xanthine oxidase system and increased free iron production.[22]

The evidence that oxygen free radicals play a role in brain injury is rapidly accumulating. Ment et al observed a decreased incidence of intraventricular hemorrhage in newborn beagle puppies treated with superoxide dismutase.[86] Palmer et al were able to show that allopurinol attenuates ischemic brain injury in newborn rats,[87] while Van Bel et al observed a protective effect of this compound on post-asphyxial free radical formation, electrical brain activity, and cerebral blood flow in newborn infants.[88] It is unclear whether this effect was mediated via allopurinol action as a xanthine oxidase inhibitor, or as an antioxidant *per se*.

It is not known whether superoxide dismutase alone reduces brain injury. Hydrogen peroxide accumulates after hypoxia-ischemia in the brain of copper-zinc superoxide dismutase (CuZn-SOD) transgenic mice, and brain injury is exacerbated in such mice.[89] On the other hand, hippocampal injury was reduced after global ischemia in CuZn-SOD transgenic mice.[90] The reason elevated activities of superoxide dismuaste may increase injury might be the fact that more hydrogen peroxide is formed. If the catalase activity is limited, the stage might be set for increased injury. However, other factors such as microvascular effects in this model might be important, since it has also been shown that CuZn-SOD transgenic mice are highly resistant to reperfusion injury after focal cerebral ischemia.[91]

Leukocytes may accumulate during hypoxemia and reoxygenation and are possible mediators of increased oxygen radical production. Cytokines mediate adherence to endothelium and influx of inflammatory cells into reperfused tissue. By blocking the neutrophil adhesion to endothelium, protection against reperfusion has been observed. Further, neutrophil accumulation in ischemic tissue is prevented by allopurinol.[92–94]

Therapeutic Considerations

The increasing evidence indicating the significance of free radicals in hypoxia-reoxygenation or ischemia-reperfusion may lead to the development of new therapeutic strategies.

Resuscitation with Room Air or 100% Oxygen

To reduce the production of oxygen radicals during post-hypoxic reoxygenation, it was suggested that resuscitation be performed with oxygen concentrations less than 100%. In subsequent animal studies, it was shown that room air resuscitation is as efficient as 100% oxygen for resuscitation.[95–97] Further, leukocytes isolated from the sagittal sinus of piglets following post-hypoxic resuscitation showed an increased production of hydrogen peroxide when resuscitation was performed with 100% oxygen compared to room air.[98] Although resuscitation can be performed efficiently with oxygen concentrations of 15– 16%, when the oxygen concentration is lower than this the metabolic acidosis and other biochemical and electrophysiologic measures deteriorate even further.[99,100] Recent data on the resuscitation of newborn piglets indicate that the recovery of the brain microcirculation is slower in room air compared to 100% oxygen; however, the recovery of the microcirculation is enhanced in the presence of hypercapnia.

Three clinical studies have demonstrated the efficacy of room air resuscitation compared to 100% oxygen.[101–103] One major finding in these studies is that the time to establish spontaneous breathing is significantly delayed by 0.5–1.5 minutes in infants resuscitated with 100% oxygen compared to room air.[102,103] Resuscitation with 100% oxygen seems to inhibit the ventilatory drive in the newborn. Vento et al[103] observed higher plasma lipid peroxidation products and DNA oxidation products as long as 30 days after resuscitation in 100% oxygen compared to room air. It is extraordinary that such changes are seen at this age, and this might suggest that even a brief exposure to high oxygen concentration may induce long-term effects on DNA. All of these aspects, including the effects on the microcirculation, must be studied further before any new resuscitation regimen with room air is introduced. More studies are needed before firm conclusions can be drawn concerning the safety of room air resuscitation in a range of clinical circumstances, and also regarding the potential long-term adverse effects of using high oxygen concentrations.

The situation is probably more complex than it appears. For example, it was found that room air reoxygenation attenuated NO production compared to 100% oxygen.[104] This, therefore, might be an effective means of reducing NO concentration in the brain during resuscitation. On the other hand, inhaled NO reduces recruitment of neutrophils in the lung[105] and has been shown to be a possible antioxidant in low concentrations.[106]

Antioxidants and Inflammatory Modulators

In several animal studies, different antioxidants in combination, or combined with other agents such as iron chelators, have been tested.[107,108] In a recent study of newborn lambs with hypoxic-ischemic encephalopathy, it was shown that allopurinol, indomethacin, and catalase had protective properties. However, no synergistic effect was gained by combining these agents.[109]

Perhaps in the future, antioxidants in combination with inflammatory modulators may be used. One problem is that, during the acute resuscitation procedure, the time might be too short to enable intervention. Administration of antioxidants antenatally or during labor is one possible solution. In one rat study, antenatal vitamin E successfully protected the animals from intrapartum asphyxia.[110] On the other hand, if it is correct that resuscitation with oxygen leads to long-lasting biochemical changes, a therapeutic window might be present, perhaps allowing for intervention with antioxidant therapy even after completion of acute resuscitation.

Conclusion

Intrapartum asphyxia and resuscitation are conditions in which a burst of free radicals may be produced. Free radicals are potentially damaging not only because of their acute effects on lipids, proteins, carbohydrates, and DNA, but also because they may induce both necrosis and apoptosis. Long-lasting effects on growth and development may also occur, since oxygen radicals act as signal transducers and second messengers. Therefore, it is highly important to elucidate these mechanisms in order to develop sensible strategies to eliminate the short- and long-term harmful effects of oxygen radicals.

References

1. Latham F: The oxygen paradox. Experiments on the effects of oxygen in human anoxia. Lancet 1951;1:77–81.
2. Gerschman R, Gilbert DL, Nyl SW, et al: Oxygen poisoning and X-ray irradiation: a mechanism in common. Science 1954;119:624–626.
3. McCord JM, Fridovich I: The reduction of cytochrome C by milk xanthine oxidase. J Biol Chem 1968;243:5753–5765.
4. Fridovich I: Quantitative aspects of the production of superoxide anion radical by milk xanthine oxidase. J Biol Chem 1970;245:4053–4057.
5. Berne RM: Cardiac nucleotides in hypoxia: possible role in regulation of coronary blood flow. Am J Physiol 1963;204:317–322.
6. Gerlach E, Deuticke B, Dreisbach RH: Zum verhalten von Nucleotiden und ihren dephosphorylierten Abbauprodukten in der Niere bei Ischemie und kurzzeitiger postischemischer Wiederdurchblutung. Pflugers Arch 1963; 278:296–315.
7. Saugstad OD: Hypoxanthine as a measurement of hypoxia. Pediatr Res 1975;9:158–161.

8. Saugstad OD, Østrem T: Hypoxanthine and urate levels of plasma during and after hemorrhagic hypotension in dogs. Eur Surg Res 1977;9:48–56.
9. Saugstad OD, Schrader H, Aasen AO: Alteration of the hypoxanthine levels in cerebrospinal fluid as an indicator of tissue hypoxia. Brain Res 1976;112:395–398.
10. Saugstad OD: Hypoxanthine as an indicator of hypoxia: its role in health and disease through free radical production. Pediatr Res 1988;23:143–150.
11. Saugstad OD, Aasen AO: Hypoxanthine in lethal canine endotoxin shock. Circ Shock 1979;6:277–283.
12. Saugstad OD, Aasen AO: Plasma hypoxanthine levels as a prognostic aid of tissue hypoxia. Eur Surg Res 1980;12:123–129.
13. Granger DN, Rutili G, McCord JM: Superoxide radicals in feline intestinal ischemia. Gastroenterology 1981;81:22–29.
14. Parks DA, Bulkley GB, Granger DN: Role of oxygen-derived radicals in shock, ischemia, and organ preservation. Surgery 1984;94:415–422.
15. McCord JM: Oxygen-derived free radicals in postischemic tissue injury. N Engl J Med 1985;312:354–364.
16. Halliwell B, Gutteridge JMC: Oxygen is poisonous: an introduction to oxygen toxicity and free radicals. In Halliwell B, Gutteridge JMC (eds): *Free Radicals in Biology and Medicine*. Clarendon Press, Oxford, 1989, pp 1–21.
17. McCord JM: Free radicals and myocardial ischemia: overview and outlook. Free Radic Biol Med 1988;4:9–14.
18. Simic MG, Taylor KA: Introduction to peroxidation and antioxidation mechanisms. In Simic MG, Taylor KA, Ward JF, von Sonntgag C (eds): *Oxygen Radicals in Biology and Medicine*. Plenum Press, New York, 1988, pp 1–10.
19. Van Zoeren-Grobben D, Lindeman JH, Houdkaamp E, et al: Postnatal changes in plasma chain-breaking antioxidants in healthy preterm infants fed formula and/or human milk. Am J Clin Nutr 1994;60:900–906.
20. Lindeman JH, Van Zoeren-Grobben D, Schrivjer J, et al: The total free radical trapping ability of cord blood plasma in preterm and term babies. Pediatr Res 1989;26:20–24.
21. Dorrepaal CA, Berger HM, Benders MJ, et al: Nonprotein-bound iron in postasphyxial reperfusion injury in the newborn. Pediatrics 1996;98:883–889.
22. Buonocore G, Zani S, Sargentini I, et al: Hypoxia-induced free iron release in the red cells of newborn infants. Acta Paediatr 1998;87:77–81.
23. Stocks J, Gutteridge JMC, Sharp RJ, et al: Assay using brain homogenate for measuring the antioxidant activity of biological fluids. Clin Sci Mol Med 1974;47:215–222.
24. Stocks J, Gutteridge JMC, Sharp J, et al: The inhibition of lipid autoxidation by human serum and its relation to serum proteins and alpha tocopherol. Clin Sci Mol Med 1974;47:223–233.
25. Biemond P, van Eijk HG, Swaak AJ, et al: Iron mobilization from ferritin by superoxide derived from stimulated polymorphonuclear leukocytes: possible mechanism in inflammation disease. J Clin Invest 1984;73:1576–1579.
26. Bolann BJ, Ulvik RJ: Release of iron from ferritin by xanthine oxidase: role of the superoxide radical. Biochem J 1987;243:55–59.
27. Bracci R, Buonocore G: The antioxidant status of erythrocytes in preterm and term infants. Semin Neonatol 1998;3:191–197.

28. Babior MB, Kipnes RS, Curnutte JT: Biological defense mechanisms: the production of superoxide: a potential bactericidal agent. J Clin Invest 1973;52:741–744.
29. Murakawara H, Bland CE, Willis WT, et al: Iron deficiency and neutrophil function: different rates of correction of the depressions in oxidative burst and myeloperoxidase activity after iron treatment. Blood 1987; 69:1464–1468.
30. Ramos CL, Pou S, Britigan BE, et al: Spin trapping evidence for myeloperoxidase-dependent hydroxyl radical formation by human neutrophils and monocytes. J Biol Chem 1992;267:8307–8312.
31. Candeias LP, Stratford MR, Wardman P: Formation of hydroxyl radicals on reaction of hypochlorous acid with ferrocyanide, a model iron (II) complex. Free Radic Res 1994;20:241–249.
32. Frank L: Development of the antioxidant defenses in fetal life. Semin Neonatol 1998;3:173–182.
33. Vina J, Vento M, Garcia-Sala F, et al: L-cysteine and glutathione metabolism are impaired in premature infants due to cystathionase deficiency. Am J Clin Nutr 1995;61:1067–1069.
34. Pallardo FV, Sastre J, Asensi M, et al: Physiological changes in glutathione metabolism in foetal and newborn rat liver. Biochem J 1991;274: 891–893.
35. Berger HM, Molicki JS, Moison RMW, et al: Extracellular defence against oxidative stress in the newborn. Semin Neonatol 1998;3:188–190.
36. Kelly FJ: Gluthathione: in defence of the lung. Food Chem Toxicol 1999; 37:963–966.
37. Almaas R, Rootwelt T, Øyasæter S, et al: Ascorbic acid enhances hydroxyl radical formation in iron-fortified infant cereals and infant formulas. Eur J Pediatr 1997;156:488–492.
38. Lubec G: The hydroxyl radical: from chemistry to human disease. J Invest Med 1996;44:324–346.
39. Halliwell B, Gutteridge JMC: Lipid peroxidation: a radical chain reaction. In Halliwell B, Gutteridge JMC (eds): *Free Radicals in Biology and Medicine*. Clarendon Press, Oxford, 1989, pp 189–276.
40. Packer JE, Slater TF, Wilson RL: Direct observation of a free radical interaction between vitamin E and C. Nature 1979;278:737–738.
41. Stadtman ER: Oxidation of free amino acids and amino acid residues in proteins by radiolysis and by metal-catalyzed reactions. Ann Rev Biochem 1993;62:797–821.
42. Jackson JH: Potential molecular mechanisms of oxidant-induced carcinogenesis. Eviron Health Perspect 1994;102:155–157.
43. Beckman JS, Beckman TW, Chen J, et al: Apparent hydroxyl radical production by peroxynitrite: implications for endothelial injury from nitric oxide and superoxide. Proc Natl Acad Sci USA 1990;87:1620–1624.
44. Beckman JS: The double-edged role of nitric oxide in brain function and superoxide-mediated injury. J Dev Physiol 1991;15:53–59.
45. Koken T, Inal M: The effect of nitric oxide on ischemia-reperfusion injury in rat liver. Clin Chim Acta 1999;288:55–62.
46. Beckman JS: Peroxynitrite versus hydroxyl radical: the role of nitric oxide in superoxide-dependent cerebral injury. Ann NY Acad Sci 1994;738:69–75.
47. Hockenbery DM, Oltvai ZN, Yin X-M, et al: Bcl-2 functions in an antioxidant pathway to prevent apoptosis. Cell 1993;75:241–251.

48. Malorni W, Rivabene R, Santini MT, et al: N-Acetylcysteine inhibits apoptosis and decreases viral particles in HIV-chronically infected U937 cells. FEBS Lett 1993;327:75–78.
49. Jacobson MD: Reactive oxygen species and programmed cell death. TIBS 1996;21:83–86.
50. Edwards AD, Yue X, Cox P, et al: Apoptosis in the brains of infants suffering intrauterine cerebral injury. Pediatr Res 1997;42:684–689.
51. Mehmet H, Yue X, Squier MV, et al: Increased apoptosis in the cingulate sulcus of newborn piglets following transient hypoxia-ischemia is related to the degree of high energy phosphate depletion during the insult. Neurosci Lett 1994;181:121–125.
52. Beilharz E, Williams CE, Dragunow M, et al: Mechanism of cell death following hypoxic-ischemic injury in the imature rat: evidence of apoptosis during selective neuronal loss. Mol Brain Res 1995;29:1–14.
53. Taylor DL, Edwards AD, Mehmet H: Oxidative metabolism, apoptosis and perinatal brain injury. Brain Pathol 1999;9:93–117.
54. Berger R, Garnier Y: Pathophysiology of perinatal brain damage. Brain Res Rev 1999;30:107–134.
55. Xu L, Koumenis IL, Tilly JL, et al: Overexpression of bcl-xL protects astrocytes from glucose deprivation and is associated with higher glutathione, ferritin, and iron levels. Anesthesiology 1999;91:1036–1046.
56. Leist M, Volbracht C, Kuhnle S, et al: Caspase-mediated apoptosis in neuronal excitotoxicity triggered by nitric oxide. Mol Med 1997;3:750–764.
57. Tate RM, Morris HG, Schroeder WR, et al: Oxygen metabolites stimulate thromboxane production and vasoconstriction in isolated saline-perfused rabbit lungs. J Clin Invest 1984;74:608–613.
58. Archer SL, Peterson D, Nelson DP, et al: Oxygen radicals and antioxidant enzymes alter pulmonary vascular reactivity in the rat lung. J Appl Physiol 1989;66:102–111.
59. Clyman RI, Saugstad OD, Mauray F: Reactive oxygen metabolites relax the lamb ductus arteriosus by stimulating prostaglandin production. Circ Res 1989;64:1–8.
60. Sanderud J, Norstein J, Saugstad OD: Reactive oxygen metabolites produce pulmonary vasoconstriction in pigs. Pediatr Res 1991;29:543–547.
61. Sanderud J, Bjøro K, Saugstad OD: Oxygen radicals stimulate thromboxane and prostacyclin synthesis and induce vasoconstriction in pig lungs. Scand J Clin Lab Invest 1993;53:447–455.
62. Suzuki YJ, Forman HJ, Sevanian A: Oxidants as stimulators of signal transduction. Free Radic Biol Med 1997;22:269–285.
63. Albrecht H, Tschopp J, Jongeneel CV: Bcl-2 protects from oxidative damage and apoptotic cell death without interfering with activation of NF-κB by TNF. FEBS Lett 1994;351:45–48.
64. Mattson MP, Culmsee C, Yu ZF, et al: Roles of nuclear factor κB in neuronal survival and plasticity. J Neurochem 2000;74:443–456.
65. Burton RH: Superoxide and hydrogen peroxide in relation to mammalian cell proliferation. Free Radic Biol Med 1995;18:775–794.
66. Nottet HS, van Asbeck BS, de Graaf L, et al: Role of oxygen radicals in self-sustained HIV-1 replication in monocyte-derived macrophages: enhanced HIV-1 replication by N-acetyl-cysteine. J Leukoc Biol 1994;56:702–777.
67. Okada Y, Copeland BR, Mori E, et al: P-Selectin and intracellular adhe-

sion molecule-1 expression after focal brain ischemia and reperfusion. Stroke 1994;25:202–211.

68. Korthuis RJ, Anderson DC, Granger DN: Role of neutrophil-endothelial cell adhesion in inflammatory disorders. J Crit Care 1994;9:47–71.

69. Fellman V, Raivio KO: Reperfusion injury as the mechanism of brain damage after perinatal asphyxia. Pediatr Res 1997;41:599–606.

70. Dammann O, Leviton A: Brain damage in preterm newborns: biological response modification as a strategy to reduce disabilities. J Pediatr 2000; 136:433–438.

71. Willam C, Schindler R, Frei U, et al: Increases in oxygen tension stimulate expression of ICAM-1 and VCAM-1 on human endothelial cells. Am J Physiol 1999;276:H2044–H2052.

72. Zadeh MS, Kolb JP, Geromin D, et al: Regulation of ICAM-1/CD54 expression on human endothelial cells by hydrogen peroxide involves inducible NO synthase. J Leukoc Biol 2000;67:327–334.

73. Redford EJ, Hall SM, Smith KJ: Vascular changes and demyelination induced by the intraneural injection of tumor necrosis factor. Brain 1995;118:869–878.

74. Saugstad OD: Role of xanthine oxidase and its inhibitor in hypoxia: reoxygenation injury. Pediatrics 1996;98:103–107.

75. Yokoyama Y, Beckman JS, Beckman TK, et al: Circulating xanthine oxidase: potential mediator of ischemic injury. Am J Physiol 1990;258:G564–G570.

76. Tan S, Yokoyama Y, Dickens E, et al: Xanthine oxidase activity in the circulation of rats following hemorrhagic shock. Free Radic Biol Med 1993; 15:407–414.

77. Grum CM, Ragsdale RA, Ketai LH, et al: Plasma xanthine oxidase in patients with adult respiratory distress syndrome. J Crit Care 1987;2: 22–26.

78. Rootwelt T, Almaas R, Øyasæter S, et al: Release of xanthine oxidase to the systemic circulation during resuscitation from severe hypoxia in newborn pigs. Acta Paediatr 1995;84:507–511.

79. Samesto A, Linder N, Raivio KO: Organ distribution and molecular forms of human xanthine dehydrogenase/xanthine oxidase. Lab Invest 1996;74: 48–56.

80. Supnet MC, David-Cu R, Walther FJ: Plasma xanthine oxidase and lipid hydroperoxide levels in preterm infants. Pediatr Res 1994;36:283–287.

81. Zweier JL, Broderick R, Kuppusamy P, et al: Determination of the mechanism of free radical generation in human aortic endothelial cells exposed to anoxia and re-oxygenation. J Biol Chem 1994;269:24156–24162.

82. Bågenholm R, Nilsson UA, Gotborg CW, et al: Free radicals are formed in the brain of fetal sheep during reperfusion after cerebral ischemia. Pediatr Res 1998;43:271–275.

83. Bågenholm R, Nilsson UA, Kjellmer I: Formation of free radicals in hypoxic ischemic brain damage in the neonatal rat, assessed by an endogenous spin trap and lipid peroxidation. Brain Res 1997;773:132–138.

84. Pourcyrous M, Leffler CW, Mirro R, et al: Brain superoxide anion generation during asphyxia and reventilation in newborn pigs. Pediatr Res 1990;28:618–621.

85. Pourcyrous M, Leffler CW, Bada HS, et al: Brain superoxide anion gener-

ation in asphyxiated piglets and the effect of indomethacin at therapeutic doses. Pediatr Res 1993;34:366–369.

86. Ment LR, Stewart WB, Duncan CC: Beagle puppy model of intraventricular hemorrhage: effect of superoxide dismutase on cerebral blood flow and prostaglandins. J Neurosurg 1985;62:563–569.

87. Palmer C, Vannucci RC, Towfighi J: Reduction of perinatal hypoxic-ischemic brain damage with allopurinol. Pediatr Res 1990;27:332–336.

88. Van Bel F, Shadid M, Moison RMW: Effect of allopurinol on postasphyxial free radical formation, cerebral hemodynamics, and electrical brain activity. Pediatrics 1998;101:185–193.

89. Ditelberg JS, Sheldon RA, Epstein CJ, Ferriero DM: Brain injury after perinatal hypoxia-ischemia is exacerbated in copper/zinc superoxide dismutase transgenic mice. Pediatr Res 1996;39:204–208.

90. Murakami K, Kondo T, Epstein CJ, et al: Overexpression of CuZn-superoxide dismutase reduces hippocampal injury after global ischemia in transgenic mice. Stroke 1997;28:1797–1804.

91. Yang G, Ghan PH, Chen J: Human copper-zinc superoxide dismutase transgenic mice are highly resistant to reperfusion injury after focal cerebral ischemia. Stroke 1994;25:165–170.

92. Vedder NB, Winn RK, Rice CL, et al: A monoclonal antibody to adherence-promoting leukocyte glycoprotein, CD18, reduces organ injury and improves survival from hemorrhagic shock and resuscitation in rabbits. J Clin Invest 1988;81:939–944.

93. Hallenbeck JM, Dutka AJ, Tanishima T, et al: Polymorphonuclear leukocyte accumulation in brain regions with low blood flow during the early postischemic period. Stroke 1986;17:246–253.

94. Mulligan MS, Varani JJ, Warren JS: Roles of β_2 integrins of rat neutrophils in complement- and oxygen radical-mediated acute lung inflammatory injury. J Immunol 1992;148:1847–1857.

95. Rootwelt T, Løberg EM, Moen A, et al: Blood pressure, acid base status, hypoxanthine concentrations, and brain morphology in hypoxic newborn piglets ventilated with either room air or 100% oxygen. Pediatr Res 1992;32:107–113.

96. Rootwelt T, Odden JP, Hall C, et al: Cerebral blood flow and evoked potentials during re-oxygenation with 21% or 100% O_2 in newborn pigs. J Appl Physiol 1993;75:2054–2060.

97. Feet BA, Xiang-Qing Y, Øyasæter S, et al: Effects of hypoxia and resuscitation with 21% and 100% O_2 in newborn piglets: extracellular hypoxanthine (Hx) in brain cortex and femoral muscle. Crit Care Med 1997;25:1384–1391.

98. Kutzsche S, Ilves P, Kirkeby OJ, et al: Hydrogen peroxide production in leukocytes during cerebral hypoxia and reoxygenation with 100% or 21% oxygen in newborn piglets. Pediatr Res 2001;49:834–842.

99. Feet BA, Medbø S, Rootwelt T, et al: Hypoxemic resuscitation in newborn piglets: recovery of somatosensory evoked potentials, hypoxanthine, and acid base balance. Pediatr Res 1998;43:690–696.

100. Feet BA, Brun NC, Hellstrom-Westas L, et al: Early cerebral metabolic and electrophysiological recovery during controlled hypoxemic resuscitation in piglets. J Appl Physiol 1998;84:1208–1216.

101. Ramji S, Ahuja S, Thirupuram S, et al: Resuscitation of asphyxic newborns with room air or 100% oxygen. Pediatr Res 1993;34:809–812.

102. Saugstad OD, Rootwelt T, Aalen AO: Resuscitation of asphyxiated newborn infants with room air or oxygen: an international trial: the Resair 2 study. Pediatrics 1998;102:e1.
103. Vento M, Asensi M, Sastre J, et al: Resuscitation with room air instead of 100% oxygen prevents oxidative stress in moderately asphyxiated term neonates. Pediatrics 2001;107:642–647.
104. Kutzsche S, Kirkeby OJ, Rise IR, et al: Effects of hypoxia and reoxygenation with 21% and 100% oxygen on cerebral nitric oxide concentration and microcirculation in newborn piglets. Biol Neonat 1999;76: 153–167.
105. Kinsella JP, Parker TA, Galan H, et al: Effects of inhaled nitric oxide on pulmonary edema and lung neutrophil accumulation in severe experimental hyaline membrane disease. Pediatr Res 1997;41:457–463.
106. Issa I, Lappalainen U, Kleinman M, et al: Inhaled nitric oxide decreases hyperoxia-induced surfactant abnormality in preterm rabbits. Pediatr Res 1999;45:247–254.
107. Vannucci RC: Current and potential new management strategies to perinatal hypoxic-ischemic encephalopathy. Pediatrics 1990;85:961–968.
108. Shadid M, Buonocore G, Groenendaal F, et al: Effect of deferoxamine and allopurinol on non-protein-bound iron concentrations in plasma and cortical brain tissue of newborn lambs following hypoxia-ischemia. Neurosci Lett 1998;248:5–8.
109. Shadid M, Van Bel F, Steendijk P, et al: Pretreatment with allopurinol in cardiac hypoxic-ischemic reperfusion injury in newborn lambs exerts its beneficial effect through afterload reduction. J Basic Res Cardiol 1999;94:23–30.
110. Inan C, Kilic I, Kilinc K, et al: The effect of high dose antenatal vitamin E on hypoxia-induced changes in newborn rats. Pediatr Res 1995;38:685–689.

PART III

Clinical Implications

CHAPTER 10

Antepartum Hypoxemia and the Developing Fetus

Donald M. Peebles, Mark A. Hanson

Introduction

When William Little first described cerebral palsy in 1862, he postulated that the cause related to abnormalities of the birth process.[1] There is now an accumulating body of evidence to suggest that events occurring during the *antenatal* period are more important and may lead to up to 70% of the cases of CP.[2,3] Despite a significant reduction in the perinatal mortality rate over the past 20 years, arising from improvements in obstetric and neonatal practice, there has not been a concomitant decrease in the rate of CP.[4] For instance, the introduction of intrapartum electronic fetal heart rate monitoring, a sensitive technique for the detection of fetal hypoxemia, has not resulted in a reduction in the incidence of long-term neurologic disability, though operative deliveries for fetal hypoxemia during labor have increased.[5] These facts are perhaps not surprising when epidemiologic studies consistently report evidence of intrapartum complications in only 10–15% of infants with either neonatal encephalopathy or cerebral palsy (see Chapter 2).[6,7] The suggestion that the cerebral insult can predate the onset of labor is supported by ultrasonographic data that show that the characteristic cysts of periventricular leukomalacia (PVL), which normally take 1–2 weeks to develop, can be found immediately after birth.[8] These, and other data, have led to a major shift in the emphasis of perinatal brain injury research, from intrapartum abnormalities to antenatal events.

Equally important is the realization that hypoxemia is only one of several factors which individually or in combination can damage the developing brain. Epidemiologic studies, for instance, highlight the importance of maternal thyroid status, and abnormalities of fetal hemostasis and immunology in the etiology of CP.[9,10] Indicators or risk factors for perinatal infection such as prolonged rupture of the mem-

From Donn SM, Sinha SK, Chiswick ML (eds): *Birth Asphyxia and the Brain: Basic Science and Clinical Implications.* © 2002, Futura Publishing Co., Inc., Armonk, NY.

branes, chorioamnionitis, or maternal fever are also associated with an increased risk of CP,[10,11] and white matter injury can be created experimentally by inducing intrauterine infection in fetal rabbits[12] or by exposing the developing brain to endotoxin.[13] Thus, while this chapter focuses mainly on the fetal response to hypoxemia, it must be recognized that the effects of an episode of hypoxemia on the immature brain will be influenced by coexisting factors. Indeed, cerebral inflammation may form a common final pathway in the response to both hypoxemia and infection.

Pathogenesis of Antepartum Fetal Hypoxemia

Interruption of the process of maternal-fetal gas exchange can occur in a variety of ways (Table 1), the chronicity and severity of which will determine the fetal response and pathologic consequences. While much is known about the causes of *chronic* hypoxemia because of its most frequent end result, fetal growth restriction, less is known about mechanisms of *acute* antepartum hypoxemia. Possible causes of episodes of hypoxemia, such as an umbilical cord accident, may not be

Table 1

Causes of Fetal Hypoxia

Acute Hypoxia
Causes of discrete antenatal episodes of fetal hypoxia:
- Umbilical cord compression
- Placental abruption
- Fetomaternal or fetofetal transfusion i.e, twin-to-twin transfusion syndrome
- Maternal hypotension

Chronic Hypoxia
Causes of chronic antenatal fetal hypoxia:
- High altitude
- Maternal disease leading to maternal hypoxia
- Abnormalities of uteroplacental blood flow
  Failed trophoblastic invasion spiral arteries
  Thrombosis
  Placental infarction/abruption
- Abnormalities of fetoplacental blood flow
  Peripheral villous maldevelopment
  Obliteration of fetal stem vessels

associated with any obvious clinical sign, and could easily be missed by antepartum fetal surveillance. The diagnosis is therefore normally a retrospective one, made when the fetus has postnatal evidence of brain injury. Ironically, the fetal response to acute hypoxemia is well understood, mainly because of the use of animal models, such as the chronically instrumented ovine fetus.

Epidemiologic and Pathologic Antecedents

In general, the data providing evidence for the contribution of acute causes of hypoxemia to cerebral palsy rates are scant. Thus, situations in which the cord is vulnerable to compression, such as a circumvallate insertion or multiple pregnancies, are associated with an increased risk of fetal morbidity. Bleeding during pregnancy, which may indicate partial placental separation, has been reported as a risk factor for both cerebral palsy and neonatal encephalopathy.[9,14] Severe examples of these mechanisms, such as umbilical cord prolapse and major placental abruption, which normally result in immediate delivery of the fetus, are clearly identifiable risk factors for CP.

The consequence on the surviving sibling of one twin dying *in utero* provides an important example of the effects of acute ischemia on the fetal brain. The risk of cerebral impairment in a live-birth co-twin of a deceased fetus is 20%, with monochorionic twins being particularly vulnerable.[15] The precise pathologic mechanisms underlying this impairment are not clear. The most likely explanation is that the death of a twin, especially the donor in a twin-to-twin transfusion, results in hemodynamic instability or hypotension in the recipient, which is sufficient to cause brain injury.[16] Alternatively, the release of either thromboplastic material from the deceased twin, leading to disseminated intravascular coagulation, or emboli, leading to brain infarction, has been implicated. Antenatal maternal administration of indomethacin, which inhibits prostaglandin synthesis and is known to cross the placenta and constrict the cerebral circulation, is associated with a higher incidence of PVL than in untreated controls, supporting the concept that acute cerebral hypoperfusion *in utero* can lead to brain injury.[17]

There are numerous pathologic studies that link abnormalities of the maternal and fetal placental circulations with abnormal Doppler ultrasound waveforms, fetal growth restriction, and chronic fetal hypoxemia. However, there is little evidence that these abnormalities of placental vascularization lead to CP. Thus, although low birthweight is a risk factor for CP, the association is less obvious when controlled for gestational age,[18] and in a preterm population, growth restriction does not carry a risk of CP.[11] The significance of these chronic abnormalities may instead be that they cause chronic hypoxemia, which could influence and detract from the ability of the fetus to respond to subsequent episodes of acute hypoxemia encountered during labor.

Fetal Responses to Hypoxemia

Hemodynamic Responses

Acute Hypoxemia

The effects of acute and chronic hypoxemia on the fetal circulation have been studied extensively in animals, particularly in sheep, and have recently been reported.[19–21] As in the adult, a plethora of factors act on the fetal circulation during acute hypoxemic episodes. Neural factors act directly on the sinoatrial node via the vagus and sympathetic nerves in the late-gestation sheep fetus.[22,23] These neural effects, which can form the efferent limb of reflex control, appear to play a relatively small role in mid-gestation. Hypoxemia does produce pronounced effects on the fetal circulation, even between 0.3 and 0.5 gestation in the sheep,[24] but the reflex/endocrine versus direct effects on the circulation at this age are not known. In late gestation, acute hypoxemia or asphyxia (resulting from maternal inhalation of hypoxic gas, cord occlusion, or restriction of uterine blood flow) produces an initial bradycardia; this is followed by a slow increase in heart rate, which returns to or exceeds its control value over the next few minutes. Arterial blood pressure increases and usually remains elevated. Cerebrovascular resistance falls and cerebral blood flow increases, while flow to carcass, muscle, kidneys, and gut decreases (Figure 1). The early bradycardia under these circumstances is chemoreflexive in origin, as it is abolished by cutting the carotid sinus nerves bilaterally,[25] or with administration of atropine,[23,26] or by vagotomy.[27] This bradycardia is not baroreflex-mediated, as it occurs before a rise in arterial pressure has time to develop, e.g., during a brief uterine artery occlusion or when the rise is prevented by α-adrenergic blockade,[28] or with transection of the spinal cord at L1-L2, interrupting descending sympathetic outflow.[29] The delayed increase in fetal heart rate results from a β-adrenergic stimulation from the rise in plasma catecholamines.[30–34] Other humoral agents released in hypoxemia or asphyxia may also be involved, but their precise role has yet to be determined. The most well known of these is arginine vasopressin, which is secreted in large amounts in hypoxemia, asphyxia, or hypotension[35] and has been reported to reduce fetal heart

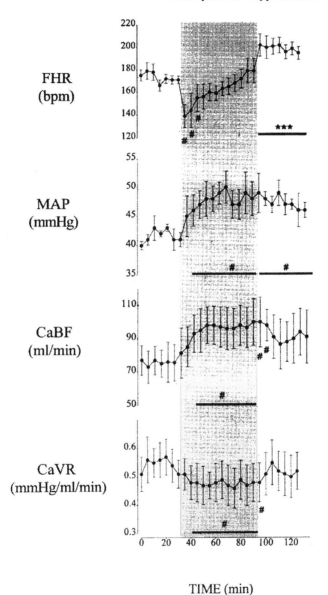

TIME (min)

Figure 1. The effect of 1 hour of isocapnic hypoxia on ovine fetal heart rate (FHR), mean arterial pressure (MAP), carotid blood flow (CaBF), and carotid vascular resistance (CaVR). The shaded area denotes the period of hypoxia. Values are means ±SEM, #p<0.05; **p<0.005, for individual time points or intervals of data (black horizontal bars). Reprinted with permission from 1998 International Pediatric Research Foundation.

rate.[36-40] However, in the fetal llama, a species in which fetal cardio-vascular responses to hypoxemia are potent even at 0.6 gestation, the cardiovascular effects of arginine vasopressin release are less vital than those of catecholamines.[41]

In the simplest terms, mean arterial pressure is determined by cardiac output (combined ventricular output in the fetus) and total peripheral resistance. These two components are under both extrinsic and intrinsic control, as is the case for heart rate alone. Indeed, the major determinant of combined ventricular output in late gestation is fetal heart rate, as the mechanical constraints on the heart permit only small changes in stroke volume. Extrinsic mechanisms affecting the peripheral arterioles form the efferent limb of reflex control, predominantly by α-adrenergic means. Thus, the rise in mean arterial pressure occurring during hypoxemia can be reduced by cutting the carotid sinus nerves,[25] or by α-adrenergic blockade with phentolamine.[28] Again, such reflexes have an indirect component via the release of catecholamines from the adrenal medulla. Many other humoral agents play a role.

Chronic Hypoxemia

More prolonged hypoxemia leads to an initial bradycardia followed by a tachycardia lasting for at least 24 hours. This prolonged increase in fetal heart rate may be related to a sustained release of catecholamines.[42] If hypoxemia is maintained, fetal blood pressure returns to normal both in the presence or absence of acidemia.[42,43] The mechanisms of this are not known but may involve both chemorecep-tor adaptation and endocrine changes.[44] Hence, blood pressure in the chronically hypoxemic, growth-restricted sheep fetus is not different from that of normally grown normoxemic fetuses.

In contrast to the minimal changes in fetal heart rate and blood pressure seen in prolonged hypoxemia, the redistribution of cardiac output that occurs in acute hypoxemia in fetal sheep appears to be maintained with prolonged hypoxemia. Hence, the increase in blood flow to the brain, heart, and adrenal glands can be maintained for up to 48 hours.[42] The increase in cerebral blood flow with prolonged hypoxemia is greatest to subcortical and brainstem structures, as is seen with acute hypoxemia.[45] A similar sustained increase in cerebral blood flow is seen during chronic hypoxemia in the sheep fetus at mid-gestation,[46] although the acute response may be blunted at earlier gestation.[47]

In-depth studies of the effects of chronic hypoxemia or repeated acute hypoxemia have focused on specific aspects of fetal homeostatic mechanisms. It appears that activation of the hypothalamic-pituitary-adrenal axis occurs, producing adrenal cortical responsiveness.[48] This may involve effects both on adrenal, steroidogenic enzyme activity, and also on glucocorticoid receptor-mediated feedback at the pituitary and hypothalamus. In addition, there are organ-specific effects on components of the insulin-like growth factor (IGF) system (including IGF peptides, their binding proteins, and their receptors), which affect organ growth and/or differentiation, as well as local blood flow.

Metabolic Responses

Some vertebrate species exposed to prolonged periods of reduced oxygen supply, such as the fresh water turtle and diving seal, have developed complex compensatory mechanisms to ensure intact brain survival.[49–52] In such "hypoxemia-tolerant" species, the traditional view that oxygen deprivation at a cellular level leads to energy depletion, and that this deficit is taken up by the activation of adenosine triphosphate (ATP)-generating anaerobic pathways, is an oversimplification. In fact, the twin strategies of reducing energy turnover and maximizing the efficiency of ATP production mean that supply and demand are balanced, and ATP levels remain stable.[53] There is abundant evidence that components of both of these strategies are adopted by the fetus to ensure intact neurologic survival after an episode of acute hypoxemia.

Interaction Between Oxygen Supply and Consumption

A number of studies in the ovine fetus have shown that overall oxygen consumption can be maintained for up to 24 hours despite a 40–50% reduction in oxygen delivery to the placenta.[54,55] This is achieved by increasing umbilical blood flow so that oxygen delivery to the fetus is not so severely reduced, as well as by increasing the percentage of oxygen extracted. However, although whole body consumption is not affected until oxygen delivery is reduced by more than 50%, there are regional differences in oxygen delivery (Vo_2), and therefore consumption (Do_2), which are consequent on the changes in regional blood flow described above. Thus, peripheral vasoconstriction, by imposing a further reduction in Do_2 to organs such as the carcass and gut, at a time when arterial Po_2 is already reduced, produces a reduction in oxidative metabolism and an increase in lactate production in those tissues. The mechanism is sensitive; Vo_2 of fetal skeletal muscles studied *in vitro* falls linearly as Po_2 is decreased over a range which is substantially higher than that at which aerobic metabolism fails in the adult.[56] The importance of this

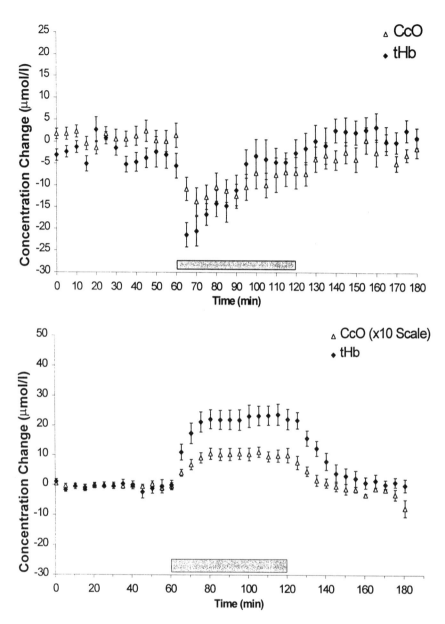

Figure 2. The effect of 1 hour occlusion of the maternal common internal iliac artery (denoted by shaded horizontal bars) on concentrations of total hemoglobin (tHb), i.e., cerebral blood volume, and oxidized cytochrome oxidase (CcO) measured by near-infrared spectroscopy simultaneously in fetal sheep hind limb muscle (**top**) and brain (**bottom**).

response in terms of limiting fetal Vo_2 is demonstrated by the finding that plasma lactate and the excretion of organic acids in the fetal urine increase less in fetal sheep after denervation of the peripheral arterial chemoreceptors[57]; this prevents the short-term reflex response to hypoxemia and leading to an increase in fetal mortality.

Data from studies in which blood flow and the redox state of cytochrome oxidase (Cu_A), the terminal enzyme of the oxidative phosphorylation pathway, were assessed simultaneously in carcass muscle, and brain of the term ovine fetus during moderately severe hypoxemia, demonstrate several ways in which the cerebral response differs.[58] First, as described above, cerebral blood flow increases, rather than decreases, which helps to maintain cerebral oxygen delivery. Second, while the severe fall in oxygen delivery to muscle resulted in decreased oxygen binding at the Cu_A center and a reduction of cytochrome oxidase (CcO) (Figure 2A), a different response was observed in the brain (Figure 2B). Despite a decrease in oxygen delivery to the brain during occlusion, there was a gradual *increase* in Cu_A, which returned to control values with normoxia. Thus, the hypothesis generated by these data would be that, as a result of a moderate reduction in fetal cerebral Do_2, cerebral metabolism decreases and ATP turnover is reduced. This could decrease oxidative phosphorylation in several ways: through an inhibitory effect of ATP on the Krebs cycle and by causing a rise in NAD^+, which in turn will inhibit the flow of reducing equivalents. If the rate of electron transfer across the mitochondrial chain falls, the Cu_A moiety will become oxidized. In addition, nitric oxide, which is known to increase in the brain during hypoxemia, has been shown to decrease oxygen consumption by inhibition of complex I and IV of the oxidative phosphorylation pathway.[59] This could have a similar effect on the CcO redox state.

A notable feature of this response is that it is observed within minutes of the onset of hypoxemia. This suggests the presence of sensitive, rapidly acting sensor mechanisms within the brain, the activation of which results in metabolic adaptations. While there are few data concerning such mechanisms within the fetal brain, there is much circumstantial evidence from other tissues that these exist.

Oxygen Sensing

In order to respond rapidly to hypoxemia, the fetal brain, in common with other tissues, is dependent on mechanisms for sensing oxygen and regulation of gene expression. One potential mechanism is through the adequacy of high-energy phosphate supply from mitochondrial oxidative phosphorylation. This type of "metabolic sensing" is partly responsible for the rapid enhancement of GLUT1 glucose transporter expression observed with hypoxemia (see Chapter 5), as it can also be caused by metabolic inhibitors such as cyanide.[60] Improved glucose transport into cells during hypoxemia is essential to meet the increased cellular demand for glucose metabolism through the glycolytic pathway. However, studies of two systems known to be involved in the hypoxemia response, the carotid body and regulation of red cell production by erythropoietin, suggest that there are other rapid, sensitive mechanisms which are widely distributed throughout many cell types.[61] Oxygen-sensitive K^+ channels, first recognized in the carotid body, have now been demonstrated in a number of vascular cells, while mechanisms involving NADPH oxidase, cytochrome P-450 (an O_2-binding heme protein), and mitochondrial reactive oxygen species have all been proposed as sensing mechanisms involved in the regulation of gene transcription.[62] There are little available data describing the function of these pathways in the fetus.

Hypoxemia-Inducible Factor

A key mediator in the induction of genes necessary for intact survival during medium- to long-term hypoxemia is hypoxemia-inducible factor-1 (HIF-1). This transcription factor has been shown to accumulate rapidly in the nucleus during hypoxemia and leads to transcriptional activation of erythropoietin, vascular endothelial growth factor, and glycolytic enzymes.[61] Taken together, these responses improve oxygen delivery to tissues and facilitate the production of glycolytic ATP. Mouse embryos with complete deficiency of HIF-1α (a subunit of HIF-1) because of homozygosity for a null allele at the Hif1a locus die at mid-gestation, while heterozygotes survive normally but have an impaired response to chronic hypoxemia, compared to wild-type litter mates.[63] HIF-1α gene expression has been demonstrated in the brain of the fetal rat as early as embryonic day 14, and mRNA transcript levels increase with hypoxemia.[64] Enhanced DNA binding of HIF-1 by iron chelators leads to upregulation of glycolytic genes and neuroprotection in embryonic neuronal cell cultures exposed to oxidative stress,[65] but the role of HIF-1 in the response of the intact fetal brain still needs to be elucidated.

Adenosine

Adenosine is a vasoactive purine metabolite, produced during the breakdown of high-energy phosphates in hypoxemia. Tissue levels of adenosine are 2 to 3 times higher in the fetus than in the adult,[66] and have been shown to rise further within minutes of the onset of hypoxemia in the ovine fetus.[67] Plasma adenosine levels are also higher in hypoxemic, acidotic, growth-restricted human fetuses than in fetuses that have grown appropriately.[68] This may be seen as a direct consequence of the hypoxemia, but there is also the possibility that elevated tissue and plasma adenosine may form part of a protective fetal adaptation aimed at matching oxygen demand to availability.[69,70] Adenosine, acting via A2 receptors, is known to cause peripheral vasodilation and an increase in cerebral blood flow, thus improving oxygen delivery to tissues.[71,72] In addition, adenosine inhibits fetal breathing and eye and body movements, depresses excitatory neurotransmission, and causes neuronal hyperpolarization, all of which will reduce fetal oxygen consumption.[73,74] Certainly, a neuroprotective role for adenosine has been proposed in the adult,[69] and potentiation of endogenous adenosine reduces cerebral injury following ischemia in the newborn rat.[70] An indication of the adenosine receptors that are important in this process is provided by data showing that treatment with nonselective and A2, but not A1, adenosine receptor antagonists reduces brain injury after hypoxia- ischemia in the immature rat.[75]

Adaptive Mechanisms and Neuronal Survival

The fetal brain at term is protected against the deleterious effects of acute hypoxemia by hemodynamic and metabolic compensatory mechanisms. If, however, the insult is of sufficient length or severity, compensatory mechanisms will be overwhelmed and neuronal loss will ensue. Complete occlusion of the umbilical cord for 10 minutes results in a fall in cerebral blood flow and arterial pressure in the sheep fetus,[76] and has been shown to result in the loss of hippocampal neurons.[77] Figure 3 shows an example of a brief period of mild fetal hypoxemia, superimposed on chronic hypoxemia in a growth-restricted sheep fetus, which resulted in immediate hypotension, a fall in cerebral blood flow, and reduction of Cu_A. This response contrasts with that of the previously normoxic fetus, in which a similar insult results in a sustained increase in both blood pressure and cerebral perfusion.[76] In a study of the fetal cerebral consequences of maternal uterine artery occlusion, Gunn et al reported a strong correlation between hypotension and the severity of neuronal loss, assessed histologically.[78] No association was seen with fetal oxygenation. Maintenance of cerebral perfusion seems to be an essential prerequisite for long-term neuronal survival.

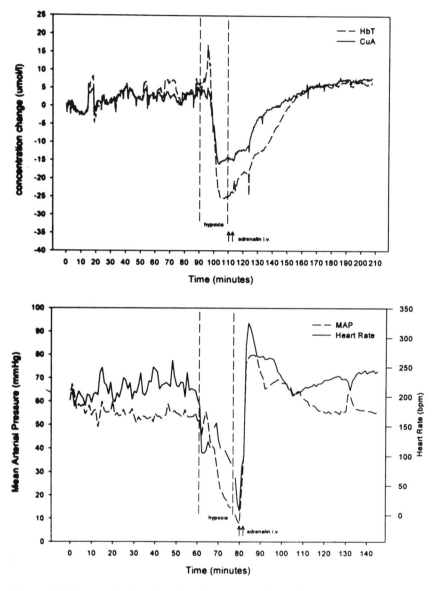

Figure 3. Changes in fetal cerebral concentrations of total hemoglobin (Hbt) and cytochrome oxidase (Cu_A) (top panel), and mean arterial pressure (MAP) and fetal heart rate (bottom panel), caused by brief exposure to isocapnic hypoxia in a chronically hypoxic fetus (Po_2 pre-insult of 15 mmHg). The response (a fall in MAP, fetal heart rate, and Hbt, and a reduction in Cu_A) is the reciprocal of that seen in normoxic fetuses exposed to hypoxia (see Figures 1 and 2).

Consequences of Fetal Hypoxemia

The effects of hypoxemia on the developing brain are influenced primarily by two factors, the stage of brain development and the duration and severity of the hypoxemic challenge.

Influence of Gestation

Early Pregnancy

It has been suggested that hypoxemia-inducible transcription factors are important for normal development. Exposure of the embryonic rat (gestational day 9–11) to a hyperoxic environment (45% oxygen) resulted in reduced apoptosis and gross morphologic abnormalities such as defective neural tube closure.[79] Embryos grown in an hypoxemic environment (5% oxygen) were small compared with controls, but were normally formed. These data suggest that a hypoxemic environment during early pregnancy may be essential for proper morphologic development.

Hypoxemia and the Preterm Brain

With improving placental function and fetal oxygenation, the fetal brain becomes dependent on oxygen; severe deprivation leads to neuronal loss, with the pattern of brain injury being related to gestation. Prior to myelination, approximately 32 weeks of gestation in the human, damage is observed mainly in white matter. The typical appearance is of small multifocal zones of necrosis in the periventricular white matter, termed periventricular leukomalacia (PVL), although others suggest that a more generalized form of white matter injury may be just as important.[80] Between 60% and 100% of preterm infants with PVL will develop CP, and although they account for only 2% of all births, infants delivered at less than 32 weeks of gestation contribute to 25% of all cases of CP.[81]

The fact that white matter injury is seen infrequently after 32 weeks of gestation suggests that aspects of cerebral development predispose white matter to injury. Two different areas have been considered. The first concerns the vulnerability of cellular components in the white matter, particularly oligodendrocytes, because of immaturity of the blood-brain barrier, incomplete myelination, and suboptimal levels of endogenous protectors such as gliotrophins or oligotrophins.[80] The second unique feature of immature white matter is its potential vulnerability to ischemia. Volpe suggests that deep white matter lies at a watershed between two arterial supplies, the ventriculopetal branches of the leptomeningeal arteries, and the ventriculofugal branches of the thalamostriate and choroidal arteries.[82] It has also been suggested that, because of immaturity of chemoreflex mechanisms, the fetus at this early gestation is unable to maintain adequate cerebral blood flow.[83] In the fetal sheep, systemic hypotension, caused by hemorrhage, can induce PVL,[84] while the white matter, in particular, remains hypoperfused after reversal of hypotension.[85]

Hypoxemia and the Term Brain

Near term, the pattern of brain injury observed after an episode of acute hypoxemia changes, and gray matter, rather than white, is affected. Acute asphyxia, caused by complete uterine artery occlusion in the sheep, results in damage to striatum, parasagittal cortex, and the CA 1/2 region of the hippocampus.[78] This is similar to the pattern of brain injury observed by Myers in the term monkey fetus after partial asphyxia, with necrosis that was restricted to the middle third of the paracentral region and basal ganglia.[86] Magnetic resonance imaging (MRI) scans in infants exposed to severe hypoxemia-ischemia at term also demonstrate the vulnerability of basal ganglia and parasagittal cortex to injury (see Chapter13). White matter injury is rarely seen at this gestation.

One reason that has been proposed for increased neuronal vulnerability at this gestation is the development of excitatory amino acid receptors (see Chapter 3). Glutamate, the principle excitatory amino acid in the brain, is released in large quantities during hypoxia-ischemia and acts via a variety of receptor subtypes to allow accumulation of toxic intracellular calcium concentrations.[87] Pharmacologic blockade of these channels, in particular the N-methyl-D-aspartate (NMDA) receptor, is neuroprotective in experimental models of hypoxic-ischemic brain injury.[88] Studies of the ontogeny of glutamate receptors in the ovine brain show higher levels of NMDA receptors at 135 days of gestation relative to 80 days of age or to the adult.[89] In addition, binding is higher in the areas particularly prone to hypoxemic injury, namely cortex and basal ganglia. Similar findings have been reported in the rat brain with increasing levels of glutamate receptor in cortex at more advanced stages of development.[90] Therefore, excess numbers of excitatory amino acid receptors and/or relative deficiency of transporters may make these areas particularly vulnerable to excitotoxic damage.

Another related factor is the increase in the cerebral metabolic rate observed with increasing maturity and development of interneuronal synapses. Immature fetal guinea pigs (0.75 gestation) do not show any increase in glucose metabolism or lactate accumulation during mild hypoxemia, a finding ascribed to the low baseline metabolic rate at this gestation.[91] With advancing gestation, cortical nitric oxide synthase activity increases, associated with higher cortical blood flow and oxygen utilization.[92] Positron emission tomography of normal infants showed high metabolic rates for glucose in the sensorimotor cortex, thalamus, cerebellum, and brainstem.[93] If ATP production is limited by depletion of metabolic substrates such as oxygen and glucose, it is apparent that the areas of brain with the highest energy requirements will be the most affected. If these coincide with areas of high NMDA receptor density, the effect of energy depletion and membrane depolarization on these "voltage-dependent" channels is to potentiate further the effect of increased glutamate levels.

Other factors that determine the susceptibility of the developing brain to hypoxemic damage are the lipid composition of brain cell membranes, the rate of lipid peroxidation, and the presence of antioxidant defenses[94] (see Chapter 9). It is therefore relevant that hypoxemia results in an increase in cerebral oxygen free radical levels that is approximately twice as large in term compared to preterm guinea pigs, suggesting that the more mature brain may be more susceptible to free radical-mediated damage.[95]

Vulnerability to Hypoxemia

With increasing gestation, the pattern of brain injury following hypoxia-ischemia shifts from white to gray matter. The overall vulnerability of the brain also changes with the stage of development, and an inverse correlation exists between gestation and resistance to hypoxic-ischemic brain injury.[96] For example, neuronal loss after 10 minutes of complete occlusion of the umbilical cord is only observed in late gestation versus preterm ovine fetuses.[77,97] Furthermore, 20 minutes of cord occlusion, which would be fatal toward term, does not result in brain injury at 0.6 gestation.[98]

Duration of Hypoxemia

Considering the different metabolic and hemodynamic responses to an episode of acute versus chronic hypoxemia, it is not surprising that the cerebral consequences of a hypoxemic insult depend on its severity, length, and recurrence.

In a classic series of experiments using term monkey fetuses, Myers observed that the pattern of brain injury differed between animals exposed to a short period (10 minutes) of complete asphyxia and those exposed to between 30 minutes and 2 hours of partial asphyxia.[86] In the former group, damage was limited almost entirely to the brainstem, while in the latter group, injury was confined to the hemispheres, with the degree of neuronal loss in cortex and basal ganglia proportional to the length of insult. The latter pattern is most commonly seen in the term infant.

Similarly, the type of damage observed in the ovine fetal brain depends on the method of induction of hypoxemia. A short period (10 minutes) of umbilical cord occlusion leads to selective loss of hippocampal neurons,[77] whereas if the period of occlusion is shorter (5 minutes) but repeated four times at 30-minute intervals, then the striatum appears to be preferentially damaged.[99] Frequent (every 2.5 minutes) 1-minute cord occlusions cause a pattern of injury similar to that observed after occlusion of the uterine artery for 30 minutes (i.e., neuronal loss in parasagittal cortex, thalamus, and cerebellum).[78,100] In the preterm fetus (0.6 gestation), white matter damage is not observed until umbilical cord occlusion is prolonged for more than 20 minutes; however, cerebral hypoperfusion following carotid clamping causes a similar degree of injury in both term and preterm fetuses, with subcortical infarcts as the predominant feature at early gestations, and selective neuronal loss in upper cortical layers at later gestations.[96]

Gross brain injury is only rarely observed in animal models after more chronic insults, perhaps because these insults infrequently result in hypotension. However, this does not mean that brain development is unaffected. Twelve hours of partial uterine artery occlusion at 0.6 gestation in the sheep fetus resulted in severe brain injury in only one of eight fetuses, but resulted in a reduction in the cross-sectional area of the cerebral cortex by 12%, and depletion of neurons in hippocampus, cerebellum, and cortex.[101] Evidence that prolonged exposure to hypoxemia *in utero* can affect human fetal brain development is provided by data showing accelerated shortening of visual-evoked potential latencies in infants who had evidence of fetal brain sparing.[102] In this situation, chronic hypoxemia appears to result in accelerated neurophysiologic maturation, possibly as a consequence of more rapid myelination. At 5 years of age, this cohort of children showed impairment of cognitive function compared to controls with normal cerebral blood flow *in utero,* suggesting that while redistribution of cardiac output might be neuroprotective in the short-term, it may result in deleterious long-term consequences.[102]

New Modalities to Assess the Fetal Brain

From the previous discussion, it is apparent that a comprehensive description of the fetal responses and consequences of an episode of hypoxemia will include information about cerebral hemodynamics, metabolism, function, and structure. Sophisticated physiologic and histologic techniques are now available to assess these parameters in instrumented animal models. However, direct antenatal access to the human fetus is limited to fetal blood sampling techniques, which are associated with a risk to the fetus, provide only one-time measurements, and are of limited clinical value in the management of the growth-restricted fetus.[103] Clinical management is hampered by a shortage of appropriate noninvasive techniques for the assessment of the fetal brain *in utero.*

Doppler Ultrasound of the Cerebral Circulation

The use of pulsed and color Doppler ultrasound techniques for assessing the fetal circulation is not novel, as early reports were available nearly two decades ago. However, both the prognostic value of analysis of waveforms from fetal intracerebral arteries, and assessment of the cerebral venous circulation, are still unclear. The value of new Doppler techniques, such as power Doppler, is also as yet unestablished. The dilation of cerebral arteries and increase in cerebral blood flow observed in the fetus during both acute and chronic hypoxemia provide the physiologic basis for studies using Doppler ultrasound. Increased diastolic velocities, described by a decrease in the pulsatility index (PI), have been described in the middle cerebral artery during labor as well as in the growth-restricted, chronically hypoxemic fetus.[104,105] Using color Doppler, it is possible to identify a variety of intracerebral arteries, all of which show decreased downstream impedance in growth-restricted fetuses; however, the middle cerebral artery is the most sensitive parameter for discriminating between growth-restricted and normal fetuses.[106] Color Doppler studies of the cerebral venous circulation have not yet proven clinically useful.[107]

The use of umbilical artery Doppler studies in high-risk pregnancies has been shown to reduce the mortality rate in normally formed newborns, and is a rare example of an obstetric intervention of proven efficacy.[108] The two important questions related to Doppler studies of the cerebral circulation are: (1) Do the studies yield better results than umbilical artery Doppler alone? (2) Does prenatal cerebral vasodilation predict future neurologic compromise? In a number of studies, the combination of middle cerebral and umbilical artery PI in a ratio appears to improve the prediction of small-for-gestational-age fetuses with sensitivities ranging from 58% to 78%.[109,110] The use of the middle cerebral artery PI may be particularly useful in the third trimester when the predictive power of umbilical artery Doppler is diminished.[111] However, the only two published studies describing neurologic follow-up in children who had antenatal evidence of increased cerebral blood flow failed to demonstrate any sign of cerebral dysfunction at 2 and 3 years of age.[109,112] It was concluded that the increase in cerebral blood flow is a protective compensatory mechanism, rather than a sign of impending brain injury. However, while fetal "brain sparing" can be viewed as a benign, even necessary, short-term response to hypoxemia, its long-term benefit is called into question by a recent study that shows a significant cognitive deficit in these children at 5 years of age. This suggests that prolonged periods of hypoxemia and/or increased cerebral blood flow can have subtle effects on brain development.[102]

Doppler ultrasound is an easy-to-use, noninvasive method of assessing the fetal cerebral circulation, and this technique is available to many clinicians. The significance of abnormalities of middle cerebral artery flow is only now becoming clear.

Magnetic Resonance Imaging

Magnetic resonance imaging is a powerful, noninvasive technique for assessing the structure of the perinatal brain. The majority of reported studies are of the neonatal brain, where MRI is a sensitive method for resolution of lesions such as PVL or more diffuse white matter injury (see Chapter 13).[113,114] Movements *in utero* complicate imaging of the fetal brain although the problem has been partially resolved by the use of rapid acquisition sequences. Normal brain development, in terms of gyral maturation and gray and white matter differentiation, has been described between 12 and 38 weeks of gestation,[115] and MRI has been used successfully to detect abnormalities not diagnosed by ultrasound.[116,117] These studies suggest that prenatal MRI may be particularly useful for the detection of ischemic and hemorrhagic lesions, neuronal migration disorders, and abnormalities of the corpus callosum.

A further development of this technique, which has the potential to provide information about fetal brain activity as well as structure, is functional magnetic resonance imaging (fMRI). Hykin et al reported a small series of four fetuses that were studied using ultra high-speed, echo-planar fMRI (each image was acquired in 130 milliseconds).[118] Auditory stimulation of the fetal brain resulted in an activation signal in the temporal cortex, reflecting a local increase in cortical blood flow and paramagnetic oxyhemoglobin. Further studies are needed to determine whether fMRI is capable of detecting abnormalities of brain function *in utero*. Other imaging techniques that have the potential to provide information about fetal cerebral metabolism and perfusion have been developed successfully in animals. Diffusion-weighted imaging reveals changes in the apparent diffusion coefficient of tissue water that correlate closely with decreases in high-energy phosphate metabolism in a neonatal piglet model of hypoxic-ischemic brain injury.[119] A noninvasive marker of abnormalities of fetal cerebral ATP metabolism is likely to be a powerful tool in understanding the effect of hypoxemia on the developing brain.

Magnetic Resonance Spectroscopy

The principle of magnetic resonance spectroscopy depends on the tendency of the nuclei of phosphorus and hydrogen atoms, among others, to align themselves in a strong magnetic field. Disturbance of this alignment by a radiofrequency pulse at the appropriate wavelength results in a magnetic resonance signal that can be detected, and which correlates in intensity with the concentration of the atom. Proton and phosphorus spectroscopy of the neonatal brain are now well-established techniques that have provided invaluable data about many aspects of perinatal brain injury. These include the phenomenon of "secondary energy failure," described in animal models and in the human infant, in which acute hypoxemia results in a temporary decrease in high-energy phosphates, which return to normal with restoration of normoxia only to fall again over the next 24–48 hours.[120,121] The secondary fall in ATP and phosphocreatine is ascribed to delayed mitochondrial damage and impairment of oxidative metabolism; it correlates strongly with both the degree of cerebral apoptosis and long-term neurologic outcome.[122,123] Hypoxemia-related changes in cerebral lactate, reflecting anaerobic metabolism, and N-acetyl aspartate, a marker of neuronal loss and mitochondrial dysfunction, have also been described using proton spectroscopy.[124] Moreover, a recent report describes spectroscopic techniques for the *in vivo* detection of apoptosis.[125]

The potential use of these techniques for the noninvasive assessment of fetal cerebral metabolism and development is apparent. However, studies are hampered by the inability to apply the radiofrequency coil directly to the head, as well as by fetal movement. Proton spectra have been obtained from the exteriorized fetal sheep brain, showing an increase in lactate concentrations during hypoxemia similar to those observed in neonatal animals.[126] Rudimentary proton spectra have also been obtained from the human fetal brain *in utero,* using a surface coil on the maternal abdomen.[127] These contain peaks ascribed to N-acetyl aspartate, creatine, and choline. Unfortunately, a signal from maternal fat obscures the potential signal from lactate. However, these data demonstrate the feasibility of obtaining proton spectra from the fetal brain, and it is hoped that technical advances will improve the results even further.

References

1. Little WJ: On the influence of abnormal parturition, difficult labours, premature birth, and asphyxia neonatorum, on the mental and physical condition of the child, especially in relation to deformities. Trans Obstet Soc London 1862;3:293–344.
2. Torfs CP, Van der Berg BJ, Oeschali FW: Prenatal and perinatal factors in the aetiology of cerebral palsy. J Pediatr 1990;116:615–619.
3. Behar R, Wozniak P, Allard M, et al: Antenatal origin of neurologic damage in newborn infants. Am J Obstet Gynecol 1988;159:357–363.
4. Stanley FJ, Watson L: Trends in perinatal mortality and cerebral palsy in Western Australia, 1967 to 1985. BMJ 1992;304:1658–1663.
5. Thacker SB: The efficacy of intrapartum electronic fetal monitoring. Am J Obstet Gynecol 1987;156:24–30.
6. Blair E, Stanley FJ: Intrapartum asphyxia: a rare cause of cerebral palsy. J Pediatr 1988;112:515–519.
7. Australian and New Zealand Perinatal Societies: The origins of cerebral palsy: a consensus statement. Med J Aust 1995;162:85–90.
8. Scher, MS, Belfar H, Martin J, Painter MJ: Destructive brain lesions of presumed fetal onset: antepartum causes of cerebral palsy. Pediatrics 1991;88:898–906.
9. Badawi N, Kurinczuk JJ, Keogh JM, et al: Antepartum risk factors for newborn encephalopathy: the Western Australian case-control study. BMJ 1998;317:1549–1553.
10. Nelson KB, Dambrosia JM, Ting TY, Phillips TM: Neonatal cytokines and coagulation factors in children with cerebral palsy. Ann Neurol 1998;44:665–675.
11. Murphy DJ, Sellers S, MacKenzie IZ, et al: Case-control study of antenatal and intrapartum risk factors for cerebral palsy in very preterm singleton babies. Lancet 1995;346:1449–1454.
12. Yoon BH, Kim CJ, Romero R, et al: Experimentally induced intrauterine

infection causes fetal brain white matter lesions in rabbits. Am J Obstet Gynecol 1997;177:797–802.

13. Gilles FH, Leviton A, Kerr CS: Endotoxin leuconencephalopathy in the telencephalon of the newborn kitten. J Neurol Sci 1976;27:183–191.

14. Hagberg G, Hagberg B, Olow I: The changing panorama of cerebral palsy in Sweden 1954–1970. III. The importance of fetal deprivation of supply. Acta Paediatr 1976;65:403–408.

15. Pharoah POD, Adi Y: Consequences of in-utero death in a twin pregnancy. Lancet 2000;355:1597–1602.

16. Larroche JC, Droulle P, Delezoide AL, et al: Brain damage in monozygous twins. Biol Neonate 1990;57:261–278.

17. Baerts W, Fetter WPF, Hop WCJ, et al: Cerebral lesions in preterm infants after tocolytic indomethacin. Dev Med Child Neurol 1990;32:910–918.

18. Ellenberg JH, Nelson KB: Birthweight and gestational age in children with cerebral palsy or seizures disorders. Am J Dis Child 1979;133:1044.

19. Giussani DA, Spencer JAD, Hanson MA: Fetal cardiovascular reflex responses to hypoxaemia. Fetal Mat Med Rev 1994;6:17–37.

20. Hanson MA: Do we now understand the control of the fetal circulation? Eur J Obstet Gynecol Reprod Biol 1997;75:55–61.

21. Hanson MA, Spencer JAD, Rodeck CH (eds): *The Circulation (Vol 1): The Fetus and Neonate, Physiology and Clinical Applications.* Cambridge University Press, Cambridge, 1993.

22. Mott, JC, Walker DW: Neural and endocrine regulation of circulation in the fetus and newborn. In: *Handbook of Physiology/Cardiovascular System III.* American Physiology Society, Bethesda, MD,1983, pp 837–883.

23. Martin MB: Pharmacological aspects of fetal heart rate regulation during hypoxia. In Kunzel W (ed): *Fetal Heart Rate Monitoring.* Springer-Verlag, Berlin, 1985, pp 170–184.

24. Kiserud T: Hemodynamics of the ductus venosus. Eur J Obstet Gynecol Reprod Biol 1999;84:139–147.

25. Giussani DA, Spencer JAD, Moore PJ, Hanson MA: The effect of carotid sinus nerve section on the initial cardiovascular response to acute isocapnic hypoxia in fetal sheep in utero. J Physiol 1990;432:33P.

26. Caldeyro-Barcia, R, Mendez-Bauer C, Poseiro JJ, et al: Control of human fetal heart rate during labor. In Cassels DE (ed): *The Heart and Circulation in the Newborn and Infant.* Grune and Stratton, New York, 1966, pp 7–36.

27. Barcroft J: *Researches on Pre-natal Life 1946.* Blackwell Scientific Publications, Oxford.

28. Giussani DA, Spencer JAD, Moore PJ, Hanson MA: Effect of phenotolamine on initial cardiovascular response to isocapnic hypoxia in intact and carotid sinus denervated fetal sheep. J Physiol 1991;438:56P.

29. Blanco CE, Dawes GS, Walker DW: Effect of hypoxia on polysynaptic hind-limb reflexes of unanaesthetized fetal and newborn lambs. J Physiol 1983;339:453–466.

30. Cohn HE, Piasecki GJ, Jackson BT: The effect of β-adrenergic stimulation on fetal cardiovascular function during hypoxaemia. Am J Obstet Gynecol 1982;144:810.

31. Jensen A, Kunzel W, Kastendieck E: Fetal sympathetic activity, transcutaneous PO_2 and skin blood flow during repeated asphyxia in sheep. J Dev Physiol 1987;9:337–346.

32. Martin AA, Kapoor R, Scroop GC: Hormonal factors in the control of heart rate in the normoxaemic and hypoxaemic fetal, neonatal and adult sheep. J Dev Physiol 1987;9:465–480.
33. Jones CT, Roebuck MM, Walker DW, Johnston BM: The role of the adrenal medulla and peripheral sympathetic nerves in the physiological responses of the fetal sheep in hypoxia. J Dev Physiol 1988;10:17–36.
34. Perez R, Espinoza M, Riquelime R, et al: Arginine vasopressin mediates cardiovascular responses to hypoxaemia in fetal sheep. Am J Physiol 1989;256:R1011–R1018.
35. Wood CE, Chen H-G: Acidemia stimulates ACTH, vasopressin, and heart rate responses in fetal sheep. Am J Physiol 1989;257:R344–R349.
36. Iwamoto HS, Rudolph AM, Keil LC, Heyman MA: Hemodynamic responses of the sheep fetus to vasopressin infusion. Circ Res 1979;44:430.
37. Courtice GP, Kwong TE, Lumbers ER, Potter EK: Excitation of the cardiac vagus nerve by vasopressin in mammals. J Physiol 1984;354:547–556.
38. Dunlap CE III, Valego NK: Cardiovascular effects of dynorphin A-(1–13) and arginine vasopressin in fetal lambs. Am J Physiol 1989;256:R1318–R1324.
39. Irion GL, Mack CE, Clark KE: Fetal hemodynamic and fetoplacental vascular response to exogenous arginine vasopressin. Am J Obset Gynecol 1990;162:1115–1120.
40. Piacquadio KM, Brace RA, Cheung CY: Role of vasopressin in mediation of fetal cardiovascular responses to acute hypoxia. Am J Obstet Gynecol 1990;163:294–300.
41. Giussani DA, Riquelme RA, Sanhueza EM, et al: Adrenergic and vasopressinergic contributions to the cardiovascular response to acute hypoxaemia in the llama fetus. J Physiol (Lond) 1999;515:233–241.
42. Bocking AD, Gagnon R, White SE, et al: Circulatory responses to prolonged hypoxaemia in fetal sheep. Am J Obstet Gynecol 1988;159:1418–1424.
43. Rurak DW, Richardson BS, Patrick JE, et al: Blood flow and oxygen delivery to fetal organs and tissues during sustained hypoxemia. Am J Physiol 1990;258:R1116–R1122.
44. Stein P, White SE, Homan J, et al: Altered fetal cardiovascular responses to prolonged hypoxia after sinoaortic denervation. Am J Physiol 1999; 276: R340–R346.
45. Ashwal S, Dale PS, Longo LD: Regional cerebral blood flow: studies in the fetal lamb during hypoxia, hypercapnia, acidosis and hypertension. Pediatr Res 1984;18:1309–1316.
46. Richardson B, Korkola S, Asano H, et al: Regional blood flow and the endocrine response to sustained hypoxemia in the preterm fetus. Pediatr Res 1996;40:337–343.
47. Matsuda Y, Patrick J, Carmichael L, et al: Effects of sustained hypoxemia on the sheep fetus at midgestation: endocrine, cardiovascular, and biophysical responses. Am J Obstet Gynecol 1992;167:531–540.
48. Green LR, Homan J, White SE, Richardson BS: Cardiovascular and metabolic responses to intermittent umbilical cord occlusion in the preterm ovine fetus. J Soc Gynecol Investig 1999;6:56–63.
49. Hochachka PW, Land SC, Buck LT: Oxygen sensing and signal transduction in metabolic defense against hypoxia: lessons from vertebrate facultative anaerobes. Comp Biochem Physiol 1997;118A:23–29.

50. Hochachka PW, Buck LT, Doll CJ, Land SC: Unifying theory of hypoxia tolerance: molecular/metabolic defense and rescue mechanisms for surviving oxygen lack. Proc Natl Acad Sci USA 1996;93:9493–9498.
51. Lutz PL, Nilsson GE: Contrasting strategies for anoxic brain survival: glycolysis up or down? J Exp Biol 1997;200:411–419.
52. Castellini MA, Kooyman GL, Ponganis PJ: Metabolic rates of freely diving Weddell seals: correlations with oxygen stores, swim velocity and diving durations. J Exp Biol 1992;165:181–194.
53. Connett RJ, Honig CR, Gayeski TEJ, Brooks GA: Defining hypoxia: a systems view of VO_2, glycolysis, energetics and intracellular PO_2. J Appl Physiol 1990;68:833–842.
54. Wilkening RB, Meschia G: Fetal oxygen uptake and acid-base balance as a function of uterine blood flow. Am J Physiol 1983;244:H749–H755.
55. Bocking AD, White J, Homan J, Richardson BS: Oxygen consumption is maintained in fetal sheep during prolonged hypoxaemia. J Dev Physiol 1992;17:169–174.
56. Braems G, Jensen A: Hypoxia reduces oxygen consumption of fetal skeletal muscle cells in monolayer culture. J Devel Physiol 1992;16:209–215.
57. Walker V, Bennet L, Mills GA, et al: Effects of hypoxia on urinary organic acid and hypoxanthine excretion in fetal sheep. Pediatr Res 1996;40: 309–318.
58. Newman JP, Peebles DM, Harding SRG, et al: Hemodynamic and metabolic responses to moderate asphyxia in brain and skeletal muscle of late-gestation fetal sheep. J Appl Physiol 2000;88:82–90.
59. Clementi E, Brown GC, Feelisch M, Moncada S: Persistent inhibition of cell respiration by nitric oxide: crucial role of S-nitrosylation of mitochondrial complex I and protective effect of glutathione. Proc Natl Acad Sci USA 1998;95:7631–7636.
60. Behrooz A, Ismail-Beigi F: Stimulation of glucose transport by hypoxia: signals and mechanisms. News Physiol Sci 1999;14:105–110.
61. Ratcliffe PJ, O'Rourke JF, Maxwell PH, Pugh CW: Oxygen sensing, hypoxia-inducible factor-1 and the regulation of mammalian gene expression. J Exp Biol 1998;201:1153–1162.
62. Chandel NS, Maltepe E, Goldwasser E, et al: Mitochondrial reactive oxygen species trigger hypoxia-induced transcription. Proc Natl Acad Sci USA 1998;95:11715–11720.
63. Yu AY, Shimoda LA, Iyer NV, et al: Impaired physiological responses to chronic hypoxia in mice partially deficient for hypoxia-inducible factor 1 alpha. J Clin Invest 1999;103:691–696.
64. Royer C, Lachauer J, Crouzoulon G, et al: Effects of gestational hypoxia on mRNA levels of Glut3 and Glut4 transporters, hypoxia inducible factor-1 and thyroid hormone receptors in developing rat brain. Brain Res 2000;856:119–128.
65. Zaman K, Ryu H, Hall D, et al: Protection from oxidative stress-induced apoptosis in cortical neuronal cultures by iron chelators is associated with enhanced DNA binding of hypoxia-inducible factor-1 and ATF-1/CREB and increased expression of glycolytic enzymes, p21 (waf1/cip1), and erythropoietin. J Neurosci 1999;19:9821–9830.
66. Sawa R, Asakura, H, Power GG: Changes in plasma adenosine during simulated birth of fetal sheep. J Appl Physiol 1991;70:1524–1528.

67. Kubonoya K, Power GG: Plasma adenosine responses during repeated episodes of umbilical cord occlusion. Am J Obstet Gynecol 1997;177: 395–401.

68. Yoneyama Y, Wakatsuki M, Sawa R, et al: Plasma adenosine concentration in appropriate and small for gestational age fetuses. Am J Obstet Gynecol 1994;170:684–688.

69. Rudolphi KA, Schubert P, Parkinson FE, Fredholm BB: Neuroprotective role of adenosine in cerebral ischaemia. Trends Pharmacol Sci 1992;13: 439–445.

70. Gidday JM, Fitzgibbons JC, Shah AR, et al: Reduction in cerebral ischaemic injury in the newborn rat by potentiation of endogenous adenosine. Pediatr Res 1995;38:306–311.

71. Kurth CD, Wagerle LC: Cerebrovascular reactivity to adenosine analogues in 0.6–0.7 gestation and near term fetal sheep. Am J Physiol 1992;262: 1338–1342.

72. Laudignon N, Farri E, Beharry K, et al: Influence of adenosine on cerebral blood flow during hypoxic hypoxia in the newborn piglet. J Appl Physiol 1990;68:1534–1541.

73. Karimi A, Ball KT, Power GG: Exogenous infusion of adenosine depresses whole body O_2 use in fetal/neonatal sheep. J Appl Physiol 1996;81:541–547.

74. de Mendonca A, Ribiero JA: Adenosine inhibits the NMDA receptor-mediated excitatory postsynaptic potential in the hippocampus. Brain Res 1993;606:351–356.

75. Bona E, Aden U, Gilland E, et al: Neonatal cerebral hypoxia-ischaemia: the effect of adenosine receptor antagonists. Neuropharmacology 1997; 36:1327–1338.

76. Bennett L, Peebles DM, Edwards AD, et al: The cerebral hemodynamic response to asphyxia and hypoxia in the near-term fetal sheep as measured by near infrared spectroscopy. Pediatr Res 1998;44:1–7.

77. Mallard C, Gunn A, Williams C, et al: Transient umbilical cord occlusion causes hippocampal damage in the fetal sheep. Am J Obstet Gynecol 1992;167:1423–1430.

78. Gunn AJ, Parer JT, Mallard EC, et al: Cerebral histologic and electrocorticographic changes after asphyxia in fetal sheep. Pediatr Res 1992;31: 486–491.

79. Chen EY, Fujinaga M, Giaccia AJ: Hypoxic microenvironment within an embryo induces apoptosis and is essential for proper morphological development. Teratology 1999;60:215–225.

80. Dammann O, Leviton A: Brain damage in preterm newborns: might enhancement of developmentally regulated endogenous protection open a door for prevention? Pediatrics 1999;104:541–550.

81. Hagberg B, Hagberg G, Olow I, van Wendt L: The changing panorama of cerebral palsy in Sweden. VII. Prevalence and origin in the birth year period 1987–1990. Acta Paediatr 1996;85:954–960.

82. Volpe JJ: Brain injury in the premature infant: neuropathology, clinical aspects and pathogenesis. Clin Perinatol 1997;24:567–587.

83. Iwamoto HS, Kaufman T, Keil LC, Rudolph AM: Responses to acute hypoxemia in the fetal sheep at 0.6–0.7 gestation. Am J Physiol 1989;256: 613–620.

84. Matsuda T, Okuyama K, Cho K, et al: Induction of antenatal periventric-

ular leukomalacia by hemorrhagic hypotension in the chronically instrumented fetal sheep. Am J Obstet Gynecol 1999;181:725–730.

85. Szymonowicz W, Walker AM, Yu VYH, et al: Regional cerebral blood flow after haemorrhagic hypotension in the preterm, near term and newborn lamb. Pediatr Res 1990;28:361–366.

86. Myers RE: Two patterns of perinatal brain damage and their conditions of occurrence. Am J Obstet Gynecol 1972;112:246–276.

87. McDonald JW, Johnston MV: Physiological and pathophysiological roles of excitatory amino acids during central nervous system development. Brain Res Rev 1990;15:41–70.

88. Hagberg H, Gilland E, Diemer NH, Andine P: Hypoxia-ischaemia in the neonatal rat brain: histopathology after post-treatment with NMDA and non-NMDA receptor anatagonists. Biol Neonate 1994;66:205–213.

89. Anderson KJ, Mason KL, McGraw TS, et al: The ontogeny of glutamate receptors and D-aspartate binding sites in the ovine CNS. Dev Brain Res 1999;118:69–77.

90. Martin LJ, Fututa A, Blackstone CD: AMPA receptor protein in developing rat brain: glutamate receptor-1 expression and localisation change at regional, cellular and subcellular levels with maturation. Neuroscience 1998;83:917–928.

91. Berger R, Gjedde A, Hargater L, et al: Regional cerebral glucose utilisation in immature fetal guinea pigs during maternal isocapnic hypoxemia. Pediatr Res 1997;42:311–316.

92. Northington FJ, Tobin JR, Harris AP, et al: Developmental and regional differences in nitric oxide synthase activity and blood flow in the sheep brain. J Cereb Blood Flow Metab 1997;17:109–115.

93. Chugani HT, Phelps ME: Maturational changes in cerebral function in infants determined by 18FDG positron emission tomography. Science 1986;231:840–843.

94. Mishra OP, Delivoria-Papadopoulos M: Cellular mechanisms of hypoxic injury in the developing brain. Brain Res Bull 1999;48:233–238.

95. Maulik D, Zanelli S, Numagami Y, et al: Oxygen free radical generation during in-utero hypoxia in the fetal guinea pig brain: the effects of maturity and of magnesium sulfate administration. Brain Res 1999;817:117–122.

96. Reddy K, Mallard C, Guan J, et al: Maturational change in the cortical response to hypoperfusion injury in the fetal sheep. Pediatr Res 1998;43:674–682.

97. Mallard EC, Williams CE, Johnston BM, Gluckman PD: Increased vulnerability to neuronal damage after umbilical cord occlusion in fetal sheep with advancing gestation. Am J Obstet Gynecol 1994;170:206–214.

98. Bennet L, Rossenrode S, Gunning MI, et al: The cardiovascular and cerebrovascular responses of the immature fetal sheep to acute umbilical cord occlusion. J Physiol 1999;517:247–257.

99. Mallard EC, Waldvogel HJ, Williams CE, et al: Repeated asphyxia causes loss of striatal projection neurons in the fetal sheep brain. Neuroscience 1995;65:827–836.

100. Ohyu J, Marumo G, Ozawa H, et al: Early axonal and glial pathology in fetal sheep brains with leukomalacia induced by repeated umbilical cord occlusion. Brain Dev 1999;21:248–252.

101. Rees S, Breen S, Loeliger M, et al: Hypoxemia near mid-gestation has

long-term effects on fetal brain development. J Neuropathol Exp Neurol 1999;58:932–945.
102. Scherjon S, Briet J, Oosting H, Kok J: The discrepancy between maturation of visual-evoked potentials and cognitive outcome at five years in very preterm infants with and without hemodynamic signs of fetal brain sparing. Pediatrics 2000;105:385–391.
103. Nicolini U, Nicolaidis P, Fisk NM, et al: Limited role of fetal blood-sampling in prediction of outcome in intrauterine growth retardation. Lancet 1990; 336:768–772.
104. Sutterlein MW, Seelbach-Gobel B, Oehler MK, et al: Doppler ultrasonographic evidence of intra-partum brain sparing effect in fetuses with low oxygen saturation according to pulse oximetry. Am J Obstet Gynecol 1999;181:216–220.
105. Rizzo G, Arduini D, Luciano R, et al: Prenatal cerebral Doppler ultrasonography and neonatal neurological outcome. J Ultrasound Med 1989;8:237–240.
106. Noordam MJ, Heydanus R, Hop WC, et al: Doppler colour flow imaging of fetal intracerebral arteries and umbilical artery in the small for gestational age fetus. Br J Obstet Gynaecol 1994;101:504–508.
107. Laurichesse-Delmas H, Grimaud O, Moscoso G, Ville Y: Color Doppler study of the venous circulation in the fetal brain and hemodynamic study of the cerebral transverse sinus. Ultrasound Obstet Gynecol 1999;13:34–42.
108. Neilson JP: Doppler ultrasound in high risk pregnancies. In Enkin MW, Keirse MJNC, Renfrew MJ, Neilson JP (eds): Pregnancy and Childbirth Module. Cochrane Database of Systematic Reviews.
109. Chan FY, Pun TC, Lam P, et al: Fetal cerebral Doppler studies as a predictor of perinatal outcome and subsequent neurologic handicap. Obstet Gynecol 1996;87:981–988.
110. Arias F: Accuracy of the middle cerebral to umbilical artery resistance index ratio in the prediction of neonatal outcome in patients at high risk for fetal and neonatal complications. Am J Obstet Gynecol 1994;171:1541–1545.
111. Hershkovitz R, Kingdom JC, Geary M, Rodeck CH: Fetal cerebral blood flow redistribution in late gestation: identification of compromise in small fetuses with normal umbilical artery Doppler. Ultrasound Obstet Gynecol 2000;15:209–212.
112. Scherjon SA, Oosting H, Smolders-DeHaas H, et al: Neurodevelopmental outcome at three years of age after fetal "brain-sparing." Early Hum Dev 1998;52:67–79.
113. Keeney SE, Adcock EW, McArdle CB: Prospective observations of 100 high-risk neonates by high field (1.5 Tesla) magnetic resonance imaging of the central nervous system. II. Lesions associated with hypoxic-ischemic encephalopathy. Pediatrics 1991;87:431–436.
114. Maalouf EF, Duggan PJ, Rutherford MA, et al: Magnetic resonance imaging of the brain in a cohort of extremely preterm infants. J Pediatr 1999;135:351–357.
115. Lan LM, Yamashita Y, Tang Y, et al: Normal fetal brain development: MR imaging with a half-fourier rapid acquisition with relaxation enhancement sequence. Radiology 2000;215:205–210.
116. Sonigo PC, Rypens FF, Carteret M, et al: MR imaging of fetal cerebral anomalies. Pediatr Radiol 1998;28:212–222.

117. D'Ercole C, Girard N, Cravello L, et al: Prenatal diagnosis of fetal corpus callosum agenesis by ultrasonography and magnetic resonance imaging. Prenat Diagn 1998;18:247–253.

118. Hykin J, Moore R, Duncan K, et al: fMRI of fetus. Lancet 1999;354: 645–646.

119. Thornton JS, Ordidge RJ, Penrice J, et al: Temporal and anatomical variations of brain water apparent diffusion coefficient in perinatal cerebral hypoxic-ischemic injury: relationships to cerebral energy metabolism. Magn Reson Med 1998;39:920–927.

120. Lorek A, Takei Y, Cady EB, et al: Delayed ("secondary") cerebral energy failure following acute hypoxia-ischaemia in the newborn piglet: continuous 48-hour studies by 31P magentic resonance spectroscopy. Pediatr Res 1994;36:699–706.

121. Hope PL, Costello AM, Cady EB, et al: Cerebral energy metabolism studied with phosphorus NMR spectroscopy in normal and birth-asphyxiated infants. Lancet 1984;2:366–370.

122. Martin E, Buchli R, Ritter S, et al: Diagnostic and prognostic value of cerebral 31P magnetic resonance spectroscopy in neonates with perinatal asphyxia. Pediatr Res 1996;40:749–758.

123. Taylor DL, Edwards AD, Mehmet H: Oxidative metabolism, apoptosis and perinatal brain injury. Brain Pathol 1999;9:93–117.

124. Penrice J, Lorek A, Cady EB, et al: Proton magnetic resonance spectroscopy of the brain during acute hypoxia-ischaemia and delayed cerebral energy failure in the newborn piglet. Pediatr Res 1997;41:795–802.

125. Hakumaki JM, Poptani H, Sandmair AM, et al: ^{1}H MRS detects polyunsaturated fatty acid accumulation during gene therapy of glioma: implications for the *in vivo* detection of apoptosis. Nat Med 1999;5:1323–1327.

126. van Cappellen AM, Heerschap A, Nijhuis JG, et al: Hypoxia, the subsequent systemic metabolic acidosis, and their relationship with cerebral metabolite concentrations: an in vivo study in fetal lambs with proton magnetic resonance spectroscopy. Am J Obstet Gynecol 1999;181:1537–1545.

127. Heerschap A, van den Berg PP: Proton magnetic resonance spectroscopy of human fetal brain. Am J Obstet Gynecol 1994;170:1150–1151.

CHAPTER 11

Intrapartum Hypoxic-Ischemic Brain Injury

Jenny A. Westgate, Laura Bennet, Alistair J. Gunn

Introduction

The focus of this chapter is impaired fetal gas exchange during labor: how it happens, how the fetus responds, and how clinicians can detect such events. The fetus is highly adapted to intrauterine conditions, which include low partial pressures of oxygen and a relatively limited supply of other substrates compared to postnatal life. The fetus cannot store significant amounts of oxygen and, for a steady supply, it is wholly dependent on placental gas exchange and transport of oxygenated blood from the placenta to the fetus, via the umbilical vein. Despite this, the normal fetus has a surplus of oxygen relative to its metabolic needs, which it can further augment or redirect, as described later in this chapter. The surplus provides a significant margin of safety when oxygen delivery is impaired.

Labor is a critical period in life. At no other time is a human being so likely to encounter such significant impairment of gas exchange. The fact that most fetuses survive labor without injury is a function of their extraordinary capacity to adapt to repeated interruptions of gas exchange related to uterine contractions. This chapter addresses only the full-term pregnancy; however, many of the same considerations apply to the preterm pregnancy.

Hypoxia and Asphyxia

Hypoxia, by definition, is a reduction in oxygen supply leading to hypoxemia (i.e., a reduction in partial pressure of oxygen in the blood).

This work has been supported by National Institutes of Health grant RO-1 HD32752, and by grants from the Health Research Council of New Zealand, Lottery Health Board of New Zealand, and the Auckland Medical Research Foundation.
From Donn SM, Sinha SK, Chiswick ML (eds): *Birth Asphyxia and the Brain: Basic Science and Clinical Implications.* © 2002, Futura Publishing Co., Inc., Armonk, NY.

In these circumstances oxygen delivery to the fetus is reduced, but overall fetal gas exchange is unaffected. The fetus is able to compensate for oxygen supply reduced to the equivalent of approximately 50% of uterine artery blood flow, by increasing blood flow and oxygen extraction and decreasing oxygen demand. Under these conditions, the fetus is able to maintain the removal of the waste products of metabolism, mainly carbon dioxide and water, and thus avoids any oxygen debt and does not become acidotic.

Stable fetal hypoxia occurs exclusively in the antenatal period but, unfortunately, it is difficult to detect clinically, especially if hypoxia occurs late in gestation so that fetal growth is not obviously slowed. Experimental studies in sheep have demonstrated the impressive ability of the late gestation fetus to adapt to prolonged mild inhalational hypoxia; after 12 hours, fetal blood pressure, acid-base status, movements, fetal heart rate (FHR) variability, and accelerations all returned to baseline levels.[1,2] Only the FHR showed a significant elevation from the original baseline.[3] With time, fetuses can improve tissue oxygen delivery during chronic hypoxia to near baseline levels by increasing hemoglobin synthesis, mediated by greater erythropoietin release.[4]

Asphyxia is defined as impaired respiratory gas exchange (i.e., hypoxia and hypercapnia) accompanied by the development of metabolic acidosis. When we consider the impact of clinical asphyxia on the brain, it is critical to keep in mind that this definition reflects much about things that can be measured relatively easily (i.e., blood gases and systemic acidosis) and essentially nothing about fetal blood pressure or perfusion, or brain metabolism and function, the factors that contribute directly to the pathogenesis of brain injury.

Asphyxia is a continuum and may be graded according to the degree of hypercapnia and metabolic acidosis. Clearly, if antenatal hypoxia is sufficient to exceed fetal compensatory mechanisms, respiratory and metabolic acidosis will develop. Once asphyxia with a progressive metabolic acidosis has developed, the fetus will not be able to continue to adapt indefinitely.[3] Further, preexisting hypoxia/asphyxia is highly likely to impair fetal ability to adapt to the additional stress of labor. Unfortunately, clinical identification of either hypoxia or developing asphyxia is difficult and is based primarily on the following information: maternal reports of reduced fetal movement; abnormal antenatal fetal heart patterns; and ultrasound assessment of fetal movement, tone, and umbilical artery Doppler waveforms. As a result, fetuses may enter labor in an unrecognized, already compromised condition with either stable, compensated hypoxia, or varying degrees of asphyxia.

The Effect of Uterine Contractions on Fetal Gas Exchange

During labor, maternal blood supply to the placenta is normally reduced by uterine contractions,[5] so that oxygen levels in fetal blood are reduced during contractions and recover once placental flow resumes.[6] Doppler studies in humans have shown an almost linear relationship between the fall in uterine artery flow and a rise in intrauterine pressure, from 0 to 60 mmHg. Median flow was reduced by 60% (range, 48–73%) when intrauterine pressure increased by 60 mmHg.[7] The direct effect of increased pressure may be augmented by compression of the umbilical cord. Normally, the cord is cushioned by amniotic fluid; however, during oligohydramnios or after rupture of the membranes the cord may be compressed between the fetus and the abdominal wall.[8,9]

Thus, the key, distinctive characteristic of labor is the development of intermittent, repetitive asphyxia. Even during normal labor, this intermittent impairment of placental gas exchange results in a fall in pH and oxygen tension, and a rise in carbon dioxide and base deficit.[10,11] Therefore, during labor, essentially all fetuses are technically exposed to "asphyxia." Fortunately, it is usually mild and well tolerated by the fetus. Unfortunately, the term "asphyxia" is often associated with the development of severe metabolic acidosis, postasphyxial encephalopathy, and other end-organ damage or death. In our haste to avoid using the term, the normal nature of labor and its effects on the fetus are often not fully appreciated.

The adaptations of the fetus to the inevitable asphyxia of labor are sufficiently effective in the majority of cases that the concept of "birth asphyxia" itself has been controversial. Indeed, the majority of cases of cerebral palsy appear to be related to antenatal events.[12] Nevertheless, studies monitoring cerebral function from birth demonstrate the existence of cases of early onset, evolving cerebral injury after birth, associated with acidosis or evidence of immediate peripartum precipitating events.[13–15] Follow-up of these children has shown that a significant number have long-term cognitive or functional sequelae, demonstrating that birth asphyxia is a true syndrome.[13]

Pathologic or Exacerbated Asphyxia

A number of events, some peculiar to labor, may result in fetal compromise during labor. These may be broadly grouped as chronic, acute catastrophic, and repeated hypoxia. Chronic hypoxia is discussed more fully in Chapter 10, and may be caused by decreased fetal hemoglobin (e.g., fetomaternal or fetofetal hemorrhage), infection, and maternal causes such as systemic hypoxia and reduced uteroplacental blood flow from hypotension. Catastrophic events include cord prolapse, cord entanglements, true knots, vasa previa, placental abruption, uterine rupture, and entrapment, such as shoulder dystocia.

Repeated asphyxia is almost entirely related in some way to uterine contractions. In turn, the effects of repeated hypoxia may be amplified by fetal vulnerability, for example, from intrauterine growth restriction and/or chronic hypoxia, or by greater severity of contractions as discussed in the following section. Even a normal fetus, with normal placental function, may not be able to fully adapt to hyperstimulation causing brief, but severe asphyxia that is repeated with excessive frequency.

Uterine Contraction Patterns

Uterine contractions have such a significant impact on fetal gas exchange during labor that it is worth examining their effect in more detail. Contraction patterns preceding and during labor have been well described.[16] Prelabor contractions occur infrequently and reach pressures of 20 to 30 mmHg. The accompanying reduction in placental perfusion may be sufficient to further compromise an already hypoxic or asphyxiated fetus. The frequency and intensity of contractions increase progressively during labor until, in the second stage, contractions of up to 60 mmHg can occur every 2.5 to 3 minutes. Thus, the second stage of normal labor is the time of greatest asphyxial stress for the fetus, and it is accompanied by a more rapid decline in pH[10,17,18] and transcutaneous oxygen tension[11,18] and a rise in transcutaneous carbon dioxide tension.[18]

Although contraction strength is important, once labor is established contraction frequency and duration are the key factors that determine the rate at which fetal asphyxia develops (Figure 1). The proportion of time the uterus spends at resting tone compared with contracting tone will determine the extent to which fetal gas exchange can be restored between contractions.[11] Studies using near-infrared spectroscopy have shown a progressive fall in cerebral oxygen saturation when contractions occur more frequently than every 2.3 minutes.[19] Any intervention that increases the frequency and/or duration of uterine contractions clearly places the fetus at increased risk of asphyxia. The dangers of uterine hyperstimulation or prolonged tonic contractions with oxytocin infusion used for induction or augmentation are well established.[5] Similarly, the use of prostaglandin preparations to induce labor also carries a risk of excessive uterine activity.[20,21]

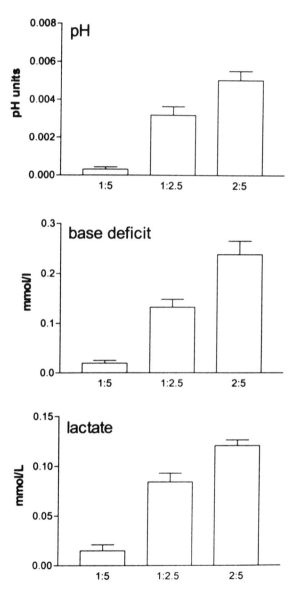

Figure 1. The rate of deterioration of acid-base status of near-term fetal sheep subjected to three different protocols of repeated umbilical cord occlusion: 1-minute occlusions repeated every 5 (1:5) or every 2.5 minutes (1:2.5), or 2-minute occlusions repeated every 5 minutes (2:5). The rise in hydrogen ion concentration (pH units), base deficit, and lactate per minute increased significantly as the intensity of the occlusion protocol increased (p<0.0001, one-way ANOVA).

Fetal Cardiovascular Responses to Hypoxia and Asphyxia

If the fetus has insufficient oxygen for its needs, even after optimizing oxygen delivery and extraction, several strategies are available. First, anaerobic metabolism can support production of high-energy metabolites for a limited time. However, the use of anaerobic metabolism is very inefficient since anaerobic glycolysis produces lactate and only 2 molecules of adenosine triphosphate (ATP), whereas aerobic glycolysis produces 38 molecules of ATP. Thus, glucose reserves are rapidly consumed, and metabolic acidosis develops with local and systemic consequences. Local tissue glycogen levels, particularly in the heart, are particularly important to support blood pressure during rapid, temporary periods of profound hypoxia.[22,23] Second, the fetus can, to some extent, reduce nonobligatory energy consumption by reducing physical activity and cellular metabolism.

Many experimental techniques have been used to study fetal responses to hypoxia and asphyxia, with most studies performed in the chronically instrumented fetal sheep. Pure hypoxia is typically induced by reducing the maternal inspired oxygen fraction to 0.1, and adding carbon dioxide to the gas mixture to maintain normocapnia. However, studies of asphyxia require a greater depth of hypoxia than is possible using maternal hypoxia and usually involve occlusion of either the maternal aorta or the fetal umbilical cord.[24] Furthermore, asphyxia can be induced relatively abruptly compared with inhalational hypoxia, limiting the time available for fetal adaptation.[25]

Hypoxia

Experimental data suggest that, during hypoxia, the normally grown fetus is very able to adapt to episodes of oxygen deficiency with cardiovascular, hormonal, metabolic, and behavioral adjustments.[26] These adaptive features include: tachycardia; left shift of the oxygen dissociation curve (which increases the capacity to carry and extract oxygen at low oxygen tensions); the ability to significantly reduce energy-consuming processes; increased anaerobic capability in many tissues; and the redistribution of blood flow toward essential organs and away from the periphery. By such adaptations, the fetus can maintain normal oxygen consumption until oxygen delivery is reduced by half. Additional structural features of the fetal circulation also augment these adaptive features. The structural features include shunts such as the ductus arteriosus, and preferential blood flow streaming within the inferior vena cava to avoid intermixing of oxygenated blood from the placenta and deoxygenated blood in the fetal venous system. These features ensure maximal oxygen delivery to essential organs such as the brain and heart. The preferential streaming patterns may be augmented during hypoxia to help maintain oxygen delivery to these organs.[27]

Asphyxia

During mild to moderate asphyxia of acute onset, there is usually an initial moderate transient bradycardia followed by tachycardia, as seen during prolonged partial cord occlusion. There is a rise in blood pressure and a redistribution of combined ventricular output, which leads to an increase in blood flow to vital organs, the brain, heart and adrenals, and a decrease in blood flow to peripheral organs.[28] Oxygen content can be reduced to as low as 1 mmol/L without compromising cerebral oxygen consumption because cerebral blood flow and oxygen extraction are increased as compensation.[29]

During acute severe asphyxia, however, the cardiovascular responses of the normal fetus are substantially different. Bradycardia is sustained and blood flow to the brain may not increase, although within the brain, blood flow is preferentially redirected to the brainstem to maintain autonomic function at the expense of areas such as the cerebrum.[25,30] When oxygen content falls below 1 mmol/L, cerebral blood flow fails to rise because of a significant increase in cerebral vascular resistance.[29,31–33] The fetus is unable to extract further oxygen, and cerebral oxygen consumption falls. During this insult, blood pressure initially increases markedly, but this rise is not sustained, and as hypoxia continues the fetus becomes hypotensive. The sustained bradycardia and increased peripheral resistance in the late gestation fetus during asphyxia are mediated by chemoreflexes, with a logarithmic rise in circulating catecholamine concentrations augmenting peripheral vasoconstriction.[34] The carotid chemoreflex that initiates the fall in FHR is very closely correlated with reduction of fetal arterial oxygen saturation,[35] whether secondary to reduced uterine blood flow or to cord compression.[36]

Hypotension is primarily related to asphyxial impairment of myocardial contractility, because of a direct inhibitory effect of profound acidosis and depletion of myocardial glycogen stores.[37] After glycogen has been depleted, there is a rapid loss of high-energy metabolites, such as ATP in mitochondria.[22] During a short episode (e.g., 5 minutes) of asphyxia, the fetus may not become hypotensive. If the insult is repeat-ed before myocardial glycogen can be replenished, successive periods of asphyxia will be associated with increasing duration of hypotension.[38,39]

Brief Repeated Asphyxia

It is particularly relevant to study fetal responses under condi-tions similar to labor. Brief repeated asphyxia can be produced in the fetal sheep by repeated occlusions of the umbilical cord at frequencies that represent different stages of labor. We have compared the effect of 1 minute of umbilical cord occlusion repeated every 5 minutes (1:5 group, consistent with early labor) and 1-minute occlusions repeated every 2.5 minutes (1:2.5 group, consistent with late first stage and sec-ond stage labor). Occlusions were continued for 4 hours or until fetal hypotension (<20 mmHg) occurred.[39,40] The FHR and blood pressure changes for these two occlusion groups are shown in Figure 2.

1:5 occlusion series (Figure 2A). The onset of each occlusion was accompanied by a variable FHR deceleration and a return to baseline levels between occlusions. Fetal mean arterial presure (MAP) rose at the onset of each occlusion and never fell below baseline levels during the occlusions. There was a sustained elevation in baseline MAP between occlusions. A small fall in pH and rise in base deficit and lac-tate occurred in the first 30 minutes of occlusions (pH 7.34 ± 0.07, base deficit 1.3 ± 3.9 mmol/L, and lactate 4.5 ± 1.3 mmol/L), but no subsequent change occurred despite a further 3.5 hours of occlusions. This experiment demonstrated the capacity of the healthy fetus to fully adapt to repeated episodes of asphyxia.

1:2.5 occlusion series (Figure 2B). Although this again produces a series of variable decelerations, the outcome in this group was sub-stantially different. The rapid occlusion frequency provided only a brief period of recovery between occlusions, which was inadequate to allow fetal reoxygenation and replenishment of glycogen stores.

Three 30-minute phases in the fetal response to occlusions have been observed. These include initial adjustment, a stable compensatory phase, and decompensation. The phases are discussed separately below.

Initial adjustment phase, first 30 minutes. A progressive tachycar-dia developed in the interval between occlusions. During the first three occlusions, there was a sustained rise in MAP during occlusions, fol-lowed by recovery to baseline once the occlusion ended. After the third occlusion, all fetuses developed a biphasic blood pressure response to successive occlusions, with initial hypertension followed by a fall in MAP, reaching a nadir a few seconds after release of the occluder. However, minimum MAP did not fall below baseline values. Over this initial 30 minutes, pH fell from 7.40 ± 0.01 to 7.25 ± 0.02, base deficit rose from 2.6 ± 0.6 to 3.3 ± 1.1 mmol/L, and lactate rose from 0.9 ± 0.1 to 3.9 ± 0.6 mmol/L.

Stable compensatory phase, mid 30 minutes. Minimum FHR during occlusions fell ($p<0.001$ compared to the first 30 minutes) and the interocclusion baseline rose ($p<0.01$ compared to the first 30 minutes). Although minimum MAP did fall at the end of each occlusion, it never fell below baseline levels. Despite a stable blood pressure response, without hypotension, the metabolic acidosis slowly worsened: pH fell from 7.14 ± 0.03 to 7.09 ± 0.03, base deficit rose from 11.8 ± 1.1 to 13.6 ± 1.2 mmol/L, and lactate rose from 8.2 ± 0.8 to 9.9 ± 0.7 mmol/L.

Decompensation, last 30 minutes. Minimum FHR during decelerations continued to fall ($p<0.001$ compared to mid 30 minutes) but there was no further rise in the interocclusion baseline FHR. Minimum MAP fell below baseline levels and the degree of hypotension became greater with successive occlusions. During the last 30 minutes all animals developed a severe metabolic acidosis, with pH 6.92 ± 0.03, base deficit 19.2 ± 1.46 mmol/L, and lactate 14.6 ± 0.8 mmol/L by the end of occlusions. The studies were stopped after a mean of 183 ± 43 min (range, 140–235 minutes). The key difference in outcome between the two groups was that the 1:2.5 group developed focal neuronal damage in the parasagittal cortex, the thalamus, and the cerebellum,[40] whereas no damage was seen in the 1:5 group. The effect of these two paradigms on a number of features of the FHR recording and fetal electrocardiogram (ECG) parameters was analyzed; these data are discussed later in this chapter.[41–44]

Acute-on-Chronic Asphyxia

Chronic antenatal asphyxia may also adversely affect the ability of the fetus to adapt to acute insults.[45] Chronic placental insufficiency leads to fetal arterial hypertension and myocardial hypertrophy with increased umbilical artery resistance. Experimentally growth-restricted fetuses exhibit sustained elevation of plasma catecholamines, cortisol, and prostaglandin E_2, with a significant fall in corticotrophin. In addition, when challenged with hypoxia, they have a blunted rise in plasma catecholamines, and cardiovascular responses in general.[45] In contrast, despite exposure to chronic hypoxia, the llama fetus does not show a blunted chemoreflex response; additional mechanisms such as increased vasopressin act to produce an intense vasoconstrictor response.[46] There is surprisingly little systematic data on the effect of

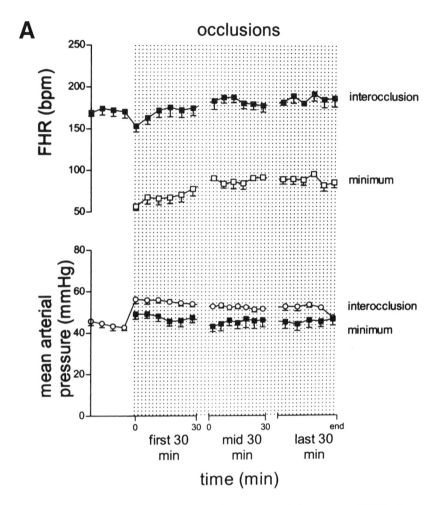

Figure 2. Fetal heart rate (FHR) and mean arterial pressure (MAP) changes occurring in near-term fetal sheep exposed to: (**A**) 1-minute umbilical cord occlusion repeated every 5 minutes for 4 hours (1:5 group), and (**B**) 1-minute occlusions repeated every 2.5 minutes (1:2.5 group) until the fetal MAP fell to less than 20 mmHg. The minimum FHR and MAP during each occlusion and the interocclusion FHR and MAP are shown. As the individual experiments in the 1: 2.5 group were of unequal duration, the data in both groups are presented for three time intervals: the first 30 minutes, the mid 30 minutes (defined as the median ±15 minutes), and the final 30 minutes of occlusions. Note that, in the 1:5 group, there was no significant change in interocclusion baseline FHR, and minimum MAP during occlusions never fell below pre-occlusion levels. In the 1:2.5 group, note that the interocclusion FHR rose in the first and mid 30 minutes. The minimum MAP fell steadily in the first 30 minutes, stabilized in the mid 30 minutes, and fell progressively in the last 30 minutes.

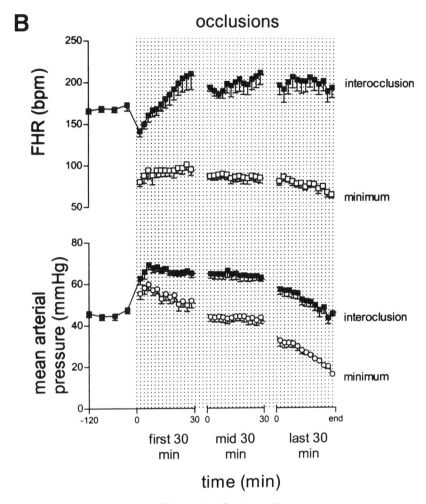

Figure 2. (Continued.)

chronic hypoxia on the response to labor-like insults. However, we can reasonably predict that such fetuses will have limited oxygen-carrying capacity and reduced glycogen levels, and thus will decompensate more quickly during repeated hypoxia.

What Initiates Neuronal Injury?

It is recognized that severe asphyxia may affect the function of many fetal organ systems.[47] However, the primary focus of attention is the effect of severe asphyxia on brain function and its role in producing neuronal injury. Though this topic has been considered in depth in the previous chapters, it is useful at this point to summarize some basic concepts relating to neuronal injury.

At the most fundamental level, injury requires a period of insufficient delivery of oxygen and substrates such as glucose (and, in the fetus, other substances, such as lactate) so that neurons (and glia) cannot maintain homeostasis. If oxygen is reduced but substrate delivery is effectively maintained (i.e., pure or nearly pure hypoxia), the cells adapt in two ways. First, they can use anaerobic metabolism to support their production of high-energy metabolites for a limited time. However, this rapidly consumes glucose reserves and a metabolic acidosis develops with local and systemic consequences. Second, neurons (and presumably other brain cells) can reduce their basal oxygen consumption. Moderate hypoxia typically induces a switch to lower frequency states, while during severe hypoxia neuronal activity ceases at a threshold above that which causes depolarization.

In contrast, when both oxygen and substrate are reduced, the options for the neuron are much more limited because there is not only less oxygen, there is also less glucose available to allow anaerobic metabolism. This may occur either during pure ischemia (reduced tissue blood flow) or, more critically, during hypoxia-ischemia (i.e., a reduction of both oxygen content and cerebral blood flow). In the fetus, hypoxia-ischemia commonly occurs because of profound hypoxic cardiac compromise.

These concepts help to explain the highly consistent observation that there is a strong correlation between either the depth or the duration of hypotension, and the amount of neuronal loss, as illustrated by Figure 3.[40,48,49] In fetal lambs exposed to prolonged severe partial asphyxia, neuronal loss occurred only in those that had had one or more episodes of acute hypotension.[49] In contrast, in a similar study in which an equally "severe" insult was induced gradually and titrated to maintain normal or elevated blood pressure throughout the insult, no neuronal loss was seen outside the cerebellum.[50] In the brief repeated occlusion paradigm shown in Figure 2, fetuses that developed cerebral infarcts were hypotensive significantly longer than were fetuses with no or minor damage.[40]

Fetal acidosis is much less important in neuronal injury. First impressions suggest that the presence of an oxygen deficit, as shown by lactate levels or base deficit, should correlate strongly with injury. Consideration of the observations noted above, however, suggests that although some acidosis must be present because of the presence of bio-

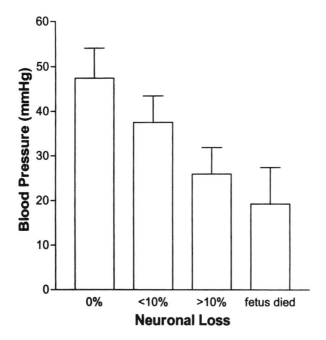

Figure 3. The proportion of neuronal loss and fetal mortality is related to the severity of hypotension following prolonged interruption of uterine blood flow in near-term fetal sheep (r = 0.69, p<0.01). From Gunn et al,[49] with permission.

chemical asphyxia, it can only have the crudest possible relationship with cerebral injury. Systemic acidosis during asphyxia is primarily related to peripheral hypoperfusion, secondary to local vasoconstriction acting to redistribute blood flow to essential organs. The contribution from cerebral acid production is relatively small. As long as sufficient glucose is available to neurons to support basal energy metabolism, injury will not occur. Thus, successful protection of the brain may accompany profound arterial metabolic acidosis, with a normal outcome. Conversely, during acute severe insults with impaired tissue perfusion, less glucose is delivered to the neurons, so less lactate is produced, and injury may occur at relatively modest levels of acidosis. Finally, acute-on-chronic insults, in which there is reduced fetal metabolic reserve, have the potential to lead to injury after shorter periods of acute asphyxia than are required to injure a healthy fetus, and consequently with relatively moderate acidosis.

Clinical Implications

Many of the conclusions drawn from experimental asphyxia have been borne out by clinical experience. For example, severe acidosis is associated with encephalopathy in only 40% of cases, while encephalopathy still occurs, although less frequently, with even moderate acidosis.[51]

As we attempt to determine methods of detecting the human fetus at risk of compromise during labor, it is necessary to consider the practical consequences that arise from these experimental data. Impaired gas exchange and mild asphyxia are part of normal labor, but the normal fetus has an enormous ability to respond to hypoxia and asphyxia and maintain the function of essential organs such as the brain and the heart. The ability to measure fetal pH or oxygenation at any one point may not tell us accurately about heart or brain function or the stage of compensation that the fetus has reached. Fetal blood pressure would be more helpful, but we are unable to measure this at present.

What sort of fetal problem are we trying to detect? If the fetus is being monitored, there is no difficulty in detecting the prolonged bradycardia that accompanies an acute, catastrophic event, such as abruption or prolapse of the umbilical cord. Such events account for approximately 25% of cases of moderate-to-severe post-asphyxial encephalopathy and are seldom predictable, or even potentially preventable.[15]

The central clinical issue is the identification of fetuses in whom adaptation to repeated asphyxia is beginning to fail. The options for doing this are limited because access to the fetus is restricted. Traditionally, we try to assess fetal condition by assessing changes in FHR and, occasionally, fetal scalp pH measurements. Newer methods for fetal surveillance include fetal pulse oximetry, near-infrared spectroscopy, and analysis of specific features of the fetal ECG. The following sections review the extent to which these techniques can provide information on fetal compensatory ability.

Fetal Heart Rate Changes During Labor

The absence of FHR decelerations, the presence of a normal baseline heart rate, and the absence of significant change in FHR variability indicate that a fetus is compensating well for mild asphyxia. The appearance of a FHR deceleration indicates that the fetal chemoreflex has responded to a hypoxic stimulus with a vagally mediated bradycardia. There are older data indicating that pressure on the fetal head in the second stage of labor can cause bradycardia[52]; however, this is likely to represent increased intracranial pressure and a reduction in cerebral perfusion. If the degree of hypoxia is severe and prolonged, the initial vagal bradycardia will, after a few minutes, be sustained by myocardial hypoxia. Fortunately, during labor most episodes of hypoxia are brief, lasting for only about a minute and thus causing only brief decelerations.

The terminology that has evolved around decelerations in labor has had a pernicious influence. When continuous electronic monitoring of the FHR during labor became possible in the late 1950s, many researchers developed classification systems based upon hours of observations of FHR recordings. Hon and Quilligan initially described three distinct types of decelerations (early, variable, and late) on the basis of both the shape and timing of decelerations relative to the contractions.[53] Caldeyro-Barcia described type 1 and type 2 deceleration on the basis of timing with respect to the contraction (type 1 with the contraction, and type 2 after the contraction).[52,54] These classifications have become ambiguous over time and many physicians, nurses, and midwives today describe decelerations only in terms of their timing with respect to contractions as "early" (type 1) or "late" (type 2). The brief shallow decelerations originally described by Hon as "early" decelerations are not associated with fetal acidosis, so it is mistakenly assumed that any deceleration that is synchronous with a contraction is innocuous, irrespective of its severity (Figure 4). In fact, true early decelerations occur infrequently during labor[55] and are probably just mild variable decelerations.[36] Similarly, true late decelerations, as described by Hon, are rarely seen in active labor, as this pattern is most commonly associated with chronically asphyxiated fetuses in early labor or in the antenatal period.

The authors propose that the terms "early," "vagal," and "hypoxic" deceleration should be abandoned, and that the term "late" deceleration should only be used in relation to antenatal recordings. In practice, all decelerations related to labor are "variable," have an abrupt fall in FHR from the baseline, and frequently vary in shape, depth, and duration. Most variable decelerations are more or less closely related to contractions. It has been assumed that any variable deceleration that occurs after a contraction (a "late" variable deceleration) indicates direct myocardial hypoxia, but this is not the case. Early clinical studies of FHR patterns during labor showed that "late" decelerations could occur for 90–100 minutes before acidosis was noted[56] and were associated with soft markers of "fetal distress" (i.e., 1 minute Apgar scores <7 or pH <7.25) in only 40–50% of cases.[57]

At present, the mechanisms responsible for "late" variable deceler-

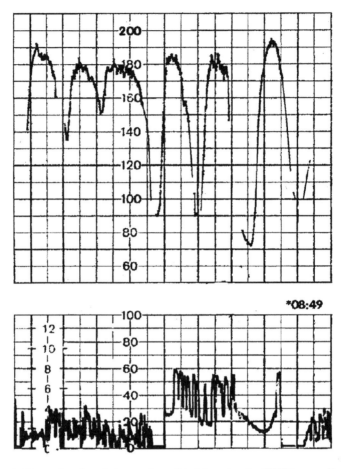

Figure 4. Example of an intrapartum fetal heart rate (FHR) recording showing severe variable decelerations that were misinterpreted as "type 1 dips."

ations (i.e., variables which occur after a contraction) are unclear. In one study, the maternal aorta was occluded, upstream from the fetus, so there was a time lag between occlusion and the reduction in fetal oxygenation, and consequently, the deceleration.[58] Another study associated "late" decelerations with background hypoxia and acidosis during induced labor in the rhesus monkey.[59] In both studies, however, the deceleration was temporally associated with actual arterial desaturation. There is some evidence that late *recovery* from variable decelerations may result from reversible subendocardial injury, although the onset was not delayed.[60] It may be relevant that partial (50%) reduction of umbilical cord blood flow is associated with a relatively slow onset of bradycardia.[36] True "late" decelerations in the antenatal or early labor period may suggest a fetus with limited oxygen/glycogen reserves, who was exposed to small reductions in blood flow that would not cause bradycardia in a healthy fetus.

Earlier emphasis on distinguishing reflex and hypoxic bradycardia has led to some misunderstanding. The chemoreflex that mediates the first few minutes of FHR deceleration is a highly sensitive indicator of hypoxemia as well as a significant component of fetal adaptation. Decelerations from true myocardial hypoxia do not occur unless hypoxia is continued for a prolonged time or unless the fetus is chronically hypoxic, with low reserves of myocardial glycogen. The depth to which the FHR falls is broadly related to the severity of the hypoxia.[36] Shallow decelerations indicate a modest reduction in utero-placental flow, while deep decelerations indicate near or total cessation in flow. Unfortunately, once deep decelerations are established, there is relatively little further change in the shape of the deceleration despite repeated decelerations and the consequent development of hypotension.[39] Thus, the typical variable deceleration in FHR can only be attributed to exposure to a brief period of asphyxia.

As the duration and frequency of contractions increase, the ability of the fetus to recover between occlusions must be reduced correspondingly, and thus these features give us more information about the potential importance of a series of decelerations. As highlighted by the studies shown in Figure 1, prolonged occlusions (more than 1 minute in duration), or very frequent contractions (occurring more often than 2.5 minutes apart) ultimately lead to decompensation even in healthy fetuses. It is must be emphasized, however, that the pre-labor condition of the fetus, which often is not easy to ascertain, will have a considerable impact. In a healthy fetus exposed to short (1 minute) variable decelerations, decompensation may be expected to take many hours. Pilot data suggest that a chronically hypoxic fetus, with low reserves of myocardial glycogen and an impaired baseline oxygen level, may be expected to deteriorate even with infrequent decelerations in early labor. The specific effects of preexisting hypoxia require further study.

Experimentally, during brief repeated asphyxia leading to progressive fetal decompensation (1:2.5 group), several features are observed in the interocclusion FHR that may distinguish them from a less severe insult (shown by the 1:5 group). First, the decelerations become deeper (Figure 2B), from both a lower nadir and the development of the second feature, intercurrent fetal tachycardia.[39] This tachycardia results from increased catecholamine activity[37] and is not seen in less frequent, well-compensated occlusions.[37,42] Third, overshoot accelerations following the deceleration were noted; these were probably related to a combination of the release of vagal inhibition and increasing catecholamine levels.[43]

Fetal Heart Rate Variability

Fetal heart rate variability is one of the classic components of FHR analysis. A stable baseline FHR with no change in FHR variability indicates adequate fetal compensation.[41] Experimentally, acute hypoxia is first accompanied by an increase in FHR variation, which is consistent with many clinical observations. For example, in a clinical case of inadvertent maternal hypoxemia in labor, an immediate increase in variability was seen.[61] In a prospective study of 394 women, Pello et al reported that FHR variation increased threefold during the second stage of labor.[62] However, this consistent experimental observation has not been emphasized adequately in training related to clinical FHR interpretation.

Chronic hypoxia is consistently associated with reduced FHR variation in both experimental[63,64] and clinical antenatal studies.[65,66] However, the FHR variation response to repeated umbilical cord occlusion was more complex than expected. After the initial increase in FHR variation, progressive hypoxia was associated with a decrease in FHR variation in two thirds of fetuses, but an additional increase was seen in the remaining third (Figure 5).[41]

Thus, there are definite FHR changes associated with progressive intermittent fetal asphyxia. These include recurrent FHR decelerations that become larger, and a progressive baseline FHR tachycardia, accompanied initially by increased FHR variation, which may subsequently become reduced. Overshoot accelerations will eventually occur in cases of umbilical cord occlusion. At any time, severe prolonged asphyxia will result in prolonged bradycardia. However, the appearance of these changes is regarded as an insensitive predictor of fetal condition because of the unique ability of the fetus to compensate for hypoxia. Both experimental[39] and clinical[56] studies show that a healthy fetus can display an abnormal FHR pattern for some time without fetal hypotension, and with only a slow deterioration in acid-base status, before entering a phase of rapid decompensation. The clinician's role is to identify the fetus under hypoxic stress and to judge whether or not spontaneous delivery is likely to occur well before fetal decompensation begins. This decision-making process requires the clinician to integrate an understanding of the physiology of fetal responses to asphyxia with a

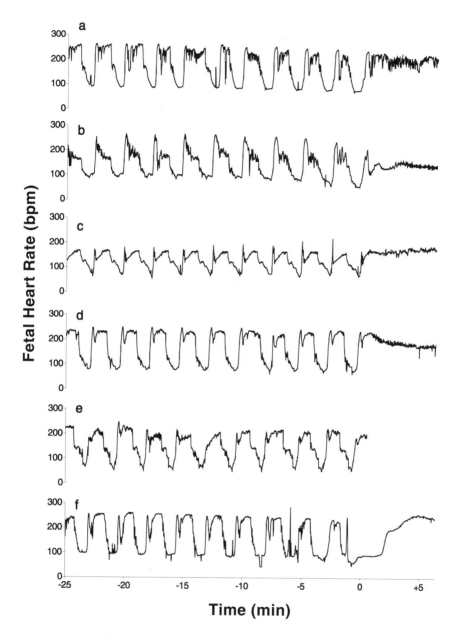

Figure 5. Fetal heart rate patterns for the last 10 occlusions (25 minutes) in a group of near-term fetal sheep undergoing 1-minute umbilical cord occlusions repeated every 2.5 minutes. Interocclusion FHR variability was increased in two fetuses (**a** and **b**) and decreased in the remaining four (**c, d, e,** and **f**). All fetuses were becoming progressively hypotensive and acidotic during this time. From Westgate et al,[41] with permission.

large number of clinical variables such as parity, past obstetric performance, and rate of progress in labor. The difficulties involved in this process have led to attempts to obtain additional information about the fetal condition during labor.

Fetal Scalp Blood Sampling

Once the cervix has dilated to approximately 3 cm, it is usually possible to draw a sample of fetal scalp blood through a capillary tube. Traditionally, this has been used to measure fetal pH and more recently, fetal lactate. Continuous measurement of pH, Pco_2, and Po_2 have all been investigated, but so far the technology has not proved reliable enough for clinical use. Scalp pH is a more direct measure of fetal state than heart rate; nevertheless, there are several intrinsic limitations that must be kept in mind, including the fact that measurements are made at single points in time. As discussed above, the capillary pH primarily reflects peripheral anaerobic metabolism, and thus is only a very crude reflection of how well the fetus has compensated or whether the brain is at risk of injury. Acid-base status is not a measure of brain function or fetal reserve, nor is its rate of decrease closely related to the rate of decrease of fetal blood pressure.

The use of fetal blood sampling (FBS) to discriminate FHR changes has been widely advocated to prevent unnecessary operative intervention.[67,68] Despite these recommendations, less than half of the obstetrical units in the U.K. have facilities for its use,[69] and in those that do, rates of use of FBS vary from 1% to 22%. The only study that has examined the efficacy of FBS use in clinical practice found that it was performed unnecessarily in 40% of cases, and was not used when indicated in 33%.[70] A new technique for measuring blood lactate levels has been developed that requires only 5 μL of blood on a test strip. In a small, randomized trial the success rate for scalp lactate sampling was higher than for scalp pH sampling, but there was no difference in the ability to predict neonatal outcome.[71] A recent retrospective study found scalp lactate measurement to be more sensitive in predicting delivery of a newborn with either a 5-minute Apgar score less than 4, or moderate-to-severe hypoxic-ischemic encephalopathy.[72] Given the relative ease of obtaining a sample, scalp lactate may prove to be an attractive alternative to pH estimation. However, the decision to perform FBS for both pH and lactate is dependent upon interpretation of the FHR pattern; if this is suboptimal, the value of a single FBS is limited. Thus, it is not surprising that, in some institutions, FBS has been replaced by scalp stimulation, vibroacoustic stimulation, or simply well-trained, experienced personnel, without any increase in the cesarean section rate or deterioration in neonatal condition at delivery.[73]

Fetal Pulse Oximetry

The feasibility of using pulse oximetry to measure fetal oxygen saturation during labor has been investigated since the late 1980s. This technique is based on the principle that oxyhemoglobin and deoxyhemoglobin absorb light at different frequencies. Light at these two frequencies is directed into the tissues and the amount of light at each wavelength that passes through the tissues without being absorbed is measured by a photodetector. This enables the proportion of hemoglobin-carrying oxygen to be calculated as the oxygen saturation percentage (SpO_2). A number of different sensor types with different fixation methods have been investigated, but only the Nellcor pulse oximetry system (N400, Nellcor Puritan Bennett, Rowland Heights, California, USA) has met the technical requirements for commercial use. The Nellcor FS14 sensor has light-emitting diodes and a photodetector placed side by side in a probe that is positioned alongside the fetal cheek and held in place by uterine pressure.

Consideration of the physiologic principles underlying asphyxia in labor suggests several factors that limit the value of this technology. Fundamentally, hypoxia occurs universally in labor. Thus, merely detecting the presence of hypoxemia is not helpful; it provides no index of the fetal condition and ability to compensate, nor is there any evidence that either the nadir, nor the recovery of oxygenation between occlusions changes significantly even after fetal decompensation. Oxygen saturation has no "memory" of previous events; it simply reports current saturation levels. The standard chemoreflex-mediated variable deceleration is an equally sensitive indicator of the acute hypoxia associated with contractions. Oximetry would theoretically be of the most value in resolving the significance of tachycardia or reduced FHR variability to the presence or absence of chronic hypoxia in the antenatal period. Although this has been attempted, practical considerations limit the use of oximetry until cervical dilation begins.

In addition to these physiologic considerations, there are a number of significant concerns that have yet to be addressed convincingly. The first is that of artifacts. The Nellcor FS14 sensor is designed to rest against the fetal cheek so that fetal hair or caput do not affect signal quality. However, optical shunting of light directly from the emitter to sensor may occur in the presence of vernix, meconium, and light-colored hair. Shunting may also occur as a result of direct pressure on the sensor during contractions. As the exact position of the probe during monitoring is unknown and may change during labor, the part of the fetal head on which it rests appears to also affect the readings that are obtained.[74]

Sensor calibration and precision is the next important area of concern. Adult oxygen saturation is typically 70–100%, but fetal oxygen saturation is much lower, in the range of 15 to 80%. Calibration of the sensors at low oxygen saturations has been performed in newborn piglets. In these studies, the standard deviation (SD) of the difference between transcutaneous SpO_2 and arterial oxygen saturation averaged 5%.[75,76] This means that the 95% confidence intervals are $\pm 10\%$ (i.e., an SpO_2 reading of 40% could indicate an arterial O_2 saturation between 30% and 50%). None of these experimental studies involved labor-like insults. Two clinical studies evaluated the precision and reproducibility of saturation values using dual sensors on a single fetus. Both have studies shown similar values for the precision of a single sensor (SD $\pm 5.4\%$,[77] and SD $\pm 5.74\%$[78]). However, the precision varied significantly at different levels of saturation; for SpO_2 between 30% and 60% the difference between two sensors was around 1%, but for SpO_2 values less than 30%, differences of more than 15% between sensors were noted.[78] When SpO_2 values were compared with O_2 saturation in fetal scalp blood measured by hemoximeter, pulse oximetry overestimated the median saturation by 6%, and 30% of values had a standard deviation of more than 15%.[74]

The critical threshold of SpO_2 that is suggested for clinical monitoring is 30% (Nellcor Puritan Bennett). This figure was determined primarily on the basis of experimental studies of the relationship between *arterial* oxygen saturation and metabolic acidosis.[79] An SpO_2 less than 30% for 10 minutes was reported as having a sensitivity of 81% and a specificity of 100% for predicting scalp pH less than 7.20 in a study of 46 fetuses.[80] Bloom et al reported that transient falls in SpO_2 less than 30% were common, but values less than 30% for longer than 2 minutes might be associated with fetal compromise.[81] However, East et al found no cases of significant acidemia in their five cases of SpO_2 less than 30% for greater than 10 minutes.[82] The sensitivity of an SpO_2 threshold of 30% to predict an umbilical artery pH less than or equal to 7.15 was 29%,[83] and to predict an umbilical artery base deficit of less than 7.5 mmol/L was 20%.[84] The authors concluded that pulse oximetry is of limited use as a diagnostic tool for predicting acidosis at birth.

Thus, it appears that SpO_2 in the normal range is associated with a good outcome but its sensitivity for detecting poor outcome is low.[85] The only randomized trial of pulse oximetry compared fetal SpO_2 in 508 cases of non-reassuring fetal status with 502 cases without SpO_2 monitoring. It is reported that fewer cesarean sections for fetal distress were performed in the SpO_2 group (5% versus 10% in the control arm), but the rate of cesarean section for failure to progress was doubled (18% versus 9%), and the overall rate of cesarean section was unchanged (29% for SpO_2 arm versus 26% in the control arm).[86] On the basis of the available data, there is no evidence that pulse oximetry is superior in any way to current methods of fetal surveillance.[74]

Near-Infrared Spectroscopy

Near-infrared spectroscopy (NIRS) is being investigated as a method for continuous monitoring of changes in fetal cerebral oxygenation and hemodynamics during labor. As the term suggests, near-infrared light is transmitted through the fetal head, the spectra for oxygenated (HbO_2) and deoxygenated hemoglobin (Hb) are extracted, and relative changes in these and total hemoglobin (tHb) are then calculated. During asphyxia, there is a fall in HbO_2 and a rise in Hb. These changes represent a fall in arterial saturation and can occur with or without changes in tHb.[87,88] Theoretically, this technique should enable us to distinguish simple hypoxia, in which cerebral oxygenation is preserved and tHb is increased, from severe hypoxia/asphyxia, in which oxygenation is compromised and tHb is little changed. This type of analysis confirmed, for example, the clinical belief that contractions every 2.3 minutes or more were associated with impaired cerebral oxygenation.[87] Nevertheless, this information does not provide direct information about the development of hypotension. Total hemoglobin did not fall during 10 minutes of complete cord occlusion in the near-term fetal sheep, despite the onset of marked hypotension.[33] There is evidence to suggest that a reduction in cerebral blood volume can reflect profound hypotension.[89] However, this is likely to reflect a situation when injury may be inevitable. Further experimental studies of NIRS during brief repeated occlusions are needed to examine more specifically the relationship between NIRS parameters and fetal decompensation.

In addition to these physiologic considerations, a number of significant technologic limitations must be overcome before the value of NIRS in clinical practice can be thoroughly evaluated. Currently, only changes in the concentrations of HbO_2 and Hb can be measured, rather than absolute values. Alterations in the optical path length as a result of pressure on the fetal head during contractions and descent through the birth canal may result in significant error in calculations.[90] Indeed, patterns of change seen in labor with a fetus who had died *in utero* while monitored with NIRS were similar to those described previously with live babies.[91] Improvements are also required in the design and fixation of fetal probes to the fetal head.

Fetal Electrocardiogram Analysis

PR-RR Interval Analysis

It has been suggested that relative changes in the PR and RR intervals of the fetal ECG may help to discriminate patterns of FHR changes during labor.[92,93] The PR interval reflects the atrioventricular conduction time and is usually positively related to the RR interval duration, (i.e., as the RR interval lengthens during bradycardia, the PR interval also lengthens); however, in some circumstances a paradoxical shortening of the PR interval may be seen (i.e., a negative relationship). Some observational studies in humans have reported that a change from a positive to a negative correlation was associated with fetal acidemia at birth,[93] whereas others studies have not confirmed this.[94] Experimentally, single brief episodes of hypoxia[95] and prolonged continuous hypoxia[96] have been associated with a negative switch.

We investigated the PR-RR relationship using brief repeated cord occlusions to reflect the typical pattern of normal labor.[42] A change in the PR-RR correlation from positive to negative was not associated with fetal hypotension and acidosis but rather with the onset of occlusions. Typically, as occlusions were continued, the correlation eventually returned to positive. These data are consistent with the clinical observation study of Luzietti et al,[94] who recently reported that a negative PR-RR relationship occurred with all decelerations of more than 40 beats/min. The immediate switch suggests that this paradoxical PR shortening with the onset of occlusions is likely to be related to reflex hypoxic cardiac stimulation.

Our study also showed that both the stable, well-compensated fetus and the severely hypoxic, hypotensive fetus may show a positive PR-RR correlation. The latter state would be erroneously identified as normal within the current model of PR-RR interpretation, in which only a persistently negative correlation is considered abnormal. Thus, PR-RR correlation in isolation is unlikely to contribute significantly to conventional clinical electronic fetal monitoring. It is not surprising, therefore, that a randomized trial comparing fetal monitoring by FHR analysis with FHR plus PR-interval analysis failed to find any significant impact on the frequency of operative intervention or neonatal outcome.[97]

ST Waveform Analysis

Monitoring of the ST waveform of the fetal ECG has also been suggested to improve the predictive value of FHR monitoring.[98] The ST segment and the T wave represent repolarization of ventricular myocardial cells, the energy-dependent part of the cardiac cycle. The shape of the ST waveform reflects the sequence of repolarization in different parts of the ventricular muscle over time. Analysis of the ST waveform of the adult ECG is a well-recognized method of assessing myocardial function during an exercise ECG.[99] Experimental studies in the fetus have shown that acute hypoxemia is accompanied by an elevation in the ST segment and a progressive increase in T wave height, quantified by the ratio between the heights of the T wave and the QRS complex (T/QRS ratio).[100] ST waveform elevation is believed to reflect altered cellular ionic currents during anaerobic myocardial metabolism, possibly augmented by catecholamine exposure.[100,101] Negative ST waveforms and ST segment depression with positive T waves (biphasic waveforms) have been observed in growth-restricted, but not normally grown, fetal guinea pigs during inhalational hypoxia.[63] It is postulated that these changes represent an ischemic pattern secondary to a failure of anaerobic metabolism.[100]

The existing experimental literature has predominantly studied the effects of continuous hypoxia/asphyxia on the ST waveform, using approaches that do not reflect the dynamic, repetitive nature of labor. The authors studied the relationship between changes in the ST waveform and the development of fetal compromise during repeated umbilical cord occlusions designed to mimic labor.[44] The pattern of ST waveform change in a 1:5 occlusion group was compared with a 1:2.5 occlusion group (as previously described, and in Figure 2). We observed an increase in ST waveform height and T/QRS ratio during each occlusion with a rapid fall between occlusions. In the 1:2.5 group, the peak T/QRS ratio during and between occlusions was greater than in the 1:5 group, reflecting the reduced time for recovery between occlusions (Figure 6). The elevation in T/QRS ratio persisted through most of the final 30-minute phase of decompensation despite progressive hypotension, reflecting that the heart is a high-priority organ and its function is preserved for as long as possible. However, negative or biphasic waveforms occurred between occlusions in all fetuses (Figure 7), suggesting that the

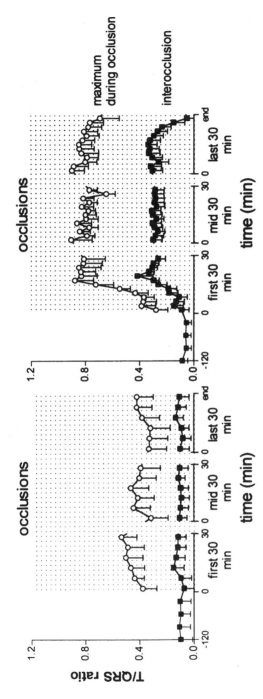

Figure 6. The time sequence of changes in T/QRS height for a group of near-term fetal sheep undergoing 1-minute umbilical cord occlusions repeated every 5 minutes (1:5 group, left panel) or every 2.5 minutes (1:2.5 group, right panel), presented as the maximum T/QRS during occlusions and the interocclusion T/QRS (see also Figure 2). The T/QRS ratio rises significantly during occlusions and falls back to baseline in the 1:5 group but never returns to baseline levels in the 1:2.5 group. Both the maximum T/QRS during and between occlusions was significantly higher in the 1:2.5 group (p<0.001), but there was some overlap in absolute values in individual fetuses. There is a significant fall in T/QRS over the last 30 minutes in the 1:2.5 group (p<0.001) because of the occurrence of biphasic and negative ST waveforms. From Westgate et al,[44] with permission.

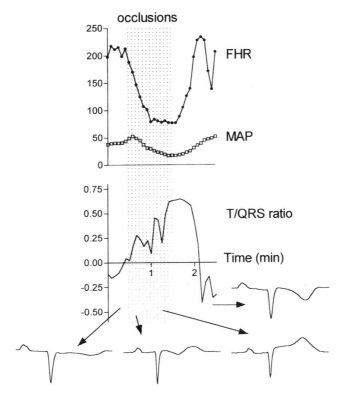

Figure 7. Examples of fetal heart rate (FHR [beats/min]), mean arterial pressure (MAP [mmHg]), T/QRS ratio, and electroencephalographic complex changes for the last occlusion in the 1:2.5 group. The occlusion is accompanied by a fall in FHR and a brief rise in MAP followed by a fall to less than 20 mmHg. There is a delay in recovery of both FHR and MAP. At the onset of the occlusion, biphasic ST changes occur with a downward-sloping ST segment and a positive T wave, but by the end of the occlusion the whole ST waveform is elevated. In recovery, the T/QRS ratio is negative because of prolonged T wave inversion. From Westgate et al,[44] with permission.

oxygen and glucose supply to the myocardium was insufficient to meet the increased demand occasioned by the recovery of heart rate and blood pressure between occlusions. The appearance of biphasic and negative waveforms between contractions may potentially be a useful marker for the development of severe fetal decompensation.

Two large randomized trials comparing FHR plus ST waveform analysis with FHR analysis alone have confirmed the ability of ST waveform analysis to discriminate FHR changes. The Plymouth study showed a 45% reduction in operative deliveries for fetal distress (p<0.001, odds ratio 0.53, 95% confidence intervals 0.38–0.74) in the ST analysis arm.[102] There was no difference in operative deliveries for other reasons. A retrospective blinded review of recordings revealed that the reduction in intervention occurred in cases with an FHR pattern that was graded as normal or intermediate. This suggests that the additional information provided by the ST waveform provided reassurance to the clinicians that intervention was not necessary in these cases. There were no significant differences in neonatal outcome, but trends toward fewer low 5-minute Apgar scores and less metabolic acidosis were apparent. This trial identified the importance of examining the whole ST waveform to identify biphasic changes that may be missed if only the T/QRS ratio is relied upon.

Following this study, an ST waveform analyzer with automatic detection of ST changes by an expert system was developed and tested in further observational studies[103] prior to its use in a multicenter Swedish randomized trial. Preliminary data from this trial suggest a 25% reduction in operative delivery for fetal distress (p = 0.004), with no change in operative deliveries for other reasons. There was a 61% reduction in the number of babies born with umbilical cord artery metabolic acidosis and a 78% reduction in babies with metabolic acidosis admitted to the neonatal unit.[104] At this stage it is not clear how much of the improvement in neonatal outcome resulted from a larger pool of subjects (4500 compared to 2400 in the Plymouth study) and how much resulted from improved detection of abnormal ST waveform patterns by the expert system.

The use of ST waveform analysis for fetal assessment offers the most significant advance in intrapartum monitoring in the last 40 years. This is the only approach that has been shown to demonstrate both a reduction in intervention and an improvement in neonatal outcome. The challenge will be to determine whether the technology can be introduced successfully into routine clinical practice. There is evidence that this has been the case in a number of Norwegian centers[103] and the technology will be tested further in a large multicenter European initiative.

Computer-Aided Support for Fetal Heart Rate Interpretation

Although electronic fetal monitoring has been associated with a significant reduction in fetal mortality, this has been accompanied by increased operative intervention in labor,[105] and the positive predictive value of changes in the FHR pattern in clinical practice is low.[106] This has led to much skepticism about the value of FHR monitoring. However, there is a large body of literature that clearly demonstrates that a significant proportion of unfavorable neonatal outcome following labor is operator-dependent. In the U.K., the 4th Annual Report of the Confidential Enquiry into Stillbirths and Deaths in Infancy (CESDI) reported that 75% of 873 intrapartum deaths from 1994–1995 had evidence of suboptimal care which could have made a difference to outcome.[107] More than half of these cases related to failures in the use and interpretation of FHR recordings. We recently reviewed the events that preceded delivery of term babies with evidence of moderate neonatal encephalopathy and acidemia.[15] A significant proportion of such babies experienced either antenatal hypoxia or catastrophic events during labor that were beyond the control of the clinician. However, suboptimal fetal monitoring practice occurred in half of the cases as a result of failure to monitor the FHR adequately, or at all, and failure to respond appropriately to gross FHR abnormalities. Similar findings have been reported in a number of other studies.[108,109]

These data suggest that one aspect of the conundrum of intrapartum fetal monitoring is the way in which it is applied. One obvious response is to recommend regular staff training and education in FHR interpretation.[107] The 7th CESDI Report found that, although 96% of surveyed hospitals in the U.K. provided FHR training to staff, evaluation of the effectiveness of training for midwives occurred in only 39%, for medical staff in only 11%.[110] Computer-based instructional packages may offer a practical solution for ensuring that all staff receive regular, effective training. The use of this type of system has been shown to be effective in improving knowledge of acid-base balance and FHR interpretation for midwifery and medical staff.[111] As more systems of this kind are developed, it will be essential that there is external review of their content and quality. Logically, the next step in the process of ensuring adequate standards of fetal monitoring practice is regular testing and accreditation of all obstetrical staff. The availability of computer-based teaching and evaluation systems improves the feasibility of this approach.

Another approach to improve the use of FHR monitoring is to utilize automatic data processing and interpretation. Until recently, computerized systems for the interpretation of FHR changes have considered FHR features in isolation from the clinical factors that affect interpretation and management. The advent of expert systems technology allows these factors to be incorporated into a computer program that simulates expert behavior to support the decision making of inexperienced staff. Such systems are used widely in industry, manufacturing, aviation, and engineering to solve complex tasks for which conventional computing approaches have failed. As these systems have the capability to explain the reasoning underlying the advice that is provided, they may also have a useful teaching role. The feasibility of this approach has been demonstrated with validation of a prototype system by a large number of external "experts."[112] In this study, the computer system recommended no unnecessary intervention in infants born in good condition, identified the same number of birth asphyxia cases as the majority of experts, and was highly consistent. Both the system and the experts performed better than clinical practice. This system is currently being developed for online use in obstetrics in preparation for further observational studies, and for eventual use in a multicenter randomized trial.

The Future

Two issues are crucial in determining the role of fetal monitoring. First, can the adequacy of fetal adaptation be assessed directly? Second, can the efficiency with which existing or new techniques are used during the intrapartum period be improved?

The critical measurements that can assess whether the fetus is compensating (i.e., retains the ability to defend itself from severe injury) are fetal arterial pressure and blood flow to essential organs. Assessment of Doppler velocity waveforms from umbilical vessels[113] and the middle cerebral artery[114] during labor is feasible. Systolic time intervals, as measured by sonography, are good indicators of myocardial contractility. Preliminary studies have suggested that these correlate with fetal acid-base status.[115] Clearly, these techniques have major practical limitations and it is striking that, after the initial enthusiasm, there have been few recent studies using these tools. Fundamentally, blood pressure is determined by cardiac output and peripheral resistance. Sophisticated modeling of the fetal circulation and imaging of the vasculature may offer the possibility of estimating these parameters noninvasively.[116,117]

It is highly probable that significant improvements in the quality of intrapartum fetal assessment are possible with more effective use of existing techniques. Attempts to improve education and training of staff must be ongoing. However, until the labor and delivery room is seen as the intensive care unit of obstetrics, necessitating highly trained and dedicated staff, these efforts are unlikely to consistently achieve the required level of expertise. The introduction of expert systems technology offers the best chance to support the consistent and optimal interpretation of fetal condition in daily practice.

References

1. Bocking AD, Gagnon R, Milne KM, White SE: Behavioral activity during prolonged hypoxemia in fetal sheep. J Appl Physiol 1988;65:2420–2426.
2. Bocking AD, White S, Gagnon R, Hansford H: Effect of prolonged hypoxemia on fetal heart rate accelerations and decelerations in sheep. Am J Obstet Gynecol 1989;161:722–727.
3. Richardson BS, Bocking AD: Metabolic and circulatory adaptations to chronic hypoxia in the fetus. Comp Biochem Physiol A Mol Integr Physiol 1998;119:717–723.
4. Kitanaka T, Alonso JG, Gilbert RD, et al: Fetal responses to long-term hypoxemia in sheep. Am J Physiol 1989;256:R1348–R1354.
5. Brotanek V, Hendricks CH, Yoshida T: Changes in uterine blood flow during uterine contractions. Am J Obstet Gynecol 1969;103:1108–1116.
6. Jansen CA, Krane EJ, Thomas AL, et al: Continuous variability of fetal PO_2 in the chronically catheterized fetal sheep. Am J Obstet Gynecol 1979;134:776–783.
7. Janbu T, Nesheim BI: Uterine artery blood velocities during contractions in pregnancy and labor related to intrauterine pressure. Br J Obstet Gynaecol 1987;94:1150–1155.
8. Grubb DK, Paul RH: Amniotic fluid index and prolonged antepartum fetal heart rate decelerations. Obstet Gynecol 1992;79:558–560.
9. Shields LE, Brace RA: Fetal vascular pressure responses to nonlabor uterine contractions: dependence on amniotic fluid volume in the ovine fetus. Am J Obstet Gynecol 1994;171:84–89.
10. Modanlou H, Yeh SY, Hon EH: Fetal and neonatal acid-base balance in normal and high-risk pregnancies: during labor and the first hour of life. Obstet Gynecol 1974;43:347–353.
11. Huch A, Huch R, Schneider H, Rooth G: Continuous transcutaneous monitoring of fetal oxygen tension during labor. Br J Obstet Gynaecol 1977; 84(suppl 1):1–39.
12. MacLennan A: The International Cerebral Palsy Task Force: Gunn AJ, Bennet L, Westgate JA. A template for defining a causal relation between acute intrapartum events and cerebral palsy: international consensus statement. BMJ 1999;319:1054–1059.
13. Roth SC, Baudin J, Cady E et al: Relation of deranged neonatal cerebral oxidative metabolism with neurodevelopmental outcome and head circumference at 4 years. Dev Med Child Neurol 1997;39:718–725.
14. Hellstrom Westas L, Rosen I, Svenningsen NW: Predictive value of early continuous amplitude integrated EEG recordings on outcome after severe birth asphyxia in full term infants. Arch Dis Child 1995;72:F34–F38.
15. Westgate JA, Gunn AJ, Gunn TR: Antecedents of neonatal encephalopathy with fetal acidaemia at term. Br J Obstet Gynaecol 1999;106:774–782.
16. Caldeyro-Barcia R: *The Cervix in Pregnancy and Labor*. Churchill Livingstone, London, 1959, pp 7–36.
17. Weber T, Hahn-Pedersen S: Normal values for fetal scalp tissue pH during labor. Br J Obstet Gynaecol 1979;86:728–731.
18. Katz M, Lunenfeld E, Meizner I, et al: The effect of the duration of the second stage of labor on the acid-base state of the fetus. Br J Obstet Gynaecol 1987;94:425–430.

19. Peebles DM, Spencer JA, Edwards AD, et al: Relation between frequency of uterine contractions and human fetal cerebral oxygen saturation studied during labor by near infrared spectroscopy. Br J Obstet Gynaecol 1994;101:44–48.
20. Gunn TR, Wright IM: The use of black and blue cohosh in labor. N Z Med J 1996;109:410–411.
21. Winkler M, Rath W: A risk-benefit assessment of oxytocics in obstetric practice. Drug Saf 1999;20:323–345.
22. Shelley HJ: Glycogen reserves and their changes at birth and in anoxia. Br Med Bull 1961;17:137–143.
23. Hokegard KH, Eriksson BO, Kjellmer I, et al: Myocardial metabolism in relation to electrocardiographic changes and cardiac function during graded hypoxia in the fetal lamb. Acta Physiol Scand 1981;113:1–7.
24. Gunn AJ, de Haan HH, Gluckman PD: Experimental models of perinatal brain injury. In Stevenson DK, Sunshine P (eds): *Fetal and Neonatal Brain Injury: Mechanisms, Management, and the Risks of Practice.* Oxford University Press, New York, 1997, pp 59–70.
25. Parer JT: Effects of fetal asphyxia on brain cell structure and function: limits of tolerance. Comp Biochem Physiol A Mol Integr Physiol 1998;119: 711–716.
26. Giussani DA, Spencer JAD, Hanson MA: Fetal cardiovascular reflex responses to hypoxemia. Fetal Maternal Med Rev 1994;6:17–37.
27. Battaglia FC, Meschia G: Principal substrates of fetal metabolism. Physiol Rev 1978;58:499–527.
28. Giussani DA, Spencer JA, Moore PJ, et al: Afferent and efferent components of the cardiovascular reflex responses to acute hypoxia in term fetal sheep. J Physiol 1993;461:431–449.
29. Jones MJ, Sheldon RE, Peeters LL, et al: Fetal cerebral oxygen consumption at different levels of oxygenation. J Appl Physiol 1977;43:1080–1084.
30. Jensen A, Hohmann M, Kunzel W: Dynamic changes in organ blood flow and oxygen consumption during acute asphyxia in fetal sheep. J Dev Physiol 1987;9:543–559.
31. Field DR, Parer JT, Auslender RA, et al: Cerebral oxygen consumption during asphyxia in fetal sheep. J Dev Physiol 1990;14:131–137.
32. Richardson BS, Carmichael L, Homan J, et al. Fetal cerebral, circulatory, and metabolic responses during heart rate decelerations with umbilical cord compression. Am J Obstet Gynecol 1996;175:929–936.
33. Bennet L, Peebles DM, Edwards AD, et al: The cerebral hemodynamic response to asphyxia and hypoxia in the near-term fetal sheep as measured by near infrared spectroscopy. Pediatr Res 1998;44:951–957.
34. Hanson MA: Do we now understand the control of the fetal circulation? Eur J Obstet Gynecol Reprod Biol 1997;75:55–61.
35. Baan JJ, Boekkooi PF, Teitel DF, Rudolph AM: Heart rate fall during acute hypoxemia: a measure of chemoreceptor response in fetal sheep. J Dev Physiol 1993;19:105–111.
36. Itskovitz J, LaGamma EF, Rudolph AM: Heart rate and blood pressure responses to umbilical cord compression in fetal lambs with special reference to the mechanism of variable deceleration. Am J Obstet Gynecol 1983;147:451–457.
37. Rosen KG, Hrbek A, Karlsson K, Kjellmer I: Fetal cerebral, cardiovascular

and metabolic reactions to intermittent occlusion of ovine maternal placental blood flow. Acta Physiol Scand 1986;126:209–216.

38. de Haan HH, Gunn AJ, Williams CE, et al: Magnesium sulfate therapy during asphyxia in near-term fetal lambs does not compromise the fetus but does not reduce cerebral injury. Am J Obstet Gynecol 1997;176: 18–27.

39. de Haan HH, Gunn AJ, Gluckman PD: Fetal heart rate changes do not reflect cardiovascular deterioration during brief repeated umbilical cord occlusions in near-term fetal lambs. Am J Obstet Gynecol 1997;176:8–17.

40. de Haan HH, Gunn AJ, Williams CE, Gluckman PD: Brief repeated umbilical cord occlusions cause sustained cytotoxic cerebral edema and focal infarcts in near-term fetal lambs. Pediatr Res 1997;41:96–104.

41. Westgate JA, Bennet L, Gunn AJ: Fetal heart rate variability changes during brief repeated umbilical cord occlusion in near term fetal sheep. Br J Obstet Gynaecol 1999;106:664–671.

42. Westgate JA, Gunn AJ, Bennet L, Gunning MI, et al: Do fetal electrocardiogram PR-RR changes reflect progressive asphyxia after repeated umbilical cord occlusion in fetal sheep? Pediatr Res 1998;44:297–303.

43. Westgate JA, Bennet L, de Haan HH, Gunn AJ: Fetal heart rate overshoot during repeated umbilical cord occlusion in sheep. Obstet Gynecol 2001; 97:454–459.

44. Westgate JA, Bennet L, Brabyn C, et al: ST waveform changes during brief repeated asphyxia in near-term fetal sheep. Am J Obstet Gynecol 2001;184:743–751.

45. Hanson MA: Role of chemoreceptors in effects of chronic hypoxia. Comp Biochem Physiol A Mol Integr Physiol 1998;119:695–703.

46. Giussani DA, Riquelme RA, Moraga FA, et al: Chemoreflex and endocrine components of cardiovascular responses to acute hypoxemia in the llama fetus. Am J Physiol 1996;271:R73–R83.

47. Perlman JM, Tack ED, Martin T, et al: Acute systemic organ injury in term infants after asphyxia. Am J Dis Child 1989;143:617–620.

48. Ikeda T, Murata Y, Quilligan EJ, et al: Physiologic and histologic changes in near-term fetal lambs exposed to asphyxia by partial umbilical cord occlusion. Am J Obstet Gynecol 1998;178:24–32.

49. Gunn AJ, Parer JT, Mallard EC, et al: Cerebral histological and electrophysiological changes after asphyxia in fetal sheep. Pediatr Res 1992;31: 486–491.

50. de Haan HH, Van Reempts JL, Vles JS, et al: Effects of asphyxia on the fetal lamb brain. Am J Obstet Gynecol 1993;169:1493–1501.

51. Low JA, Cox MJ, Karchmar EJ, et al: The prediction of intrapartum fetal metabolic acidosis by fetal heart rate monitoring. Am J Obstet Gynecol 1981;139:299–305.

52. Caldeyro-Barcia R, Medez-Bauer C, Poseiro J, et al: Control of the human fetal heart rate during labor. In Cassels D (ed): *The Heart and Circulation in the Newborn and Infant.* Grune & Stratton, New York, 1966, pp 7–36.

53. Hon E, Quilligan EJ: The classification of fetal heart rate. II. A revised working classification. Conn Med 1967;31:779–784.

54. Goodlin RC: History of fetal monitoring. Am J Obstet Gynecol 1979;133: 323–352.

55. van Geijn HP, Copray FJ, Donkers DK, Bos MH: Diagnosis and manage-

ment of intrapartum fetal distress. Eur J Obstet Gynecol Reprod Biol 1991;42(suppl):S63–S72.

56. Fleischer A, Schulman H, Jagani N, et al: The development of fetal acidosis in the presence of an abnormal fetal heart rate tracing. I. The average for gestational age fetus. Am J Obstet Gynecol 1982;144:55–60.

57. Thomas G: The aetiology, characteristics and diagnostic relevance of late deceleration patterns in routine obstetric practice. Br J Obstet Gynaecol 1975;82:121–125.

58. Harris JL, Krueger TR, Parer JT: Mechanisms of late decelerations of the fetal heart rate during hypoxia. Am J Obstet Gynecol 1982;144:491–496.

59. James LS, Morishima HO, Daniel SS, et al: Mechanism of late deceleration of the fetal heart rate. Am J Obstet Gynecol 1972;113:578–582.

60. Gunn AJ, Maxwell L, de Haan HH, et al: Delayed hypotension and subendocardial injury after repeated umbilical cord occlusion in near term fetal lambs. Am J Obstet Gynecol 2000;183:1–9.

61. Thaler I, Timor-Tritsch IE, Blumenfeld Z: Effect of acute hypoxia on human fetal heart rate: the significance of increased heart rate variability. Acta Obstet Gynecol Scand 1985;64:47–50.

62. Pello LC, Rosevear SK, Dawes GS, et al: Computerized fetal heart rate analysis in labor. Obstet Gynecol 1991;78:602–610.

63. Widmark C, Jansson T, Lindecrantz K, Rosen KG: ECG waveform, short term heart rate variability and plasma catecholamine concentrations in response to hypoxia in intrauterine growth retarded guinea-pig fetuses. J Dev Physiol 1991;15:161–168.

64. Murotsuki J, Bocking AD, Gagnon R: Fetal heart rate patterns in growth-restricted fetal sheep induced by chronic fetal placental embolization. Am J Obstet Gynecol 1997;176:282–290.

65. Dawes GS, Moulden M, Redman CW: Short-term fetal heart rate variation, decelerations, and umbilical flow velocity waveforms before labor. Obstet Gynecol 1992;80:673–678.

66. Odendaal HJ, Steyn W, Theron GB, et al: Does a nonreactive fetal heart rate pattern really mean fetal distress? Am J Perinatol 1994;11:194–198.

67. Saling E, Schneider D: Biochemical supervision of the foetus during labor. J Obstet Gynaecol Br Common 1967;74:799–811.

68. Beard RW, Morris ED, Clayton SG: pH of foetal capillary blood as an indicator of the condition of the foetus. J Obstet Gynaecol Br Common 1967;74:812–822.

69. Wheble AM, Gillmer MD, Spencer JA, Sykes GS: Changes in fetal monitoring practice in the UK: 1977–1984. Br J Obstet Gynaecol 1989;96:1140–1147.

70. Westgate J, Greene K: How well is fetal blood sampling used in clinical practice? Br J Obstet Gynaecol 1994;101:250–251.

71. Westgren M, Divon M, Horal M, et al: Routine measurements of umbilical artery lactate levels in the prediction of perinatal outcome. Am J Obstet Gynecol 1995;173:1416–1422.

72. Kruger K, Hallberg B, Blennow M, et al: Predictive value of fetal scalp blood lactate concentration and pH as markers of neurologic disability. Am J Obstet Gynecol 1999;181:1072–1078.

73. Goodwin TM, Milner Masterson L, Paul RH: Elimination of fetal scalp blood sampling on a large clinical service. Obstet Gynecol 1994;83:971–974.

74. Luttkus AK, Dudenhausen JW: Fetal pulse oximetry. Baillieres Clin Obstet Gynaecol 1996;10:295–306.
75. Nijland R, Jongsma HW, Nijhuis JG, Oeseburg B: Accuracy of fetal pulse oximetry and pitfalls in measurements. Eur J Obstet Gynecol Reprod Biol 1997;72(suppl):S21–S27.
76. Nijland R, Jongsma HW, Nijhuis JG, Oeseburg B: The accuracy of a fiberoptic oximeter over a wide range of arterial oxygen saturation values in piglets. Acta Anaesthesiol Scand Suppl 1995;107:71–76.
77. East CE, Colditz PB, Dunster KR, Khoo SK: Human fetal intrapartum oxygen saturation monitoring: agreement between readings from two sensors on the same fetus. Am J Obstet Gynecol 1996;174:1594–1598.
78. Davies MG, Greene KR: Fetal pulse oximetry: a preliminary report on sensor precision determined by dual sensor studies. Eur J Obstet Gynecol Reprod Biol 1997;72(suppl):S35–S41.
79. Nijland R, Jongsma HW, Nijhuis JG, et al: Arterial oxygen saturation in relation to metabolic acidosis in fetal lambs. Am J Obstet Gynecol 1995; 172:810–819.
80. Kuhnert M, Seelbachgoebel B, Butterwegge M: Predictive agreement between the fetal arterial oxygen saturation and fetal scalp pH: results of the German multicenter study. Am J Obstet Gynecol 1998;178:330–335.
81. Bloom SL, Swindle RG, McIntire DD, Leveno KJ: Fetal pulse oximetry: duration of desaturation and intrapartum outcome. Obstet Gynecol 1999; 93:1036–1040.
82. East CE, Dunster KR, Colditz PB, et al: Fetal oxygen saturation monitoring in labor: an analysis of 118 cases. Aust N Z J Obstet Gynaecol 1997;37: 397–401.
83. Carbonne B, Langer B, Goffinet F, et al: Multicenter study on the clinical value of fetal pulse oximetry. II. Compared predictive values of pulse oximetry and fetal blood analysis. The French Study Group on Fetal Pulse Oximetry. Am J Obstet Gynecol 1997;177:593–598.
84. Alshimmiri M, Bocking AD, Gagnon R, et al: Prediction of umbilical artery base excess by intrapartum fetal oxygen saturation monitoring. Am J Obstet Gynecol 1997;177:775–779.
85. Luttkus AK, Friedmann W, Homm-Luttkus C, Dudenhausen JW: Correlation of fetal oxygen saturation to fetal heart rate patterns: evaluation of fetal pulse oximetry with two different oxisensors. Acta Obstet Gynecol Scand 1998;77:307–312.
86. Garite TJ, Dildy GA, McNamara H, et al. A multicenter controlled trial of fetal pulse oximetry in the intrapartum management of nonreassuring fetal heart rate patterns. Am J Obstet Gynecol 2000;183:1049-1058.
87. Peebles DM, Spencer JA, Edwards AD, et al: Relation between frequency of uterine contractions and human fetal cerebral oxygen saturation studied during labor by near infrared spectroscopy. Br J Obstet Gynaecol 1994;101:44–48.
88. Nomura F, Naruse H, Duplessis A, et al: Cerebral oxygenation measured by near infrared spectroscopy during cardiopulmonary bypass and deep hypothermic circulatory arrest in piglets. Pediatr Res 1996;40:790–796.
89. Bennet L, Rossenrode S, Gunning MI, et al: The cardiovascular and cerebrovascular responses of the immature fetal sheep to acute umbilical cord occlusion. J Physiol (Lond) 1999;517:247–257.

90. Hamilton RJ, Hodgett SG, O'Brien PM: Near infrared spectroscopy applied to intrapartum fetal monitoring. Baillieres Clin Obstet Gynaecol 1996;10: 307–324.

91. Hamilton RJ, O'Brien PM, Wickramasinghe YA, Rolfe P: Intrapartum fetal cerebral near infrared spectroscopy: apparent change in oxygenation demonstrated in a nonviable fetus. Br J Obstet Gynaecol 1995;102:1004–1007.

92. Murray HG: The fetal electrocardiogram: current clinical developments in Nottingham. J Perinat Med 1986;14:399–404.

93. Mohajer MP, Sahota DS, Reed NN, et al: Cumulative changes in the fetal electrocardiogram and biochemical indices of fetal hypoxia. Eur J Obset Gynecol Reprod 1994;55:63–70.

94. Luzietti R, Erkkola R, Hasbargen U, et al: European Community Multi-center Trial "Fetal ECG Analysis During Labor": the P-R interval. J Perinat Med 1997;25:27–34.

95. Widmark C, Lindecrantz K, Murray H, Rosen KG: Changes in the PR, RR intervals and ST waveform of the fetal lamb electrocardiogram with acute hypoxemia. J Dev Physiol 1992;18:99–103.

96. van Wijngaarden WJ, de Haan HH, Sahota DS, et al: Changes in the PR interval: fetal heart rate relationship of the electrocardiogram during fetal compromise in chronically instrumented sheep. Am J Obstet Gynecol 1996;175:548–554.

97. Strachan BK, van Wijngaarden WJ, Sahota D, et al: Cardiotocography only versus cardiotocography plus PR-interval analysis in intrapartum surveillance: a randomized, multicenter trial. FECG Study Group. Lancet 2000;355:456–459.

98. Westgate J, Harris M, Curnow JSH, Greene KR: Plymouth randomized trial of cardiotocogram only versus ST waveform plus cardiotocogram for intrapartum monitoring in 2400 cases. Am J Obstet Gynecol 1993;169: 1151–1160.

99. Miranda CP, Lehmann KG, Froelicher VF: Correlation between resting ST segment depression, exercise testing, coronary angiography, and long-term prognosis. Am Heart J 1991;122:1617–1628.

100. Greene KR, Westgate JA: The fetal ECG with particular reference to the ECG waveform. RCOG (Royal College of Obstetrics and Gynaecology) Press, London, 1994, pp 281–294.

101. Greene KR, Rosen KG: Long-term ST waveform changes in the ovine fetal electrocardiogram: the relationship to spontaneous labor and intrauterine death. Clin Phys Physiol Meas 1989;10(suppl B):33–40.

102. Westgate JA, Harris M, Curnow JS, Greene KR. Randomized trial of cardiotocography alone or with ST waveform analysis for intrapartum monitoring. Lancet 1992;340:194–198.

103. Rosen KG, Luzietti R: Intrapartum fetal monitoring: its basis and current developments. Prenat Neonat Med 2000;5:1–14.

104. Amer-Wåhlin, I: Randomized controlled trial of CTG versus CTG+ST analysis of the fetal ECG. FIGO World Congress 2000, Washington DC.

105. Vintzileos AM, Nochimson DJ, Guzman ER, et al: Intrapartum electronic fetal heart rate monitoring versus intermittent auscultation: a meta-analysis. Obstet Gynecol 1995;85:149–155.

106. Nelson KB, Dambrosia JM, Ting TY, Grether JK: Uncertain value of

electronic fetal monitoring in predicting cerebral palsy. N Engl J Med 1996;334:613–618.

107. Confidential Enquiry into Stillbirths and Deaths in Infancy. 4th Annual Report by Maternal and Child Health Research Consortium, London, 1997.

108. Murphy KW, Johnson P, Moorcraft J, et al: Birth asphyxia and the intrapartum cardiotocograph. Br J Obstet Gynaecol 1990;97:470–479.

109. Gaffney G, Sellers S, Flavell V, et al: Case-control study of intrapartum care, cerebral palsy, and perinatal death. BMJ 1994;308:743–750.

110. Confidential Enquiry into Stillbirths and Deaths in Infancy. 7th Annual Report, 2000. Maternal and Child Health Research Consortium, London, 2000.

111. Beckley S, Stenhouse E, Greene K. The development and evaluation of a computer-assisted teaching programme for intrapartum fetal monitoring. Br J Obstet Gynaecol 2000;107:1138–1144.

112. Keith RD, Beckley S, Garibaldi JM, et al: A multicenter comparative study of 17 experts and an intelligent computer system for managing labor using the cardiotocogram. Br J Obstet Gynaecol 1995;102:688–700.

113. Damron DP, Chaffin DG, Anderson CF, Reed KL. Changes in umbilical arterial and venous blood flow velocity waveforms during late decelerations of the fetal heart rate. Obstet Gynecol 1994;84:1038–1040.

114. Yagel S, Anteby E, Lavy Y, et al: Fetal middle cerebral artery blood flow during normal active labor and in labor with variable decelerations. Br J Obstet Gynaecol 1992;99:483–485.

115. Lewinsky RM: Cardiac systolic time intervals and other parameters of myocardial contractility as indices of fetal acid-base status. Baillieres Clin Obstet Gynaecol 1994;8:663–681.

116. Menigault E, Berson M, Vieyres P, et al: Feto-maternal circulation: mathematical model and comparison with Doppler measurements. Eur J Ultrasound 1998;7:129–143.

117. Mori A, Iwabuchi M, Makino T: Fetal haemodynamic changes in fetuses during fetal development evaluated by arterial pressure pulse and blood flow velocity waveforms. Br J Obstetr Gynaecol 2000;107:669–677.

CHAPTER 12

Clinical Management of the Asphyxiated Newborn

Malcolm I. Levene, Sunil K. Sinha

Introduction

Despite improvements in our understanding of the pathogenesis of hypoxic-ischemic cerebral injury, there have been few innovative treatments that have been shown to improve the neurodevelopmental outcome of newborn infants who have suffered severe intrauterine injury. It is likely that our expanding knowledge of the basic science of hypoxic-ischemic brain damage, as described in many of the chapters in this book, will lead to such treatments in the future. In the meantime, the approach to the asphyxiated infant should be one that emphasizes high-quality supportive care, as well as the avoidance of potentially harmful interventions.

Clinical Concept of Birth Asphyxia

The term "birth asphyxia" is an imprecise term, but it is now deeply embedded in medical terminology. It is commonly used to describe infants with depressed vital signs at birth following a period of severe intrauterine hypoxemia. However, careful consideration must be given to the use of this term because intrauterine hypoxemia may simply *coexist* with other conditions that cause depression at birth, and which require specific treatments (Table 1). In this chapter, birth asphyxia will be used to describe depression of vital signs at birth caused by significant prior impairment of fetal gas exchange. Asphyxia should be defined biochemically by the concomitant presence of hypoxemia, hypercapnia, and excess hydrogen ion concentration (acidosis). Alternatively, it can be defined functionally as a failure of the organ of respiration.

From Donn SM, Sinha SK, Chiswick ML (eds): *Birth Asphyxia and the Brain: Basic Science and Clinical Implications.* © 2002, Futura Publishing Co., Inc., Armonk, NY.

Table 1

Causes Other Than Fetal Hypoxemia of Depression of Vital Signs at Birth

- Maternal analgesia and anesthesia
- Severe intrapartum hypoxia
  Maternal circulatory collapse
  Placental pathology (e.g., abruption)
  Cord accidents
- Severe fetal hemorrhage
  Fetomaternal
  Twin-to-twin
- Severe birth trauma (cerebral, spinal)
- Neuromuscular disorders (e.g., myotonic dystrophy)
- Severe infection (e.g., intrauterine group B streptococcal)

The Physiologic Basis of Birth Asphyxia

Dawes described the sequence of events that occurs following a total asphyxial insult induced immediately *after birth* in rhesus monkeys[1] (Figure 1). After the period of asphyxia, there is an episode of regular small-volume breaths followed by a fall in the heart rate and cessation of breathing. This is termed *primary apnea,* and it is accompanied by cyanosis. With no intervention, the period of primary apnea lasts for a minute or so and is followed by a period of spontaneous gasping. The last gasp heralds the onset of a second period of apnea known as *secondary or terminal apnea.* In monkeys, the time interval from the asphyxial insult to the last gasp is around 8 or 9 minutes. The heart rate and blood pressure fall progressively during gasping and continue to do so into terminal apnea. If resuscitation is not undertaken promptly within a few minutes of terminal apnea, death will ensue.

In human newborns, it is very rare for an acute total asphyxial event to occur *de novo* immediately *after* birth, and in this respect the experimental model differs from the human newborn experience. However, close parallels can be drawn with the sequence of events described above, albeit with modified timing.

Labor is normally accompanied by some degree of hypoxemia, and most infants who do not breathe immediately at birth are born in primary apnea and can be considered as having undergone a period of primary apnea in the womb. The clinical features of primary apnea that distinguish it from terminal apnea are shown in Table 2. Infants in primary apnea respond to minimal external stimulation; indeed the nor-

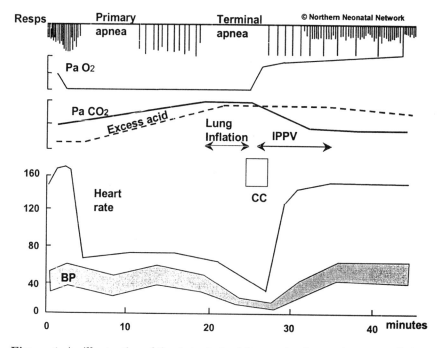

Figure 1. An illustration of the data derived from animal experiments outlining the response of a newborn subjected to hypoxia at birth. Initially, the conscious baby's breathing movements (Resps) become deeper and more rapid. During this time, the PO_2 falls, the $PaCO_2$ rises, the baby begins to lose consciousness, and within a few minutes regular breathing movements cease. Up to this point, the heart rate has remained unchanged but now falls to about half its normal rate, though blood pressure (BP) is hardly altered. If the insult continues and the baby is not delivered, then after a variable period of primary apnea, agonal gasping respiration begins. This is easily distinguishable from normal breaths as these breaths occur every 10–20 seconds and involve all the accessory muscles of respiration, in a maximal inspiratory effort. The baby then enters terminal apnea when circulation falters, and heart rate and blood pressure fade away. A baby who has entered terminal apnea will die without resuscitation, and may die in spite of it. However, a brief period of intermittent positive pressure ventilation (IPPV) and external cardiac compression (CC) can sometimes produce a rapid recovery, as shown. From Richmond,[97] with permission.

mal bombardment with sensory stimuli that accompanies birth is often enough to stimulate spontaneous breathing. The history of neonatology is punctuated by descriptions of many different and allegedly successful resuscitation techniques; the reason for this is that the infants were simply in primary apnea, and thus the success of these techniques was assured.

Fetuses who experience more severe intrauterine hypoxemia lead-

Table 2

Distinguishing Features of Primary and Secondary Apnea

Primary apnea
- Skin dusky, or blue
- Heart rate greater than 60 beats/min and accelerating
- Some muscle tone
- Some spontaneous movement
- Preserved gag reflex
- Gasps in response to lung inflation (Head's reflex)
- Spontaneous breathing before skin becomes pink

Secondary apnea
- Skin pale
- Heart rate less than 60 beats/min, sometimes decelerating
- No muscle tone
- No spontaneous movement
- No gag reflex
- No Head's reflex on lung inflation
- Heart rate and color improve before spontaneous breathing

ing to true asphyxia (i.e., hypoxemia, hypercapnia, and acidemia) commence gasping in the womb and may be born gasping, or they may be in terminal apnea at birth. These infants are conceptually "beyond the last gasp," and death will occur if resuscitation is not started.

Thus, although the Apgar score is a helpful "shorthand" way of assessing an infant's status at birth, it is more meaningful to consider the distinction between primary and terminal apnea. Gasping infants should always be treated as though they are in terminal apnea.

Resuscitation

Risk factors that predict the need for resuscitation at birth are well known, but in a Swedish national survey of babies who required resuscitation, the need occurred unpredictably in 19%.[2] All professional staff working in an environment where babies are delivered must be regularly trained in appropriate resuscitation techniques. All equipment must be checked regularly to ensure that it is in working order. In a Chinese study, the introduction of standard neonatal resuscitation program guidelines developed by the American Academy of Pediatrics and the American Heart Association has been shown to result in a threefold reduction in perinatal mortality.[3]

The immediate management of birth asphyxia is directed towards rapid and efficient resuscitation followed by stabilization of the infant's condition. At birth, all infants should be gently but thoroughly dried and efforts made to prevent excessive heat loss. Only broad principles will be addressed here, and details including the management of complications such as meconium aspiration and pulmonary hypertension can be found in many standard textbooks on neonatology.

Suspected Primary Apnea

Most infants who do not cry or breathe spontaneously at birth are in primary apnea. They are often centrally cyanotic but they normally have a heart rate of greater than 100 beats/min. *Gentle* suction applied to the mouth and nose is traditional and harmless as long as it *is* gentle. Together with tactile stimulation and oxygen blown across the nostrils, it is usually sufficient to generate spontaneous breathing without the need for further intervention. However, if it is not sufficient, and the infant's circulatory signs remain favorable, a brief period of bag and mask ventilation will normally induce spontaneous breathing. In primary apnea, the first artificial inflation induces a gasp known as Head's paradoxical reflex – it is paradoxical because, in other circumstances, stimulation of stretch receptors within the lungs triggers cessation of inspiration. In recovery from primary apnea, spontaneous breathing is first established, and is rapidly followed by an accelerating heart rate and a generalized pink appearance.

The transplacental passage of opiate analgesics may prolong primary apnea in the newborn. If this is suspected, the infant should be treated with the specific opioid antagonist, naloxone (100 micrograms/kg), after ventilation has been established, either by positive pressure or spontaneously. The dose may be repeated if necessary. (It should be avoided, however, if maternal substance abuse is known or suspected.)

Suspected Secondary Apnea

Infants who were thought to have been in primary apnea but who fail to respond to the simple measures outlined above, as well as those who are apneic at birth, pale, and with a heart rate below 100 beats/ min, are presumed to be in secondary apnea; prompt resuscitation is required in these cases. Laryngoscopy should be performed immediately, and any mucus obstructing the view of the vocal cords should be removed by gentle suction. The infant should then be intubated and positive pressure ventilation should be given as a priority. Most infants in secondary apnea will respond to positive pressure ventilation that is administered effectively through an endotracheal tube. The sequence of response differs from that seen in primary apnea. A prompt increase in the heart rate and improvement in the infant's color *precedes* the onset of spontaneous breathing. In broad terms, the time interval between the start of positive pressure ventilation and the onset of regular spontaneous breathing is a guide to the severity of the intrauterine hypoxemic insult.

If there is severe bradycardia (<60 beats/min), external cardiac massage should be given. If severe bradycardia persists after approximately 1 minute of cardiac massage, it is reasonable to infer that the infant has a significant metabolic acidemia and sodium bicarbonate can be given through an umbilical venous catheter (2–3 mEq/kg), provided ventilation is adequate. Infants who remain pale with a persisting severe bradycardia despite adequate positive pressure ventilation, cardiac massage, and treatment with sodium bicarbonate might have another problem that requires consideration (Table 1). If other problems are considered unlikely, and the cause is severe intrauterine hypoxemia, the situation is perilous. There is a range of options traditionally used to improve cardiac activity and circulation, including epinephrine (through the endotracheal tube or intravenously), atropine, calcium gluconate, and volume expansion by colloid or crystalloid. It is probably not justified to continue with active resuscitation beyond the age of 15 minutes in infants with persisting circulatory failure if all attempts to correct this have failed.

Resuscitation Controversies

Air Versus Oxygen

It is standard practice in many delivery rooms to resuscitate babies with 100% oxygen. There is evidence from animal experiments and also from several human studies to suggest that this is unnecessary and also potentially harmful.[4,5] (These data are summarized in Chapter 9.) None of the experimental data sheds lights on whether there are long-term harmful effects of resuscitation with 100% oxygen. Furthermore, the resuscitation needs of individual infants are not identical, and firm conclusions cannot yet be drawn about the safety of resuscitation with room air.

Hypothermia

Accidental hypothermia is a common complication during resuscitation, but cold stress may be associated with increased energy utilization of oxygen to maintain body temperature, and therefore should be avoided if at all possible. Planned and controlled hypothermia may be a therapeutic strategy in the future (see Chapter 14), but it cannot be recommended at present.

Correction of Metabolic Acidosis

Metabolic acidemia is a feature of severe intrapartum asphyxia, but there is no justification for the *routine* use of buffer agents at resuscitation. The use of sodium bicarbonate in infants with prolonged bradycardia who are receiving cardiac massage was mentioned earlier. After resuscitation, infants who have good circulation and effective ventilation should be able to correct spontaneously a mild or moderate acidemia. Early assessment of arterial pH is helpful as a baseline, and a further measurement should be made an hour later. If the pH has not significantly improved by the second measurement, it is reasonable to use a buffer agent. The choice between sodium bicarbonate and tris-hydroxyaminomethane (THAM) should probably be influenced by the adequacy of ventilation and the potential for worsening respiratory acidemia. Sodium bicarbonate, in large doses or infused too rapidly, has been implicated as a risk factor for intracranial hemorrhage.[6]

The routine use of albumin in neonatal resuscitation is controversial; there is no evidence that this practice is beneficial for the baby and it may be associated with additional myocardial compromise.[7] A recent systematic review of albumin infusion has suggested that it may increase mortality,[8] but this report included both adult and infant studies.

Intravenous Glucose

Glucose is often given during routine resuscitation to avoid hypoglycemia, which is a common complication of asphyxia. It has been known for many years that glucose infusion resulting in hyperglycemia is associated with adverse effects on asphyxial cerebral injury in the adolescent or mature animal.[9] This association has been extrapolated by some investigators to the fetus and newborn, but evidence to support it is very limited.

More recently, published reports have shown conclusively that there is a fundamental difference between the way the immature and mature brains respond to glucose infusion. (These differences are described in Chapter 5.) In experimental situations, the immature brain appears to be protected by elevated blood glucose levels immediately prior to asphyxia compared with animals that were not exposed to additional glucose.[10] The evidence that administration of glucose *after* asphyxia in immature animals is beneficial remains controversial. Hattori and Wasterlain have shown that glucose treatment following hypoxic-ischemic insult in 7-day-old rat pups protects against neuropathologic damage compared to controls.[11] However, another study in immature rat pups found that treatment with glucose immediately after hypoxic-ischemic insult caused more severe neuronal damage than in animals exposed to a similar insult without glucose infusion.[12]

Animal models are useful in extending our knowledge about the effects of substrate manipulation in hypoxic-ischemic injury. However, our ability to evaluate the benefit for asphyxiated human newborn infants is still a long way off. Until then, well-established principles must be relied upon, i.e., following birth asphyxia, the development of hypoglycemia should be monitored and treated, and the use of additional glucose to induce hyperglycemia should be avoided.

Neonatal Encephalopathy

Neonatal encephalopathy is a disturbance in cerebral function that manifests as a cluster of signs, including a disturbed level of

Table 3

Other Causes of Neonatal Encephalopathy

Intracranial pathology
- Stroke (cerebral infarction)
- Intracranial hemorrhage/ischemia
- Congenital cerebral malformation/dysgenesis

Infectious disorders
- Early onset meningitis
- Congenital infections (bacterial, TORCH)

Metabolic disorders
- Hypoglycemia, hypocalcemia, hypo/hypernatremia
- Hyperammonemia
- Amino acid disorders
- Organic acid disorders
- Pyridoxine dependency

Toxic disorders
- Neonatal abstinence syndrome following maternal drug addiction

TORCH = toxoplasmosis, other (syphilis, hepatitis, zoster), rubella, cytomegalovirus, and herpes simplex (maternal infections).

arousal, altered muscle tone, brainstem dysfunction, seizures, and raised intracranial pressure. However, all of these features need not be present to warrant the term encephalopathy. The term *hypoxic-ischemic encephalopathy* (HIE) specifically refers to infants in whom encephalopathy is caused by a severe asphyxial insult. Other causes of neonatal encephalopathy that may be confused with HIE are shown in Table 3. It is inappropriate to label an encephalopathy as HIE simply because the clinical course was consistent with the occurrence of fetal hypoxia or because the newborn is encephalopathic. An early and accurate assessment and documentation of the factors thought to have causally contributed to neonatal encephalopathy is essential from both the clinical and medico-legal perspectives (see Chapter 15).

Hypoxic-Ischemic Encephalopathy

The onset of HIE following intrapartum asphyxia is within 24 hours of birth, most commonly within 12 hours of brain insult. Among those infants with moderate or severe HIE, the neurologic signs typically worsen during the first 3 or 4 days after birth and then gradually improve among survivors. Severe HIE may be accompanied by signs of secondary organ dysfunction from ischemia, which may involve the heart, kidneys, bowel, liver, and the hemostatic system. The extent to which secondary organ dysfunction is manifested clinically is variable, but the features include low-output cardiac failure, oliguria, and other

Table 4

Simplified Clinical Assessment of Encephalopathy

Level of arousal (consciousness)
- Lethargy: arouses spontaneously, but not maintained
- Obtundation: arouses on stimulation, not maintained
- Stupor: aroused only by painful stimulus
- Coma: not arousable

Spontaneous movements
- Frequency and type

Seizure activity
- Frequency and type

Posture
- Posture at rest, and abnormal posturing

Muscle tone
- Increased, decreased, or variable

Anterior fontanel and suture tension

Table 5

Suggested Chart for Recording Daily Clinical Assessment*

Assessment Items		Days of Week						
Tonic neck reflex	Slight							
	Strong							
	Absent							
Pupils	Dilated							
	Constricted							
	Poorly reactive							
Gut motility	Decreased							
	Normal							
	Increased/diarrhea							
Seizures	None							
	Focal or multifocal							
	Decerebrate posturing							
Drugs (dose)	Paralysis							
	Sedation							
	Anticonvulsants							

*Modified from Sarnat and Sarnat,[13] with permission.

signs of renal impairment, necrotizing enterocolitis, and disseminated intravascular coagulation.

Serial clinical assessment and documentation of the encephalopathy is important because its severity and duration reflect the magnitude of the hypoxic-ischemic brain injury, and, to some extent, predict neurodevelopmental outcome. Another cogent reason for serial assessment is that it reminds us to consider causes other than asphyxia. A simplified neurologic examination in these circumstances can be done quite quickly and is not difficult, but it is often a neglected aspect of the neonatal examination, and is often poorly documented in the medical record. The key elements are shown in Table 4. In some neonatal units, a more detailed daily clinical assessment of the infant's neurologic status is used; an example of such a protocol is shown in Table 5.

The grading of HIE as mild, moderate, or severe, as originally described by Sarnat and Sarnat in 1976, remains helpful (Table 6).[13] This can be simplified as follows: the distinguishing features of mild HIE are a hyperalert state, the absence of seizures, and normal muscle tone; these manifestations appear during the first 24 hours of life, and then

Table 6

Severity of Neonatal Encephalopathy*

	Stage I (Mild)	Stage II (Moderate)	Stage III (Severe)
Sensorium	Jitteriness Hyperalert Irritability	Lethargic Dulled sense	Stuporous
Muscle tone	Normal	Hypotonia at rest Hypertonia on stimulation	Flaccid Unresponsiveness
Posture	Mild distal flexion	Strong distal flexion	Intermittent decerebrate
Stretch reflexes	Overactive	Decreased	Absent
Moro reflex	Strong Low threshold	Incomplete High threshold	Absent
Suck reflex	Normal	Weak	Absent
Seizures	None	Focal or multifocal	Decerebrate posturing

*Modified from Sarnat and Sarnat,[13] with permission.

progressively diminish. Moderate HIE is characterized by seizures, and the infant is lethargic or obtunded with mild hypotonia. The clinical situation remains severely abnormal for 48 to 72 hours or longer, and following this, improvement is usual. Severe HIE is characterized by stupor or coma, with flaccid muscle tone; seizures may be frequent, and may occur against a background of abnormal posturing suggestive of decerebrate rigidity. Signs of increased intracranial pressure with a tense fontanel and loss of pupillary and oculo-vestibular reflexes may develop after 24 to 72 hours, and these signs are characterized as ominous. There is a relationship between the severity of HIE and outcome. In a meta-analysis comprising more than 400 infants with HIE with an overall mortality of 12.5%, Peliowski and Finer concluded that the predicted risk of death in severe HIE is 61%, in moderate HIE, 5.6%, and in mild HIE, the risk is virtually zero.[14]

Obviously, the use of anticonvulsants may suppress seizure activity, and when given in large doses or combined with opioids, the infant's level of arousal will be affected. This does not negate the role of neurologic assessment, and in Sarnat and Sarnat's original classification, depression of the background electroencephalogram (EEG) pattern was a feature in those infants with severe (stage III) encephalopathy.[13]

Care of Infants with Hypoxic-Ischemic Encephalopathy

Infants with severe HIE often have multisystem derangements of function. The management of these infants is directed toward: (1) the provision of supportive care; (2) strategies that are aimed, at least in theory, at protecting the brain from further damage; and (3) a consideration of the ethical implications of decisions to continue intensive care in babies who are critically ill and who have underlying extensive brain damage.

Respiratory Support

Some infants who develop HIE have received assisted ventilation that commenced with their initial resuscitation in the delivery room. In others, respiratory support may be started because of respiratory depression, frequent and refractory convulsions, or because of deranged blood gases resulting from persistent pulmonary hypertension, meconium aspiration syndrome, or some other parenchymal lung disease.

Babies with hypercapnia ($Paco_2$ >50 mmHg, 7 kPa) should be intubated and ventilated promptly because, with an underlying condition of severe HIE, hypercapnia often becomes progressively worse in the spontaneously breathing infant. This especially applies to those infants with frequent or prolonged seizures. Respiratory support may also be needed to combat respiratory depression in infants who need relatively large doses of anticonvulsant therapy to control their seizures. Control of seizures is a priority, and fear that the infant might require mechanical ventilation cannot be considered justification for inadequate anticonvulsant treatment.

The potentially harmful effects of raised carbon dioxide tension in infants with HIE are: (1) the development of tissue acidosis; (2) an increase in cerebral blood flow and possibly a risk of cerebral hemorrhage; (3) the loss of autoregulation of cerebral perfusion; and (4) possible induction of an intracerebral "steal" phenomenon, in which perfusion of undamaged brain occurs at the expense of damaged but potentially viable brain tissue.

In adults, for every 1 mmHg (0.13 kPa) change in $Paco_2$, there is approximately a 3% change in cerebral blood flow over the physiologic range for $Paco_2$.[15] This proportional change diminishes for levels of $Paco_2$ below 20 mmHg (2.7 kPa). A similar relationship has been shown in the newborn infant.[16] However, following intrapartum asphyxia, the arteriolar response may be less sensitive to changes in $Paco_2$, and in some infants there may be a paradoxical increase in cerebral blood flow with controlled hyperventilation.[17]

Hypocapnia ($Paco_2$ <22.5 mmHg or <3.0 kPa) has been reported to be associated with periventricular leukomalacia in the preterm newborn by a presumed mechanism of inducing regional cerebral ischemia.[18] As cerebral ischemia is an important component of the pathophysiology of post-asphyxial injury, it is possible that severe hyperventilation may exacerbate impaired reperfusion to the compromised brain. This is particularly relevant when high-frequency ventilation is being used, as it has the propensity to produce hypocapnia if ΔP (amplitude) is not adjusted properly.

The precise influence of carbon dioxide tension on cerebral blood flow and perfusion in infants with HIE is likely to be complex, with many other confounding factors. For example, Ferriero and Ashwal (see Chapter 8) have drawn attention to the complementary role of nitric oxide. In the absence of clinical trials of hyperventilation in asphyxiated newborn infants, and in light of the current knowledge, the recommendation is to maintain normocapnia.

Persistent pulmonary hypertension of the newborn (PPHN) has been reported to be a specific complication of birth asphyxia.[19] It can pose a particular problem in ventilated infants who are severely hypoxemic and who have HIE. In order to control the hypoxemia, the temptation exists to use excessively high ventilatory pressures. Many of these infants do not have parenchymal lung disease and are exposed to the risk of raised intrathoracic pressure, which might impair venous return and thus reduce cardiac output. Raised cerebral venous pressure and reduced arterial blood pressure result in impaired cerebral perfusion. The management of PPHN is beyond the scope of this chapter, but other methods should be used to control PPHN while keeping distending pressure, tidal volume delivery, and positive endexpiratory pressure to a necessary minimum.

PPHN may coexist with meconium aspiration syndrome; in this case, there is the potential for gross derangements in pulmonary mechanics and blood gases, which impact adversely on the cerebral circulation.

Hypotension

Asphyxia may cause myocardial ischemia and, more rarely, myocardial necrosis.[20,21] Myocardial dysfunction detected by Doppler ultrasound studies has been reported in 28–50% of asphyxiated infants.[19,22,23]

Evidence for myocardial ischemia may also be present on echocardiography.[24,25] Compromise of myocardial contractility may reduce cardiac output because of decreased stroke volume with subsequent systemic hypotension. In extreme cases, cardiogenic shock and heart failure may occur.[26,27] Acute cardiac dilation associated with asphyxia may cause functional tricuspid insufficiency, thereby further impairing cardiac function.[28] In a group of infants with low Apgar scores and acidosis (pH <7.10), blood pressure, cardiac output, and stroke volume were found to be lower than in a similar but nonacidotic group.

As hypotension is a common and anticipated complication of asphyxiated infants, continuous or very frequent monitoring of arterial blood pressure is essential.[29] Volume expansion is often ineffective in restoring normotension, and the use of albumin carries the risk of an additional volume load on an already compromised myocardium. Dopamine (5–20 microgram/kg/min) or dobutamine (5–20 microgram/kg/min) is usually necessary to raise the blood pressure to the normal range.

Renal Impairment

In experimental fetal and neonatal animal models, asphyxia causes a marked reduction in renal blood flow with a significant increase in the vascular resistance of the kidney,[30] and renal failure is a relatively common complication of a severe asphyxial insult.[31] In human infants, Doppler studies of renal hemodynamics after birth asphyxia have shown an increase in apparent renal vascular resistance with a reduction in renal systolic flow velocity,[32] which has been used to predict the development of acute renal failure.[33]

The incidence of renal impairment following birth asphyxia varies from 23% to 55% in different reports.[34,35] Acute renal failure was reported in 19% of asphyxiated infants born at ≥ 34 weeks gestation.[36] Full-term asphyxiated newborns have impaired renal tubular function compared with controls,[37] and the severity is related to the magnitude of the insult.

Oliguria from renal compromise is managed by maintenance of careful fluid balance, and the infant should receive only the volume of fluid necessary to maintain adequate hydration. It is often helpful to measure serum osmolality, and urinary osmolality or specific gravity, with the objective of maintaining the serum osmolality near 290 mOsm/L and/or the urinary specific gravity at 1.010.

Daily measurement of the plasma creatinine level is the most sensitive clinical method of assessing renal function. Measurement of central venous pressure in severely oliguric patients may help with the fluid management of acute renal failure but is fraught with practical difficulties. The decision to undertake dialysis or hemofiltration is based on the patient's clinical condition, biochemical data, and on the extent of the predicted course of brain injury. There are sensitive issues involved in this decision, which must be resolved by the parents, neonatologists, and nephrologists.

Gastrointestinal Complications

Birth asphyxia is associated with abnormalities of gastrointestinal motility detected by low-compliance perfusion manometry,[38] and an increased risk of necrotizing enterocolitis.[19,39,40] Abnormal liver function tests are also described in asphyxiated infants.[41] The management of suspected necrotizing enterocolitis is expectant with the avoidance of enteral feeds and the provision of intravenous nutrition and broad spectrum antibiotics. Severe necrotizing enterocolitis or perforation of the bowel requires pediatric surgical assessment and intervention.

Altered Hemostasis

Disseminated intravascular coagulation is relatively common after intrapartum asphyxia, and bleeding as a result of this condition may cause severe secondary complications, including intracranial hemorrhage.[42–45] Management of disseminated intravascular coagulation is supportive, and there is no role for systemic heparinization. The infant should receive additional vitamin K and may require either fresh frozen plasma for replacement of clotting factors, platelet transfusions, or both. Regular hematologic checks of clotting function should be performed in all infants with severe birth asphyxia.

Metabolic Abnormalities

Metabolic problems, including hyponatremia, hypoglycemia, hypocalcemia, metabolic acidosis, and hyperammonemia, are commonly seen in asphyxiated infants. Hyponatremia may be the result of fluid retention secondary to intrinsic renal compromise, or it may be caused by the syndrome of inappropriate antidiuretic hormone secretion (SIADH), which is associated with elevated levels of antidiuretic hormone, resulting in fluid retention.[46,47] SIADH is suspected by the observation of dilute plasma and concentrated urine. Fluids should be restricted until the serum osmolality and the serum sodium concentration have returned to normal.

An association between transient hyperammonemia and severe perinatal asphyxia has been described.[48] The reason for this association is unclear, but it may be related to increased protein breakdown superimposed upon impaired liver function. Some of the clinical features in these infants that are attributed to asphyxia, including hyperthermia, hypertension, and lack of beat-to-beat variability, may in fact be caused by hyperammonemia.

Many other metabolic constituents may be raised in the blood or cerebrospinal fluid of infants with birth asphyxia.[49] These include the lactate/pyruvate ratio,[50] brain-specific creatine kinase,[51] neuron-specific enolase,[52] hypoxanthine,[53] hydroxybutyrate dehydrogenase, beta-endorphin, and various inflammatory markers.[54] None of the aforementioned are reliable predictors of outcome; however, they are interesting in that they reinforce basic science research on the mechanisms of hypoxic-ischemic brain damage, and because their presence serves to generate new research hypotheses that can be tested in animals.

Brain-Oriented Management Strategies

Although the idea of brain-oriented management sounds innovative, all medical and nursing strategies in neonatal intensive care, regardless of the underlying condition of the infant, should take into account the potential effects on the cerebral circulation and brain oxygenation. Earlier in this chapter, for example, attention was drawn to the implications of assisted ventilation on the cerebral circulation.

In the last decade, research in the field of neurobiology has enhanced the understanding of the biochemical consequences of an asphyxial event, as discussed in other chapters in this volume. The research points toward the use of specific neuroprotective strategies for asphyxiated infants in the hope of improving their chances of survival without major neurodevelopmental disability. Despite optimism regarding treatments such as hypothermia, antioxidants, and inflammatory modulators, the results of well-designed clinical trials are necessary before these treatments are implemented.

Traditionally, management of the asphyxiated infant has been directed toward achieving a stable condition, adequate treatment of seizures, and the prevention or control of cerebral edema. Increased awareness of subtle seizures or asymptomatic electroconvulsive activity in infants given neuromuscular relaxing agents has led to the wider use of continuous EEG monitoring with a cerebral function monitor (CFM). However, seizures and brain swelling are the *results* of the original brain injury rather than its cause, thus reinforcing the previously mentioned concern regarding the development of treatment strategies that target pathophysiologic mechanisms operating at a very early stage after the acute asphyxial event.

Management of Seizures

Seizures or electroseizure activity occur as the result of a variety of brain insults, and approximately 5–8 per 1000 newborn babies have clinically apparent seizures. In full-term infants, approximately 50% of clinical seizures are the result of birth asphyxia. Evidence from animal models suggests that prolonged seizures may cause additional neuronal damage by increasing metabolic demands and perturbing blood flow, as well as by contributing to the primary injury through the release of neurotoxic chemicals.

These observations, however, probably have only indirect relevance to the human newborn. Animal studies have induced seizures by pharmacologic or electrical means that are not directly comparable to the human situation. In addition, the seizure duration in these studies is prolonged and continuous, which also may not be relevant to the majority of neonatal convulsions. The effect of multiple anticonvulsant therapy may itself cause neuronal compromise; thus, the risk/benefit analysis of the use of anticonvulsants following neonatal post-asphyxial convulsions is difficult to determine.

Principles that underlie the occurrence of seizures in the newborn are listed in Table 7. These principles suggest the following treatment strategies:

1. A high suspicion should be maintained that unusual motor or autonomic activity might be a seizure.
2. Asphyxiated babies with abnormal movements should have an abbreviated EEG or CFM assessment to identify frequent or prolonged cortical seizure activity out of proportion with clinical observations.
3. Short-lived or infrequent convulsions (either clinical or electroseizure) may not require anticonvulsant treatment. It may not be necessary to eliminate all seizures, but treatment should be given if they are frequent (3 or more per hour), or prolonged (clinical or electroseizures lasting more than 2 minutes).

Table 7

Principles for the Management of Seizures

- Physiologic characteristics of the immature brain make the expression of seizures different from that in adults.
- Clinically evident movements interpreted as "seizures" may not be associated with cortically generated seizure activity on an EEG.
- Partial or fragmentary seizures that are evident clinically may grossly underestimate the electroseizure activity on EEG.
- Frequent or prolonged seizures require pharmacologic treatment.
- Approximately 50% of infants with "post-asphyxial convulsions" do not show severe neurodevelopmental sequelae.

EEG = electroencephalogram.

4. Once a decision has been made to treat seizures, the minimum number of anticonvulsants should be used to achieve acceptable control. Again, this does not mean that all seizures must be stopped.

5. One anticonvulsant at a time should be used to maximum tolerance before introducing a second. A more vigorous attempt should be made to treat seizures if the abnormal EEG is continuous (status epilepticus).

6. If the infant is pharmacologically paralyzed, motor activity cannot be evaluated. In such cases, the EEG should be repeated at regular intervals or continuous monitoring should be used to determine evidence of electrical seizure activity.

7. Anticonvulsants can be stopped once the infant is neurologically normal on clinical examination.

Barbiturates

Phenobarbital is historically the first-line anticonvulsant in the management of neonatal convulsions. The dosage of phenobarbital (20–30 mg/kg loading dose, followed by 3–6 mg/kg/day) should be carefully monitored in asphyxiated infants as toxicity may easily occur. With this dosage regimen, one can expect to achieve a serum level in microgram/mL that corresponds to the number of mg/kg given, since the volume of distribution is approximately 1.0 L/kg. Gal et al showed that asphyxiated infants require about half of the maintenance dose compared with nonasphyxiated infants to achieve a similar plasma concentration.[55] If frequent or prolonged convulsions continue, additional phenobarbital can be given. The half-life may be quite prolonged (up to 200 hours), so accumulation may occur even at maintenance dosing.

Barbiturates have multiple actions which are dose-related and may be specific to the particular type of barbiturate (Table 8).[56-61] Both human and animal studies have shown a benefit of barbiturates in the management of hypoxic-ischemic injury, but only when the drug was administered *before* the asphyxial event.[62-64] A number of randomized clinical trials assessing the cerebral protective effects of barbiturate (phenobarbital or thiopentone) administration in human newborns after resuscitation from birth asphyxia have shown no significant differences in outcome.[65-67]

The short-acting barbiturate, thiopentone, is associated with unacceptable side effects. In one study, 14 of the 17 infants given thiopentone treatment required inotropic support for hypotension compared with only 7 of 15 controls.[65] Eyre and Wilkinson reported the use of thiopentone in six severely asphyxiated infants.[66] The dosage was sufficient to produce an isoelectric EEG. In two infants, the infusion was stopped because of hypotension, and in all six the outcome was death or severe handicap.

Svenningsen et al recommended the routine use of phenobarbital (10 mg/kg) within 1 hour of delivery in all severely asphyxiated infants.[68] Using this strategy, as well as others, they claim to have reduced the mortality and incidence of neurodevelopmental disability. It seems unlikely, however, that the effect of phenobarbital in this low dose (by modern standards) would have any significant protective effect on the brain. It is more likely that these authors observed an improved outcome by paying closer attention to all aspects of the care of asphyxiated infants.

More recently, a randomized (nonblinded) controlled trial of phe-

Table 8

Actions of Barbiturates

- Reduction in cerebral metabolic rate (thiopentone reduces this by up to 50%).[56]
- Depression of cerebral function, including suppression of the EEG to the point at which it becomes isoelectric.[56]
- Reduction in cerebral blood flow from an increase in cerebral vascular resistance.[57,58]
- Reduction of cerebral edema.[59]
- Oxygen free radical consumption.[60]
- Biochemical modification of cells, including stabilization of lysosomal membranes, reduction in intracellular calcium concentrations, and modified neurotransmitter release.[61]

EEG = electroencephalogram.

nobarbital (40 mg/kg over 1 hour) prior to the onset of seizures in 20 severely asphyxiated babies showed that the outcome at 3 years was significantly better than in a similar group of babies in whom phenobarbital was given only after onset of seizures.[67] However, a meta-analysis of barbiturate treatment in asphyxia has not shown an overall benefit when all studies were considered together.[69]

Phenytoin

Phenytoin is widely used in the treatment of post-asphyxial convulsions. If phenobarbital monotherapy at a serum concentration of 40–60 micrograms/mL is not effective, a loading dose of phenytoin (20 mg/kg by slow intravenous injection) may be used to achieve control of frequent seizures. This will generally achieve a serum level of 20 micrograms/mL. Although an additional bolus of 10 mg/kg may be given, too high a dose of phenytoin (serum level above 25 micrograms/mL) should be avoided because neurotoxicity may develop. Maintenance therapy with phenytoin is also difficult to control because of the unpredictable pharmacokinetics of the drug. This unpredictability, together with the risk of toxic accumulation, reduces its value and margin of safety in the newborn. In a recent randomized controlled trial among 59 newborns with EEG-confirmed seizures, who were given either phenobarbital or phenytoin intravenously in a dose to achieve appropriate serum levels, both drugs were equally but incompletely effective in controlling seizures (43% versus 45%, respectively).[70] Phenytoin does not appear to be reliably absorbed in the newborn and the oral route is not acceptable for maintenance therapy. Its use is contraindicated with lignocaine (lidocaine).

Benzodiazepines

Four members of this group of drugs have been used to treat neonatal convulsions: diazepam, clonazepam, lorazepam, and midazolam. Diazepam is rapidly acting, with major side effects including respiratory depression, hypotension, and hypotonia. Loading doses as high as 1 mg/kg may be necessary to achieve therapeutic plasma concentrations. In view of the long half-life of this drug in the body, its use in the newborn is not recommended.

Lorazepam is relatively short-acting and is better than diazepam at bringing acute seizure activity under sustained control.[71] Lorazepam is also a better anticonvulsant than diazepam because it is not as rapidly cleared from the brain after intravenous administration. The half-life in the neonatal period is 30–50 hours. There is only limited information on the use of this drug in the neonatal period. The recommended dosage is 100 micrograms/kg once every 24 hours intravenously or intramuscularly, for 2 to 3 days in babies resistant to routine anticonvulsant medication.

Clonazepam is used by some as a second-line anticonvulsant (100 micrograms/kg loading dose by slow intravenous injection) followed by an intermittent dosage regimen every 24 hours. In intractable seizures, clonazepam has been used by continuous intravenous infusion in doses of 10–60 micrograms/kg/hour, but this is not recommended by the manufacturer and may be associated with severe hypotension. Drug tolerance becomes a problem if treatment is continued for any extended period, and increasing seizure activity may occur if the serum level exceeds 125 micrograms/mL.

Midazolam is a very short-acting benzodiazepine that is becoming more widely used as an anticonvulsant, although there is limited pharmacokinetic or pharmacodynamic data as to its effects on the newborn. It also has important sedative actions. The recommended regimen is 0.05 mg/kg as a loading dose followed by 0.15 mg/kg/hour. It is suggested that midazolam may have a synergistic effect with lignocaine (lidocaine) (see below). High-dose intravenous neonatal medication may cause respiratory depression, hypotension, and a fall in cerebral blood flow.

Lignocaine

In Scandinavian countries, lignocaine (lidocaine) is a commonly used second-line anticonvulsant. The recommended anticonvulsant dosage is 2 mg/kg as a loading dose followed by 6 mg/kg/hour by continuous infusion. There may be synergism between lignocaine and midazolam, and this combination may be useful in babies with refractory seizures. The potentially cardiotoxic effects of lignocaine are rarely seen, but are more common if phenytoin has been given prior to starting the infusion of lignocaine.

Paraldehyde

Paraldehyde has a very short-acting effect and is largely excreted by the lungs. It may be useful as an intermittent bolus while waiting for the first- or second-line anticonvulsants to have an effect if the baby continues to have frequent or prolonged convulsions. The dosage is 0.15 mL/kg given by deep intramuscular injection every 4–6 hours as required. It should generally be administered by a glass syringe. Its use in the U.S. has largely been abandoned.

Cerebral Edema

Brain swelling (cerebral edema) occurs as the result of an acute brain insult. Edema has been described as either cytotoxic (cell swelling) or vasogenic, which occurs secondary to leaking of the arteriolar endothelial barrier, with accumulation of water in the interstitial space around the cells. In practice, it is likely that both processes occur. In a fetal monkey model, evidence of cerebral edema both macroscopically and microscopically has been reported within 2 hours of a severe asphyxial insult.[72] The median time for severe intracranial hypertension (intracranial pressure >15 mmHg) to develop in the human newborn following asphyxia is 26 hours (Levene, unpublished data).

The physiologic response to cerebral edema that is severe enough to cause an increase in intracranial pressure is a rise in the systemic blood pressure and a slowing of the heart rate (Cushing's response). If the blood pressure rises in the same proportion as the intracranial pressure, then there will be no change in perfusion pressure. Therefore, maintenance of adequate blood pressure, as mentioned earlier in this chapter, is very important at least in the early stages of cerebral edema.

Cerebral edema that is severe enough to cause secondary cerebral hypoperfusion is a potential complication of asphyxia, and adequate treatment of intracranial hypertension will not prevent brain injury per se. Levene et al analyzed the results of monitoring and treating raised intracranial pressure in full-term asphyxiated infants.[73] Intervention to control intracranial hypertension had a significant beneficial effect on outcome in less than 10% of the babies studied.

There is no convenient, noninvasive way of accurately measuring intracranial pressure in newborns. Increase in intracranial pressure may be detected clinically by palpation of the anterior fontanel, but this method is neither sensitive nor specific. Acute deterioration in neurologic state may be another feature of significantly raised intracranial pressure, and strong suspicion of this condition is often considered to be an indication for treatment. None of the proposed treatments discussed below is unequivocally effective, since cerebral edema appears to be associated with brain destruction and cellular water overload.

Corticosteroids

Corticosteroids have been widely used in the management of the asphyxiated newborn infant based on their alleged property of reducing brain swelling, but there are no data from either newborn humans or animal models to support their use. Studies on 5-day-old rats showed that pretreatment with dexamethasone before asphyxia resulted in less severe cerebral effects than in untreated animals.[74] The use of steroids following neonatal asphyxia was ineffective in treating or preventing cerebral edema.[75] Levene and Evans found no improvement in cerebral perfusion pressure within 6 hours of administering dexamethasone.[76]

It has been suggested that the main benefit of dexamethasone is in treating vasogenic edema and it is less effective in cytotoxic edema[77]; however, in clinical practice, both types of brain swelling probably occur. The major role of corticosteroids is in the treatment of focal cerebral edema associated with brain tumor or abscess, neither of which bears a close resemblance to the generalized brain swelling that is likely to occur following intrapartum asphyxia. There is now considerable evidence that suggests an adverse effect of corticosteroids on the developing brain even when they are used over short periods of time. Thus, there is no convincing evidence of the beneficial effect of steroids after birth asphyxia, and their use is not recommended.

Osmotic Agents

One approach to reduce brain swelling is to increase the osmotic pressure in the systemic circulation in order to cause a shift of water from the brain across the semi-permeable blood-brain barrier. A theoretical hazard of this is that the osmotic agent will enter into the brain through the damaged blood-brain barrier, causing a rebound effect of brain swelling. A number of osmotic agents, including mannitol, glycerol, and urea, have been used to try to shrink the swollen neonatal brain.

In a neonatal animal model, mannitol has been shown to significantly reduce the water content of the brain when given immediately after an asphyxial event,[78] but it did not reduce the severity or distribution of brain damage in treated versus untreated animals. Mannitol is also the only osmotic agent for which published data exist on its use in the newborn. Marchal et al, in an uncontrolled study, administered mannitol to 225 babies with the diagnosis of asphyxia, although the precise indications for treatment varied.[79] Early treatment was defined as mannitol infusion (1 g/kg) before the baby was 2 hours of age.

There were significantly fewer deaths (p=0.005), and the survivors had a better neurologic outcome (p=0.014) in the early treatment group compared with those who were treated after 2 hours.

In a nonrandomized study monitoring the effects of mannitol on intracranial pressure in a group of severely asphyxiated babies, a reduction in intracranial pressure and an improvement in cerebral perfusion pressure was found on each occasion when mannitol (1 g/kg over 20 minutes) was infused intravenously.[76] This appears to be the only agent that is of proven value in treating intracranial hypertension in the asphyxiated newborn. Despite reduction in intracranial pressure in many babies, follow-up data did not suggest any difference in the long-term outcome. In view of this finding, there is no rationale for the routine use of mannitol in the management of asphyxiated infants.

Predicting Outcomes in Birth Asphyxia

Various clinical observations or investigations have been applied at different stages of birth asphyxia to determine their predictive value, if any. There are three variables that have been involved in this determination: the time of the test, the nature of the test, and the outcome that is being predicted.

There is no measurement or marker of intrapartum asphyxia that reliably predicts the outcome for the baby, except perhaps for the relatively clear indicator that, if the fetus has a grossly abnormal electronic fetal heart rate tracing for approximately 20 minutes or more before birth, and if this is associated with a scalp pH level of less than 7.0, it is likely that the baby will have depressed vital signs at birth and require resuscitation. This type of prediction is, however, of little clinical value.

Prediction of Outcomes Related to Condition at Birth

Even if it is the case that vital sign depression at birth was indeed caused by fetal hypoxemia alone, neither the degree of birth depression, nor the intensity of the infant's metabolic acidemia are reliable predictors of neurodevelopmental outcome. However, *prolonged* depression at birth in term infants, as reflected, for example, by an Apgar score of less than 3 at 20 minutes is associated with a poor outcome. A cord blood pH of less than 7.0 is also likely to be associated with an increased risk of neonatal death, or cerebral palsy among survivors.

Notwithstanding the recent promise of neuroprotective interventions soon after birth, it is arguable that there is little to be gained *practically* by a very early prediction of outcome. It is clinically obvious in the delivery room when a baby is critically depressed, severely acidemic, and requiring extensive resuscitation. The clinical status of the baby, rather than any predictive test, will normally dictate whether resuscitation should be discontinued. If resuscitation is continued, then predictions about outcome will normally be made later, based on further clinical observations and investigations. The difficulty is that the condition of the baby and the cord blood pH level are unreliable predictors of hypoxic-ischemic encephalopathy. *Early* prediction of a poor neurologic outcome before intracerebral secondary energy failure has advanced (see Chapter 6) may allow for the testing of different neuroprotective interventions, such as hypothermia, anti-inflammatory agents, and antioxidants.

The CFM, a simplified version of continuous EEG monitoring, provides an overall impression of cerebral activity. The CFM, usually referred to as the amplitude integrated EEG (aEEG), is easy to use and has a high concordance with the standard EEG. Burst suppression or paroxysmal activity has been reported to be associated with a poor neurodevelopmental outcome,[80] and these abnormalities may be present within 4 hours of birth.[81] At present, the aEEG is considered to be the best test to select infants shortly after delivery for neuroprotective interventional studies.

Prediction of Death and/or Disability

The predictive value of grading the clinical severity of HIE was addressed earlier in this chapter. Although it is often useful as a starting point for discussion with parents, this predictor and others used alone or in combination, do not provide the certainty that parents often seek. For example, even if it is determined that an infant has a 90% risk of surviving with significant disability, parents often want to know whether their baby will be among the 90% who are disabled or the 10% without significant impairment.

Electroencephalography

Although CFM is now widely used in neonatal care, comparison with a standard EEG should be performed, when possible, to confirm the aEEG data and to provide more detailed information than that obtained from the compressed one-channel EEG.

The EEG abnormalities seen in mature asphyxiated infants and associated with a poor prognosis include isoelectric recordings and periodic patterns,[13,82-84] and persistent low voltage states.[82] A normal EEG in asphyxiated infants is usually associated with an excellent prognosis.[13,83-86] A meta-analysis on four studies in which early EEG assessment could be correlated with outcome in groups of asphyxiated mature newborns showed that the overall risk of death or handicap is 95% for a severely abnormal EEG, 64% for a moderately abnormal EEG, and 3.3% for a normal or mildly abnormal EEG.[14] Further studies published since this meta-analysis have confirmed these findings.[83,84]

Doppler Assessment

Doppler ultrasound evaluation of cerebral hemodynamics has been shown to be a useful prognostic indicator in full-term asphyxiated newborns.[87-91] The low Pourcelot's resistance index of less than 0.55 predicts adverse outcome in full-term asphyxiated infants with an accuracy of 86%, sensitivity of 100%, and specificity of 81%.[87] The advantage of Doppler assessment is that abnormalities become apparent within 12–60 hours after birth.[87,88,91]

Brain Imaging

Early magnetic resonance (MR) brain scans offer some help with prognostication (see Chapter 13), although there are very limited data from babies scanned within the first 48 hours of life. Abnormality of signal intensity within the posterior limb of the internal capsule (PLIC), seen most clearly on inversion recovery sequences, is the best predictor of a poor neurodevelopmental outcome in MR scans taken within the first 10 days.[92] Abnormal or equivocal signal intensity within the PLIC predicted abnormal outcome with a sensitivity of 90%, specificity of 100%, and positive predictive value of 100%.

Withdrawal of Support

An integral part of the management strategy for severely asphyxiated newborns is a consideration of the justification for continuing intensive care. This applies particularly to assisted ventilation, insofar as supporting the breathing of infants with respiratory failure is life sustaining. This area of medical ethics requires the active involvement of the parents, and in the context of the term "asphyxiated infant," there are some particularly sensitive issues. While most parents appreciate the inherent risk of prematurity, it is understandably another matter to comprehend why full-term infants who are normally formed may face death or disability. It is even more difficult for parents to participate in "end-of-life" decisions when they suspect that the medical professionals themselves may have caused the problem (see Chapter 15).

The most common reason for withdrawing ventilatory support is based on the perception that an infant has entered the process of dying, and that assisted ventilation is prolonging death rather than saving life. It implies the occurrence, over a period of days, of multi-organ system failure that is not responding to appropriate treatments.

A rather different reason for withdrawing assisted ventilation is the notion that the infant *might well* survive with continuing care, but that substantial neurodevelopmental disability will severely limit the child's "quality of life," and will result in ongoing dependence on a caregiver for everyday living needs. This approach is fraught with ethical, moral, and medical difficulties, normally requiring appraisal and discussion between parents and staff. In addition, these discussions may, of necessity, occur within a short period of time. One scenario might be a baby with *persisting* abnormal neurologic signs, including an impaired level of consciousness, or seizures, and in whom there is obvious white matter damage shown on a brain scan. Sometimes, by the time a decision is ready to be made, the infant no longer requires assisted ventilation and can breathe spontaneously, albeit with a reduced level of consciousness. As noted, true quality of life decisions in neonatal intensive care units may be confounded by other ethical and legal implications.

One approach used for the early detection of irreversible brain damage is to perform an EEG (or CFM) at 6 hours, and to reassess the EEG together with a Doppler study at the age of 24 hours. If these tests at 6 and 24 hours are all abnormal, the term "irreversible brain injury" is used, and the parents are advised that the prognosis is extremely poor. When speaking to the parents, the terms "irreversible" and "massive brain injury" are more accurate than "brain death" (see next section), because of its misleading implication that the infant will not survive without the mechanical ventilator. Many of these babies do breathe once disconnected from the ventilator, and this may cause considerable distress to the parents if they are not warned about this in advance.

Limitations of Neonatal Criteria of Brain Death

The concept of "brain death" in full-term asphyxiated infants is not particularly useful. Criteria for the diagnosis of brain death in children have been published in the U.S.[93] and U.K.[94] Both documents state that brain death cannot be diagnosed in premature infants, but there is some disagreement as to the diagnosis of brain death in the mature newborn. The British Paediatric Association states that, in infants of 37 weeks gestation to 2 months of age, "given the state of knowledge it is rarely possible to diagnose confidently brainstem death at this age," and in infants below 37 weeks gestation "the concept of brainstem death is inappropriate for infants of this age group."[94] In the U.S., the Special Task Force of the American Academy of Pediatrics concluded that "in term newborns (>38 weeks gestation), the criteria (for diagnosing brain death) are useful 7 days after the neurologic insult."[93]

These differences arise because of the rapid developmental changes seen in the later stages of gestation and the early weeks of life. This means that there cannot be absolute reliance placed on the presence or absence of brainstem reflexes at this developmental age. Volpe describes two infants (one at 35 weeks gestation and one full-term) who survived after apparent brain death including coma, absent respiration, loss of pupillary responses to light, and loss of other brainstem responses.[95] The 35 weeks gestation infant showed near-normal development at 1 year of age. The full-term infant regained brainstem reflexes 24 hours following the first examination and left the hospital alive, although in a persistent vegetative state.

The American guidelines include laboratory data (EEG and radio-nuclide angiography). The natural history of the isoelectric EEG in the neonatal period is now well established in terms of predicting poor outcome, but many babies with this abnormality survive despite irreversible brain injury. A limited experience with radionuclide angiography in the neonatal period in confirming brain death makes its routine use questionable.

Ashwal and Schneider described the clinical course of 18 premature and full-term infants, who showed the features of brain death including coma, apnea, and absent brainstem reflexes.[96] About half of these infants had no evidence of cerebral blood flow on radionuclide scanning, and/or an isoelectric EEG on the first examination, although serum levels of phenobarbital greater than 25 micrograms/mL were thought to suppress the EEG and make the investigation unreliable. They concluded that, in full-term infants, the persistence of clinical signs of brainstem death was inconsistent with survival, and in premature infants the persistence of these signs for 3 days was inconsistent with survival without assisted ventilation. They also report that an isoelectric EEG in the absence of factors known to suppress the EEG was associated with inevitable death if the clinical signs of brain death persisted for 24 hours. Although all the babies in this study died, some survived for a time in a persistent vegetative state.

In summary, when a baby has multi-organ system failure resistant to treatment, associated with altered consciousness, little purpose is served by seeking confirmation of "brain death" (however defined) before withdrawing assisted ventilation. In other asphyxiated infants whose main features are coma and *clinical signs* consistent with brainstem death, formal confirmation of brain death by EEG and radionuclide angiography can still be associated with persisting brainstem function such as respiratory activity, despite the fact that the brain has been massively and irreparably damaged. These infants may survive for some time in a persistent vegetative state even when assisted ventilation has been withdrawn.

References

1. Dawes G: *Fetal and Neonatal Physiology.* Year Book, Chicago, 1968.
2. Palme-Kilander C: Methods of resuscitation in low-Apgar-score newborn infants: a national survey. Acta Paediatr Scand 1992;81:739–744.
3. Zhu XY, Fang HQ, Zeng SP, et al: The impact of the neonatal resuscitation programme guidelines (NRPG) on the neonatal mortality in a hospital in 1997. Singapore Med J 1997;38:485–487
4. Lundstrom K, Pryds O, Greisen G: Oxygen at birth and prolonged cerebral vasoconstriction in preterm infants. Arch Dis Child 1995;73:F81–F84.
5. Saugstad OD: Resuscitation with room-air or oxygen supplementation. Clin Perinatol 1998;25:741–756.
6. Levene MI, Fawer CL, Lamont RF. Risk factors in the development of intraventricular haemorrhage in the premature neonate. Arch Dis Child 1982;57:410–417.
7. Roberton NR: Use of albumin in neonatal resuscitation. Eur J Pediatr 1997;156:428–431.
8. Cochrane Injuries Group Albumin Reviewers: Human albumin administration in critically ill patients: systematic review of randomised controlled trials. BMJ 1998;317:235–240.
9. Wagner KR, Kleinholz M, de Courten-Myers GM, Myers RE: Hyperglycemic versus normoglycemic stroke: topography of brain metabolites, intracellular pH, and infarct size. J Cereb Blood Flow Metab 1992;12:213–222.
10. Vannucci RC, Mujsce DJ: Effect of glucose on perinatal hypoxic-ischemic brain damage. Biol Neonate 1992;62:215–224.
11. Hattori H, Wasterlain CG: Posthypoxic glucose supplement reduces hypoxic-ischemic brain damage in the neonatal rat. Ann Neurol 1990;28:122–128.

12. Sheldon RA, Partridge C, Ferriero DM: Postischemic hyperglycemia is not protective to the neonatal rat. Pediatr Res 1992;32:489–493.

13. Sarnat HB, Sarnat MS: Neonatal encephalopathy following fetal distress: a clinical and electroencephalographic study. Arch Neurol 1976;33:696–705.

14. Peliowski A, Finer NN: Birth asphyxia in the term infant. In Sinclair JC, Bracken MB (eds): *Effective Care of the Newborn Infant.* Oxford University Press, Oxford, 1992, pp 249–279.

15. Bruce DA: Effects of hyperventilation on cerebral blood flow and metabolism. Clin Perinatol 1984;11:673–680.

16. Greisen G. Cerebral blood flow and energy metabolism in the newborn. Clin Perinatol 1997;24:531–546.

17. Sankaran K: Hypoxic-ischemic encephalopathy: cerebrovascular carbon dioxide reactivity in neonates. Am J Perinatol 1984;1:114–117.

18. Gannon CM, Wiswell TE, Spitzer AR: Volutrauma, $Paco_2$ levels, and neurodevelopmental sequelae following assisted ventilation. Clin Perinatol 1998;25:159–175.

19. Perlman JM, Tack ED, Martin T, et al: Acute systemic organ injury in term infants after asphyxia. Am J Dis Child 1989;143:617–620.

20. DeSa DJ, Donnelly WH: Myocardial necrosis in the newborn. Perspect Pediatr Pathol 1984;8:295–311.

21. Donnelly WH, Bucciarelli RL, Nelson RM: Ischemic papillary muscle necrosis in stressed newborn infants. J Pediatr 1980;96:295–300.

22. van Bel F, Walther FJ: Myocardial dysfunction and cerebral blood flow velocity following birth asphyxia. Acta Paediatr Scand 1990;79:756–762.

23. Bennhagen RG, Weintraub RG, Lundstrom NR, et al: Hypoxic-ischemic encephalopathy is associated with regional changes in cerebral blood flow velocity and alterations in cardiovascular function. Biol Neonate 1998;73:275–286.

24. Daga SR, Prabhu PG, Chandrashekhar L, et al: Myocardial ischemia following birth asphyxia. Indian Pediatr 1983;20:567–571.

25. Primhak RA, Jedeikin R, Ellis G, et al: Myocardial ischemia in asphyxia neonatorum. Acta Paediatr Scand 1985;74:595–600.

26. Burnard ED, James LA: Failure of the heart after undue asphyxia at birth. Pediatrics 1961;28:545–547.

27. Cabal LA, Devaskar U, Siassi B, et al: Cardiogenic shock associated with perinatal asphyxia in preterm infants. J Pediatr 1980;4:705–710.

28. Bucciarelli RL, Nelson RM, Egan EA, et al: Transient tricuspid insufficiency of the newborn: a form of myocardial dysfunction in stressed newborns. Pediatrics 1977;59:330–334.

29. Diprose GK, Evans DH, Archer LNJ, et al: Dinamap fails to detect hypotension in very low birthweight infants. Arch Dis Child 1986;61:771–773.

30. Cohn HE, Sacks EJ, Heymann MA, Rudolph AM: Cardiovascular responses to hypoxemia and acidemia in fetal lambs. Am J Obstet Gynecol 1974;120:817–824.

31. Dauber IM, Krauss AN, Symchych PS, et al: Renal failure following perinatal asphyxia. J Pediatr 1976;88:851–855.

32. Akinbi H, Abbasi S, Hilpert PL, et al: Gastrointestinal and renal blood flow velocity profile in neonates with birth asphyxia. J Pediatr 1994;125:625–627.

33. Luciano R, Gallini F, Romagnoli C, et al: Doppler evaluation of renal blood flow velocity as a predictive index of acute renal failure in perinatal asphyxia. Eur J Pediatr 1998;157:656–660.

34. Fernandez F, Barrio V, Guzman J, et al: Beta-2-microglobulin in the assessment of renal function in full term newborns following perinatal asphyxia. J Perinat Med 1989;17:453–459.

35. Perlman JM, Tack ED: Renal injury in the asphyxiated newborn infant: relationship to neurologic outcome. J Pediatr 1988;113:875–879.

36. Roberts DS, Haycock GB, Dalton RN, et al: Prediction of acute renal failure after birth asphyxia. Arch Dis Child 1990;65:1021–1028.

37. Willis F, Summers J, Minutillo C, et al: Indices of renal tubular function in perinatal asphyxia. Arch Dis Child 1997;77:F57–F60.

38. Berseth CL, McCoy HH: Birth asphyxia alters neonatal intestinal motility in term neonates. Pediatrics 1992;90:669–673.

39. Caplan MS, Hedlund E, Adler L, Hsueh W. Role of asphyxia and feeding in a neonatal rat model of necrotizing enterocolitis. Pediatr Pathol 1994; 14:1017–1028.

40. Goldberg RN, Thomas DW, Sinatra FR: Necrotizing enterocolitis in the asphyxiated full-term infant. Am J Perinatol 1983;1:40–42.

41. Zanardo V, Bondio M, Pesini G, et al: Serum glutamic-oxaloacetic transaminase and glutamic-pyruvic transaminase activity in premature and full-term asphyxiated newborns. Biol Neonate 1985;47:61–69.

42. Chessells JM, Wigglesworth JS: Secondary haemorrhagic disease of the newborn. Arch Dis Child 1970;45:539–543.

43. Chadd MA, Elwood PC, Gray OP, et al: Coagulation defects in hypoxic full-term newborn infants. BMJ 1971;iv:516–518.

44. Anderson JM, Belton NR: Water and electrolyte abnormalities in the human brain after severe intrapartum asphyxia. J Neurol Neurosurg Psychiatr 1974;37:514–520.

45. Suzuki S, Morishita S: Hypercoagulability and DIC in high-risk infants. Semin Thromb Hemost 1998;24:463–466.

46. Daniel SS, Husain MK, Milliez J, et al: Renal response of the fetal lamb to complete occlusion of the umbilical cord. Am J Obstet Gynecol 1978;131: 514–519.

47. Speer ME, Gormon WA, Kaplan SL, et al: Elevation of plasma concentrations of arginine vasopressin following perinatal asphyxia. Acta Paediatr Scand 1984;73:610–614.

48. Goldberg RN, Cabal LA, Sinatra FR, et al: Hyperammonemia associated with perinatal asphyxia. Pediatrics 1979;64:336–341.

49. Volpe JJ. *Neurology of the Newborn.* 4th ed. W.B. Saunders Co, Philadelphia, 2001, pp 335–336.

50. Chou YH, Tsou Yau KI, Wang PJ: Clinical application of the measurement of cord plasma lactate and pyruvate in the assessment of high-risk neonates. Acta Paediatr 1998;87:764–768.

51. Sweet DG, Bell AH, McClure G, et al: Comparison between creatinine kinase brain isoenzyme (CK-BB) activity and Sarnat score for prediction of adverse outcome following perinatal asphyxia. J Perinat Med 1999;27:478–483.

52. Thornberg E, Thiringer K, Hagberg H, Kjellmer I: Neuron specific enolase in asphyxiated newborns: association with encephalopathy and cerebral function monitor trace. Arch Dis Child 1995;72:F39–F42.

53. Ruth V, Fyhrquist F, Clemons G, Raivio KO: Cord plasma vasopressin, erythyropoetin, and hypoxanthine as indices of asphyxia at birth. Pediatr Res 1988;24:490–494.

54. Oygur N, Sonmez O, Saka O, Yegin O. Predictive value of plasma and cere-

brospinal fluid tumour necrosis factor-α and interleukin-1β: concentrations in outcome of full term infants with hypoxic-ischemic encephalopathy. Arch Dis Child 1998;79:F190–F193.

55. Gal P, Toback J, Erkan NV, et al: The influence of asphyxia on phenobarbital dosing requirements in neonates. Dev Pharmacol Ther 1984;7:145–152.

56. Michenfelder JD: The interdependency of cerebral function and metabolic effects following massive doses of thiopental in the dog. Anesthesiology 1974;41:231–236.

57. Pierce EC, Lambertson CJ, Deutsch S, et al: Cerebral circulation and metabolism during thiopental anesthesia and hyperventilation in man. J Clin Invest 1962;41:1664–1671.

58. Hanson J, Anderson R, Sundt T: Influence of cerebral vasoconstricting and vasodilating agents on blood flow in regions of cerebral ischemia. Stroke 1975;6:642–648.

59. Simeone FA, Frazer G, Lawner P: Ischemic brain oedema: comparative effects of barbiturates and hypothermia. Stroke 1979;10:8–12.

60. Flamm ES, Demopoulos HB, Seligman ML, et al: Free radicals in cerebral ischemia. Stroke 1978;9:445–447.

61. Steen PA, Michenfelder JD: Mechanisms of barbiturate protection. Anesthesiology 1980;53:183–190.

62. Campbell AGM, Milligin JE, Talner NS: The effect of pretreatment with pentobarbital, meperidine or hyperbaric oxygen on the response to anoxia and resuscitation in newborn rabbits. J Pediatr 1968;72:518–527.

63. Cockburn F, Daniel SS, Dawes GS, et al: The effect of pentobarbital anesthesia on resuscitation and brain damage in fetal rhesus monkeys asphyxiated on delivery. J Pediatr 1969;75:281–291.

64. Goodlin RC, Lloyd D: Use of drugs to protect against fetal asphyxia. Am J Obstetr Gynecol 1970;107:227–231.

65. Goldberg R, Moscoso P, Bauer C, et al: Use of barbiturate therapy in severe perinatal asphyxia: a randomized controlled trial. J Pediatr 1986;109:851–856.

66. Eyre JA, Wilkinson AR: Thiopentone-induced coma after severe birth asphyxia. Arch Dis Child 1986;61:1084–1089.

67. Hall RT, Hall FK, Daily DK: High-dose phenobarbital therapy in term newborn infants with severe perinatal asphyxia: a randomized, prospective study with three year follow up. J Pediatr 1998;132:345–348.

68. Svenningsen NW, Blennow G, Lindroth M, et al: Brain-orientated intensive care treatment in severe neonatal asphyxia: effects of phenobarbitone protection. Arch Dis Child 1982;57:176–183.

69. Evans DJ, Levene MI. Anticonvulsants for preventing mortality and morbidity in full term newborns with perinatal asphyxia (Cochrane Review). In The Cochrane Library. Issue 1. Update Software, Oxford, 1998.

70. Painter MO, Scher MS, Stein AD, et al: Phenobarbital compared with phenytoin for the treatment of neonatal seizures. N Engl J Med 1999;341:485–489.

71. Maytal J, Novak GP, King KC: Lorazepam in the treatment of refractory neonatal seizures. J Child Neurol 1991;6:319–323.

72. Brann AW, Myers RE: Central nervous system findings in the newborn monkey following severe in utero partial asphyxia. Neurology 1975;25:327–338.

73. Levene MI, Evans DH, Forde A, et al: The value of intracranial pressure monitoring in asphyxiated newborn infants. Dev Med Child Neurol 1987; 29:311–319.
74. Adlard BPF, De Souza SW: Influence of asphyxia and of dexamethasone on ATP concentrations in the immature rat brain. Biol Neonate 1976;24: 82–88.
75. De Souza SW, Dobbing J: Cerebral oedema in developing brain. III. Brain water and electrolytes in immature asphyxiated rats treated with dexamethasone. Biol Neonate 1973;22:388–397.
76. Levene MI, Evans DH: Medical management of raised intracranial pressure after severe birth asphyxia. Arch Dis Child 1985;60:12–16.
77. Yamaguchi M, Shirakata S, Yamasaki S, et al: Ischemic brain edema and compression brain edema. Stroke 1976;7:77–83.
78. Mujsce DJ, Towfighi J, Stern DR, Vannucci RC: Mannitol therapy in perinatal hypoxic–ischemic brain damage in rats. Stroke 1990;21:1210–1214.
79. Marchal C, Costagliola P, Leveau PH, et al: Traitement de la souffrance cerebrale neonatale d'origine anoxique par le mannitol. Revue de Pédiatrie 1974;9:581–589.
80. Thornberg E, Ekstrom-Jodal B: Cerebral function monitoring: a method of predicting outcome in term neonates after severe perinatal asphyxia. Acta Paediatrica 1994;83:596–601.
81. Eken P, Toet MC, Groenendaal F, et al: Predictive value of early neuroimaging, pulsed Doppler and neurophysiology in full term infants with hypoxic-ischemic encephalopathy. Arch Dis Child 1995;73:F75–80.
82. Holmes G, Rowe J, Hafford J, et al: Prognostic value of the electroencephalogram in neonatal asphyxia. Electroencephalogr Clin Neurophysiol 1982;53:60–72.
83. Wertheim D, Mercuri E, Faundez JC, et al: Prognostic value of continuous electroencephalographic recording in full term infants with hypoxic ischemic encephalopathy. Arch Dis Child 1994;71:F97–F102.
84. Selton D, Andre M: Prognosis of hypoxic-ischemic encephalopathy in full term newborns: value of neonatal electroencephalography. Neuropediatrics 1997;28:276–280.
85. Rose AL, Lombroso CT: A study of clinical, pathological and electroencephalographic features in 137 full-term babies with a long term follow-up. Pediatrics 1970;111:133–141.
86. Watanabe K, Miyazaki S, Hara K, et al: Behavioural state cycles, background EEGs and prognosis of newborns with perinatal hypoxia. Electroencephalogr Clin Neurophysiol 1980;49:618–625.
87. Archer LNJ, Levene MI, Evans DH: Cerebral artery Doppler ultrasonography for prediction of outcome after perinatal asphyxia. Lancet 1986;ii: 1116–1118.
88. Levene MI, Fenton AC, Evans DH, et al: Severe birth asphyxia and abnormal cerebral blood-flow velocity. Dev Med Child Neurol 1989;31:427–434.
89. Low JA, Galbraith RS, Raymond MJ, et al: Cerebral blood flow velocity in term newborns following intrapartum fetal asphyxia. Acta Paediatr 1994; 83:1012–1016.
90. Liao HT, Hung KL: Anterior cerebral artery Doppler ultrasonography for prediction of outcome after perinatal asphyxia. Zhonghua Min Guo Xiao Er Ke Yi Xue Hui Za Zhi 1997;38:208–212.

91. Ilves P, Talvik R, Talkvik T: Changes in Doppler ultrasonography in asphyxiated term infants with hypoxic-ischemic encephalopathy. Acta Paediatr 1998;87:680–684.
92. Rutherford MA, Pennock JM, Counsell SJ, et al: Abnormal magnetic resonance signal in the internal capsule predicts poor neurodevelopmental outcome in infants with hypoxic ischemic encephalopathy. Pediatrics 1998;102: 323–329.
93. Task Force: Guidelines for the determination of brain death in children. Pediatrics 1987;80:298–300.
94. British Paediatric Association: *Diagnosis of Brain Stem Death in Infants and Children: A Working Party Report of the British Paediatric Association.* British Paediatric Association, London 1991.
95. Volpe JJ: Brain death determination in the newborn. Pediatrics 1987;80: 293–297.
96. Ashwal S, Schneider S: Brain death in the newborn. Pediatrics 1989;84: 429–437.
97. Richmond S. *Principles of Resuscitation at Birth.* Northern Neonatal Network. Hindson Print, Ltd, Newcastle upon Tyne, 1996, pp 8–9.

CHAPTER 13

Neuroimaging of Hypoxic-Ischemic Encephalopathy

Mary Rutherford

Introduction

Infants with neurologic signs consistent with hypoxic-ischemic encephalopathy (HIE) require a thorough assessment, which should include brain imaging. Imaging will determine whether the anatomy of the brain is normal and identify any acquired abnormalities that are consistent with a perinatal hypoxic-ischemic insult. In addition, early imaging may identify signs of antenatal damage, distinct from intrapartum abnormalities. The pattern of injury seen on imaging may be used not only for immediate management, but also to predict neurodevelopmental outcome following HIE. Of critical importance is the timing of the imaging examination, as serial imaging has shown that perinatally acquired lesions evolve rapidly. It is possible to image both too early and too late to obtain maximum benefit from the study.

Imaging Modalities

Infants with signs of HIE may be scanned with three different techniques during the neonatal period: cranial ultrasound, computed tomography (CT), and magnetic resonance imaging (MRI).

Cranial Ultrasound

Cranial ultrasound has the advantage of being portable and easily used on the neonatal intensive care unit. It is ideal for doing daily scans to follow the evolution of changes within the brain. Expertise is needed to obtain the correct angles and levels for viewing brain structures and to interpret the results. Image interpretation is most easily

From Donn SM, Sinha SK, Chiswick ML (eds): *Birth Asphyxia and the Brain: Basic Science and Clinical Implications.* © 2002, Futura Publishing Co., Inc., Armonk, NY.

done at the time of scanning, although video replay provides a suitable method of retrospective review. It may be very difficult to interpret paper reprints, particularly when these are obtained by a different operator.

Cranial ultrasound is a powerful technique for identifying cerebral edema, and parenchymal or intraventricular hemorrhage. However, areas of parenchymal infarction may take several days to be visualized as an echodensity, and it may be impossible to detect lesions near the periphery of the brain. Cranial ultrasound is excellent for identifying cystic lesions within the parenchyma, but these usually take at least 10 days to develop from the time of insult. The ability of cranial ultrasound to detect pathology within the neonatal brain may be increased by using different frequency transducers. A 5-MHz transducer increases penetration of the brain compared to a 7.5-MHz transducer, and echodensities within the basal ganglia may be more easily visualized, although they may also take several days to become apparent.[1] Hyperechogenicity of the colliculi may be seen occasionally and is indicative of brainstem necrosis in infants with severe asphyxia. A 10-MHz transducer allows identification of areas of cortical echodensity and developing subcortical white matter infarction.[2,3] Using the posterior fontanel or the lambdoid sutures in the preterm infant improves the ability of cranial ultrasound to detect lesions within the posterior fossa following HIE.[4] Cranial ultrasound is not as effective as MRI in determining the exact site and extent of parenchymal lesions. However, cranial ultrasound will provide an excellent method for screening and monitoring the evolution of lesions. Magnetic resonance will not have these capabilities in the foreseeable future, and the combination of cranial ultrasound and MRI is thus recommended as the best approach for a thorough assessment of the term neonatal brain.

An additional benefit of cranial ultrasound is that Doppler studies may be used to estimate cerebral artery blood flow. A reduced resistance index of less than 0.55 (peak systolic velocity − end-diastolic velocity/ peak systolic velocity) is associated with an abnormal outcome following perinatal asphyxia.[5] An abnormal cerebral blood flow velocity (<2 SD or >3 SD), though more difficult to measure, is also a good predictor of abnormal outcome. These measurements are useful, although the abnormalities are transient even in the presence of significant brain damage. Usually an abnormal resistance index is at its lowest between 24 and 48 hours after the asphyxial insult. It is important to ensure that both the blood pressure and the blood carbon dioxide tension are normal at the time the measurements are taken.

Computed Tomography

Computed tomography has the advantage of being available in many hospitals, at relatively low cost. However, the equipment is usually located at a distance from the neonatal intensive care unit, as are MR scanners, which is problematic for its use with critically ill or unstable infants. Scanning involves exposure to a significant amount of radiation and it is therefore not an appropriate technique for serial studies to monitor the evolution of lesions. Computed tomography is an excellent tool for identifying acute hemorrhage, although modern MRI sequences are proving to be just as sensitive. However, hemorrhage is not usually a major feature in HIE and with the wider availablity of MRI, it is becoming less justifiable to use CT to image neurologically abnormal infants.

In addition, while CT has been used to study infants with HIE, there are very few recent studies in the literature. Decreased attenuation in the white matter during the second week of life has been associated with an abnormal outcome.[6] A more recent study documented the presence of cortical abnormalities consistent with cortical "highlighting" on MRI (see below) in infants with HIE.[7] Computed tomography may be unable to detect significant basal ganglia and thalamic lesions. The technique is sensitive, however, to the presence of calcification, which produces less obvious and more variable signal intensity on MRI. Computed tomography may therefore be useful when the presence of calcification is suspected in infants who have already undergone cranial ultrasound and/or MRI. Calcium may be deposited in the basal ganglia following HIE, but it is not usually found in other sites, and its presence would therefore implicate other or additional pathologies such as congenital infection.

Magnetic Resonance Imaging

Magnetic resonance imaging relies on the presence of protons (hydrogen nuclei) within body water. A proton can be regarded as a small, freely suspended bar magnet, which spins rapidly around its own axis. When placed in a static magnetic field (B0), the magnetization of the protons within the body lines up with the applied field. As a result, in a strong magnetic field there is a net nuclear magnetization, with the protons rotating or "precessing" about the direction of the main magnetic field. If a pulse of radiofrequency magnetic field, rotating at the same frequency as the protons (B1) generated by a coil, is then applied to these protons, there is a strong resonance *or* interaction. This can be used to rotate the net magnetization, which is parallel to the main magnetic field through any angle depending on the strength and duration of the applied pulse. The usual choice is 90° or 180°, so that the net nuclear magnetization becomes perpendicular or opposite in direction to the original static magnetic field. Once the applied pulse is switched off, the protons tend to realign with the main magnetic field; the changing magnetization, perpendicular to B0, induces a small voltage in a receiver coil that is placed around the patient. This electrical signal (voltage or current) is known as free induction decay (FID). The initial magnitude of FID is determined by the number of protons within the tissue. It decays with the constant T2, the transverse relaxation time, which reflects the interaction of nuclei with one another. After the net magnetization has been rotated into the transverse plane, the longitudinal magnetization parallel to B0 recovers with the time constant T1, the longitudinal relaxation time. There is a wide range of values of T1 and T2 for different tissues but, in general terms, there is a relationship with viscosity; liquids have long T1s and long T2s, soft tissues have shorter T1s and T2s, and solids have very short T2 and very long T1 values.

Magnetic resonance pulse sequences consist of radiofrequency pulses and gradient magnetic fields that are applied to nuclei within the main static magnetic field in a systematic way, with the FID signal (or a variant of it) collected at specific times. The pulse sequence incorporates methods of localizing the signal to specific voxels. Changes to tissues can often be detected as a result of changes to T1 and T2 and other parameters. (For further detail, see references 8 and 9.)

Technical Details

Most MR scanners have been designed to image adults and also perform effectively for older children. It is usually necessary to modify the approach when imaging the newborn. Adjustments need to be made to coils, sequences, and monitoring equipment to ensure good quality images with maximum safety. Many different magnet systems may be used. Most commercially available scanners have strengths of 1 or 1.5 Tesla, although open 0.7 Tesla systems are now being produced, and three Tesla systems are being developed for clinical use. Signal-to-noise ratios are approximately proportional to field strength, but with increasing strength there are increased artifacts from chemical shift, patient motion, susceptibility, and flow.

The signal-to-noise ratio of an MR image is greatly improved by using the smallest receiver coil appropriate for the body part being examined. Preterm and term newborns can be imaged in an adult knee coil (typical internal diameter, 19 cm). A head coil with an internal diameter of 24 cm is ideal for infants aged 2 months to 2 years. A dedicated infant coil will improve signal-to-noise ratio, shorten scanning times, and allow easier positioning of the infant.

Determination of Pulse Sequences

Sequences need to be adjusted to allow for the different composition of the immature brain. The neonatal brain is approximately 92–95% water. This decreases over the first 2 years of life to adult values of 80–85%. The increased water content of the neonatal brain is associated with a marked increase in T1 and T2 and the standard sequences used for adults are not always appropriate. The choice of sequences used for an evaluation is also limited by their availability within an MR system and their duration. Infants may be clinically unstable or sedation may wear off; for those reasons, faster sequences are preferred, although image quality and anatomic detail must still be acceptable. We have routinely used a conventional T1-weighted spin echo sequence (SE 860/20 [time to repetition/time to echo, TR/TE), a conventional T2-weighted spin echo sequence (SE 3000/120 [TR/TE]), or a fast spin echo T2-weighted sequence (FSE 3000/208$_{eff}$ [TR/TE]), and an inversion recovery sequence (IR 3800/30/950 [time to repetition/time to echo/time to inversion, TR/TE/TI). Diffusion-weighted imaging is now being used more frequently. It is the method of choice for identifying areas of acute white matter infarction, but spatial resolution using fast diffusion-weighted imaging may be limited. Many abnormalities identified by diffusion-weighted imaging decrease with time from the insult and are usually no longer evident during the second week of life. Diffusion-weighted imaging has been disappointing for identifying early changes within the basal ganglia and thalami. Imaging with three different sensitization directions may show abnormalities within the posterior limb of the internal capsule; however, these changes may not be apparent earlier than with conventional images.

Measurements of apparent diffusion coefficients within different regions of the brain may provide earlier detection of injury and also help to characterize its nature. Protocols that provide fast diffusion and perfusion sequences are available and have been used with good results in adult stroke patients, but the role of perfusion-weighted imaging in the newborn has yet to be established.

Contrast enhancement is of considerable value in adults, but there is little information available about its use in infants with HIE. The appearances of the normal neonatal brain following contrast have been described.[10] Contrast administration may enhance changes within the cortex, the so-called "cortical highlighting" in HIE. As the diagnosis of HIE is not always clear, there is justification for using contrast agents more frequently. The fluid attenuated inversion recovery sequence (FLAIR) has been used to identify both subarachnoid and intraventricular hemorrhage in adult patients,[11,12] and it is frequently used in infants with suspected nonaccidental brain injury. There are few reports on the use of the FLAIR sequence in newborns with HIE,[13] but it is often used after the first year of life for identifying abnormally increased T2 consistent with glial tissue.

Proton density images may be useful in the first few days after delivery, as abnormalities within the basal ganglia and thalami may be detected earlier than with other sequences.[14] The proton density sequence may also provide early information on "cortical edema" or loss of gray/white matter differentiation.[14]

Timing of Imaging

The ideal time to image depends on the information required and is often constrained by the resources available for imaging sick newborns (Table 1). Conventional scans performed within the first 24 hours may appear normal even when there has been severe injury to the brain. Further studies to evaluate the role of early diffusion-weighted imaging and the use of contrast and the FLAIR sequence are needed, but investigation is hampered by the difficulties of transferring acutely ill infants into the scanner very soon after delivery.

There are several well-documented MRI findings during the first week of life in newborns with HIE. These imaging abnormalities "mature" and become easier to identify by the end of the first week. A scan performed between 1 and 2 weeks of age is optimal for obtaining information on the exact pattern of injury. After 2 weeks of age, there may be signs of cystic breakdown and atrophy, which may make the initial pattern of injury more difficult to define. Imaging at other times usually provides valuable information if the images are interpreted with knowledge of both the spectrum of lesions seen following perinatal events and their evolution. A normal scan following HIE is indicative of a good prognosis, but in an infant with an atypical clinical course, suggestive of a metabolic disorder, a normal scan may not have the same implications.

Table 1

Guidelines for Magnetic Resonance Imaging of Newborns with HIE

- Infants with neurologic signs should undergo MRI.
- Imaging should be performed at 24–48 hours of age for early prognostic information.
- Use diffusion-weighted imaging during the first week to detect white matter infarction.
- Conventional sequence imaging between 7 and 14 days can be used to determine the pattern of injury and type of abnormality.
- MRI can confirm or exclude congenital brain malformations, identify injury, and help establish timing and etiology.
- Miscellaneous:
  1. Absence of acquired lesions on MRI in a neurologically abnormal infant may suggest more serious pathology such as metabolic disease.
  2. All available clinical information should be used in interpretation and prognostication.
  3. Abnormalities may be related more to type of insult than its timing.
  4. Lesions evolve quickly; some may disappear, then reappear later with different characteristics.

HIE = hypoxic-ischemic encephalopathy; MRI = magnetic resonance imaging.

Patterns of Brain Injury

During the first week after delivery there are several abnormalities that may be identified on MRI in infants who fulfill all the criteria for HIE.[15] For the purposes of this discussion, these criteria are identified as: (1) fetal distress on electronic monitoring, late decelerations, or bradycardia, with or without meconium-stained amniotic fluid; (2) low Apgar scores with a need for resuscitation; (3) an encephalopathy from birth; and (4) absence of congenital malformations, metabolic disorder, or congenital infection. While one particular site may predominate, in many infants there are widespread changes throughout the brain.

Magnetic resonance imaging has been used widely to investigate the asphyxiated infant.[1,10,14,16–25] The abnormalities identified on imaging vary with field strength and the sequences used, as well as with the postnatal age of the infant at the time of the scan. However, the pattern of injury seen on MRI is most closely related to the type and severity of the insult. Severe acute asphyxia is associated with lesions in the basal ganglia, thalami, brainstem, hippocampus, and the corticospinal tracts around the central fissure.[26–29] This pattern has been termed central cortico-subcortical involvement,[30] and is the most common pattern of injury following acute fetal distress during labor and delivery. Severe basal ganglia injury may be associated with subcortical white matter infarction or with multicystic leukomalacia. The latter is relatively rare, and in the author's experience, occurs in about 5% of infants with HIE.

White matter damage may occur with preservation of the basal ganglia and thalami in infants who have a history suggestive of chronic or repetitive insults. Infants with white matter lesions may fulfill all the criteria for HIE, but often the clinical condition of the infant and the extent of damage apparent on imaging are disproportional to the documented degree of fetal distress. Repeated antenatal insults in these infants are thought to "prime" the white matter by diverting blood to the metabolically more active parts of the developing brain, such as the basal ganglia and thalami, so that the white matter becomes more vulnerable. A comparatively small insult may therefore result in extensive damage to the white matter and cortex. The white matter injury may have a classic parasagittal distribution, involving territory at the border zones between the circulations of major arteries.[31] Infants with white matter injury but normal basal ganglia and thalami may have a good neurodevelopmental outcome despite developing a secondary microcephaly.

Major white matter infarction may also be seen in infants who have other predisposing factors such as hypoglycemia.[32–35] This is usually seen as parasagittal infarction, and is most marked posteriorly. In the author's experience, multiple small hemorrhagic lesions within the white matter of patients with a history of persistent hypoglycemia have been observed, which may represent a milder form of the same injury. Hypoglycemia may be the primary insult, or perhaps exacerbate the effects of other factors (e.g., chronic or repetitive hypoxemia). This may be the case, for example, in infants with intrauterine growth restriction who are particularly susceptible to postnatal hypoglycemia.

Infants with primarily white matter damage may have a hemorrhagic component to their lesions. The author has found an incidence of approximately 5% of parenchymal hemorrhagic lesions in infants with apparent HIE. These infants may also show other metabolic abnormalities during the neonatal period, such as hypoglycemia and conjugated hyperbilirubinemia.They tend to have a worse neurodevelopmental outcome than those without a hemorrhagic component. The outcome in these infants may depend on other concurrent pathology (e.g., a metabolic or thrombotic disorder), and thus caution is advised in making predictions from imaging alone. Of interest is that later imaging in these infants resembles periventricular leukomalacia, although the injury has occurred at term, rather than preterm.

Early Magnetic Resonance Imaging Findings

Brain Swelling

Abnormalities consistent with swelling of the brain appear during the first 24–48 hours following an asphyxial episode, usually mirroring changes identified on ultrasound. These signs are best identified on T1-weighted spin echo sequences (Figures 1A and 1B). Five signs of

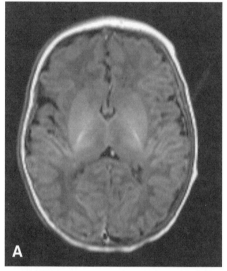

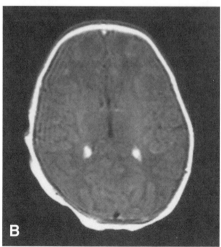

Figure 1. T1-weighted spin echo sequence (SE 860/20). **(A)** Normal brain. **(B)** Post-contrast image showing severe brain swelling at 2 days of age in an infant with stage II hypoxic-ischemic encephalopathy (HIE). This infant developed widespread cortical and white matter abnormalities on later imaging.

brain swelling may be demonstrated: (1) loss of extracerebral space; (2) loss of sulcal markings; (3) closure of the Sylvian fissures; (4) tightening of the interhemispheric fissure; and (5) slit-like anterior horns of the lateral ventricles. Loss of the normal anatomic detail may also be evident. Infants with severely swollen brains often have all the signs. More severe swelling may be associated with underlying severe white matter and cortical damage. Mild degrees of brain swelling may be seen in infants who have not had documented asphyxia. Conversely, infants with severe acute insults leading to primarily basal ganglia and thalamic injury may have no obvious brain swelling.

Evolution

Brain swelling of any degree is usually transient. It is generally no longer evident by the end of the first week.

Pathology

Swelling is likely to result from brain edema, but it is not easy to differentiate between vasogenic and cytotoxic edema on conventional scans alone. If the swelling is associated with loss of gray/white matter differentiation, it is likely to be cytotoxic edema. Diffusion-weighted imaging during the first week of life is of value in distinguishing cytotoxic edema from vasogenic edema.

Clinical Outcome

The presence of brain swelling makes assessment of the brain more difficult. However, if the underlying brain is normal in appearance at the end of the first week once the swelling has disappeared, the clinical outlook is good. Follow-up scans in these infants may show patchy increased signal intensity in the periventricular white matter on T2-weighted images. These periventricular changes may just represent terminal zones of immature unmyelinated white matter, but are usually more marked than in "normal" children and are not confined to the posterior periventricular white matter.

The Posterior Limb of the Internal Capsule

The normal term infant will have evidence of myelination in approximately one-third to one-half of the posterior limb of the internal capsule (PLIC). This can be seen as high signal intensity on T1-weighted spin echo or inversion recovery images and low signal intensity on T2-weighted spin echo images (Figures 2A and 2B). The inversion recovery sequence is the best for demonstrating myelination within the internal capsule in the neonatal period. Using a fast spin echo T2-weighted image, the low signal intensity myelin may be seen almost as clearly as the high signal intensity on inversion recovery images. The appearances with conventional T2-weighted spin echo images are more subtle.

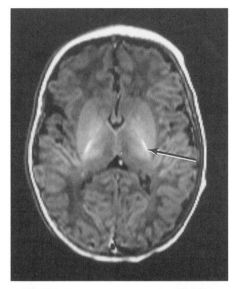

Figure 2A. Normal term infant at age 2 days, born at 40 weeks gestation. Inversion recovery sequence (IR 3800/30/950). Myelin is demonstrated in the posterior third of the posterior limb of the internal capsule (arrow).

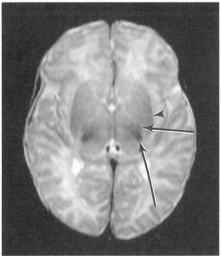

Figure 2B. Same infant as in Figure 2A. T2-weighted spin echo sequence (SE 2700/120). The low signal intensity from myelin is less obvious (short arrow). The unmyelinated fibers of the posterior limb of the internal capsule are seen as high signal intensity. There is a thin region of low signal intensity along the lateral border of the lentiform nucleus (arrowhead). The ventrolateral nuclei are seen as low signal intensity (long arrow).

A complete loss of the normal signal intensity from myelin may be seen following perinatal asphyxia (Figure 2C). This may take 1 to 2 days to develop; therefore, if the first scan is done very early, the signal intensity from myelin may appear to be normal (Figures 2D and 2E). The signal intensity from myelin may be diminished or asymmetrical prior to its loss. In association with the loss of normal signal intensity from within the limb, there may be abnormal signal intensities running

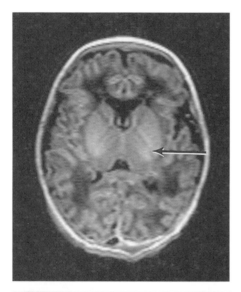

Figure 2C. Infant with stage II HIE, at age 2 days. Inversion recovery sequence (IR 3800/30/950). Abnormal appearance to the posterior limb of the internal capsule with loss of the normal high signal intensity from myelin (arrow).

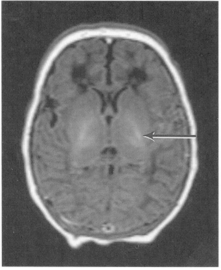

Figure 2D. Delayed loss of signal intensity in an infant with stage III HIE who subsequently died. At 2 days of age, there is a normal appearance to the myelin (arrow).

parallel to the posterior limb in the lentiform nucleus. These should not be confused with the normal signal from myelin (Figure 2F).

Evolution

The normal signal intensity from myelin may return after some weeks or months, although it is often irregular in outline. The rate of return depends on the severity of injury to the basal ganglia and thalami. In the presence of gross atrophy of the basal ganglia and thalami, the

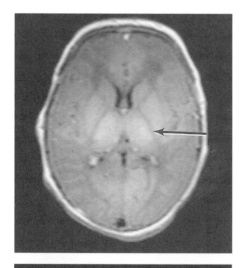

Figure 2E. Same infant as in Figure 2D. At 4 days, there is a complete loss of signal intensity (arrow).

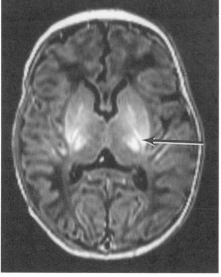

Figure 2F. Infant with stage II HIE, at age 5 days. Inversion recovery sequence (IR 3800/30/950). There is loss of the normal signal from myelin in the PLIC, but there are areas of abnormal high signal intensity running parallel to the internal capsule (arrow).

corticospinal tracts appear to be irreversibly damaged. When myelination subsequently appears it is often irregular and discontinuous.

Pathology

The increased T1 within the PLIC is consistent with edema or infarction (Figures 2G and 2H). The finding of an increased signal in this

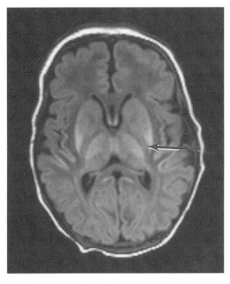

Figure 2G. Infant with stage III HIE who died at 14 days of age. Inversion recovery sequence (IR 3800/30/950) at age 12 days. There is loss of the normal high signal intensity from myelin (arrow). Additional abnormal high signal intensity areas are within the basal ganglia and thalami. (Continued in Figures 2H and 2J.)

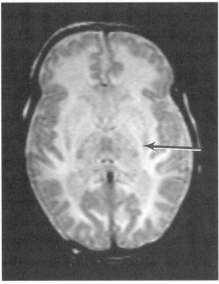

Figure 2H. (Continued.) T2-weighted spin echo sequence (SE 2700/120). There is loss of the normal low signal intensity from myelin within the PLIC (arrow). This is seen as abnormally high signal intensity throughout. There are abnormal low and high signal intensities throughout the basal ganglia and thalami.

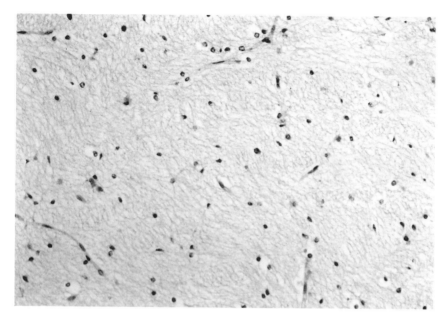

Figure 2I. Normal histologic appearances of the posterior limb of the internal capsule.

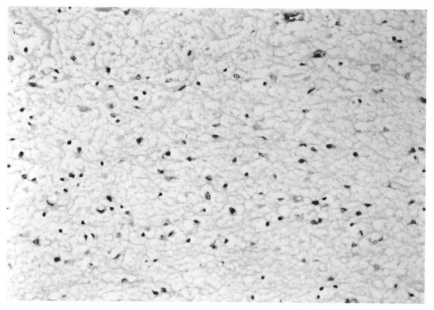

Figure 2J. The same infant as in (G) and (H) who died at 14 days of age. There is edema throughout the internal capsule. Photomicrograph courtesy of W. Squier, Oxford, with permission.

region on diffusion-weighted imaging in all three directions of sensitization is consistent with the presence of cytotoxic edema. Infants who have had abnormal signal intensity within the posterior limb and who have died in the acute phases of HIE have shown histologic signs of edema in this region (Figures 2I and 2J).[36]

Outcome

Most term infants with HIE who show abnormal signal intensity within the PLIC have an abnormal neurodevelopmental outcome (sensitivity 0.91, specificity 1.0, positive predictive value 1.0).[25] It is important to have a correct estimate of gestation, as the absence of myelin on MRI is a normal finding below 37 weeks gestation. In addition, infants with a primary metabolic disorder may have delayed myelination, which would include an absence of myelin within the posterior limb at term (nonketotic hyperglycinemia). Certain metabolic disorders that present in the neonatal period may mimic HIE both clinically and on imaging,[37] so that a metabolic screen is always warranted in any asphyxiated infant.

The Basal Ganglia and Thalami

The basal ganglia include the caudate nucleus as well as the globus pallidum and the putamen, which together form the lentiform nucleus. The normal MR appearance of the basal ganglia and thalami at term is shown in Figure 3A.

Using T1-weighted spin echo imaging, there is a high signal within the PLIC and some high signal within the ventrolateral nuclei of the thalami. Some residual high signal may be seen in the globus pallidum at term, and this may be exaggerated in infants with asphyxia.

Using T2-weighted spin echo imaging, the ventrolateral nuclei of the thalami have a low signal intensity. Myelin within the posterior limb is seen as a small area of low signal intensity. There may be a thin region of low signal intensity along the lateral borders of the lentiform nucleus (Figure 2B).

Abnormalities within the basal ganglia and thalami are a frequent finding following severe acute asphyxia. This is thought to result from the increased metabolic rate of this region which is actively myelinating at term.[38] In addition, the structures contain a high proportion of excitatory amino acid receptors. These abnormalities are frequently accompanied by abnormalities within the corticospinal tracts around the central fissure, and the hippocampus and brainstem.[30] Abnormalities within the hippocampal region usually are not evident until the second week of life, when a generalized high signal intensity is seen with T1-weighted spin echo images (Figure 3B). This is associated with later atrophy and dilation of the temporal horns of the lateral ventricles.

Abnormal signal intensity is most frequently seen within the pos-

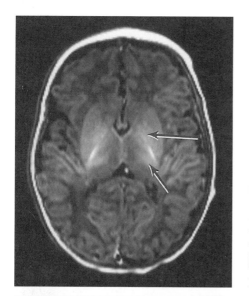

Figure 3A. Inversion recovery sequence (IR 3800/30/950). Normal appearances of the basal ganglia and thalami at term. There is high signal in the posterior limb of the internal capsule and diffuse high signal in the globus pallidum (long arrow). High signal is also apparent in the region of the ventrolateral nuclei of the thalami (short arrow). The normal appearances on T2-weighted imaging are shown in Figure 2B.

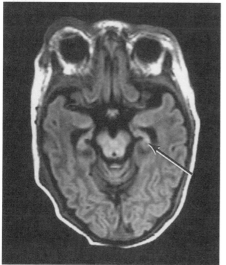

Figure 3B. Hippocampal abnormalities. Infant with stage III HIE (as in Figures 2G and 2H), at age 12 days. Inversion recovery sequence (IR 3800/300/950). There is abnormal high signal intensity in the hippocampal region (arrow), and some dilation of the temporal horn of the lateral ventricle suggestive of atrophy. This infant had diffuse changes throughout the basal ganglia and thalami on imaging and at postmortem examination.

terior and lateral part of the lentiform nucleus and in the region of the ventrolateral nuclei of the thalami (Figures 2F, 3C, 3D, 3E, and 3F). In severe injury, there may be diffuse abnormalities throughout the structures. Abnormalities are usually less obvious on T2-weighted images than on the T1-weighted images during the first week of life (Figures 2G and 2H).

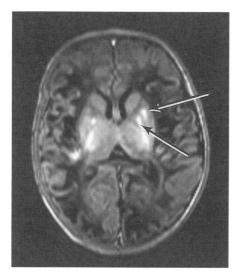

Figure 3C. Abnormal signal intensity within the basal ganglia and thalami. Moderate abnormalities with equivocal signal intensity in the posterior limb of the internal capsule (PLIC). Bilateral abnormal increased signal intensity is apparent in the lentiform nuclei (arrows). There is slight asymmetry in the myelination of the PLIC with less myelin on the left.

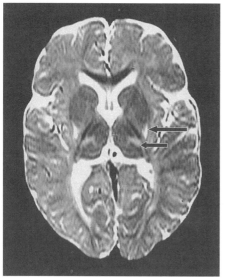

Figure 3D. Late T2-weighted imaging (SE 2700/120). There is abnormal high signal intensity within the lateral lentiform nuclei (long arrow) and the ventrolateral nuclei of the thalami (short arrow).

Evolution

Abnormal signal intensity gradually increases over the first week of life. By 2 and 4 weeks it is at its most obvious. From 2 weeks onward there may be focal or diffuse atrophy with or without the formation of cysts (Figure 3G). The high signal intensity on T1-weighted spin echo

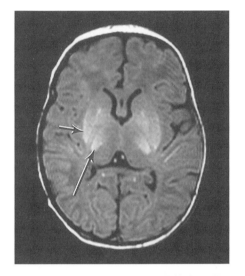

Figure 3E. Moderate abnormalities with focal lesions having abnormal signal intensity in the posterior limb of the internal capsule. There are focal abnormal high signal intensity areas in the lentiform nucleus (short arrow) and an exaggeration of the normal high signal in the lateral thalami (long arrow).

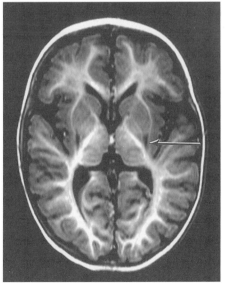

Figure 3F. At 1 year of age, there are very characteristic focal low signal intensity cysts in the posterior part of the putamen (arrow).

imaging gradually decreases over the first year of life when the basal ganglia and thalami may show varying degrees of atrophy. They may be replaced by low signal intensity lesions on T1-weighted imaging and more obvious abnormal high signal intensity regions on T2-weighted images (Figure 3D). In some infants, there may be no obvious lesions between 3 and 9 months of age despite very obvious focal abnormalities during the first months of life and at the end of the first year (Figure

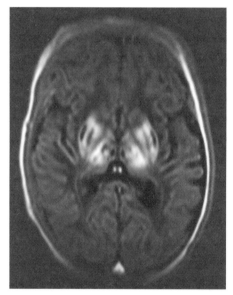

Figure 3G. Severe abnormalities with widespread abnormal low and high signal intensity throughout the basal ganglia and thalami in an infant with stage II HIE at age 18 days. There is no obvious myelin within the posterior limb of the internal capsule. The high signal intensity is probably from capillary proliferation.

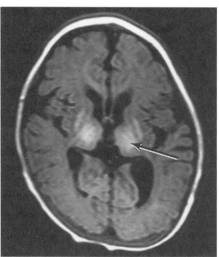

Figure 3H. The same infant as in Figure 3G at age 7 months. Inversion recovery sequence (IR 3600/30/70). Marked atrophy of the basal ganglia and thalami is seen. There is abnormal high signal intensity, which is most obvious in the thalami (arrow). This may represent abnormal myelination, or "status marmoratus." There is additional white matter atrophy. The child developed microcephaly and a severe extensor spastic quadriplegia. She had persistent convulsions and made no real developmental progress. At 3 years of age, the child died from respiratory complications.

3F). These infants may still develop major motor impairments with athetoid and dystonic movements. With very severe lesions, there may be residual abnormal high signal intensity on T1-weighted images after the first year of life which may represent abnormal myelination or "status marmoratus" (Figure 3H).[39] Infants with multifocal or diffuse lesions within the basal ganglia and thalami also have progressive white matter atrophy (Figure 3H). The white matter may have an initial "streaky" or homogenous appearance but it does not become cystic. It is

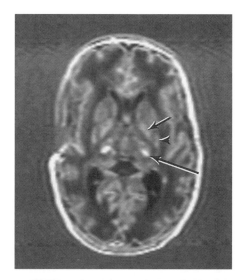

Figure 3I. A preterm infant of 28 weeks gestation, who had a cardiorespiratory arrest at 2 weeks of age in association with clinical deterioration presumed to be septic in origin. Inversion recovery sequence (IR FSE 3500/30/950) at 32 weeks. This is an artifacted image. There is abnormal high signal intensity in the lateral thalamus (long arrow), the lateral lentiform (arrowhead), and the globus pallidum (short arrow). This was found to be infarction on postmortem examination. The very bright signal intensity within the thalami (long arrow) corresponded to areas of neuronal mineralization.

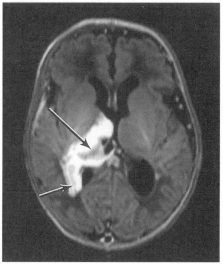

Figure 3J. Term infant who presented with convulsions. Inversion recovery sequence (IR 3800/30/850). There is unilateral high signal intensity in the thalamus consistent with primary hemorrhage or hemorrhagic infarction (long arrow). There is additional hemorrhage within the right lateral ventricle (short arrow).

unclear whether this atrophy results from the initial insult or is secondary to severe damage to the basal ganglia.

Pathology

Lesions with a short T1 and short T2 are widely assumed to be hemorrhagic but we have not demonstrated macroscopic hemorrhage in

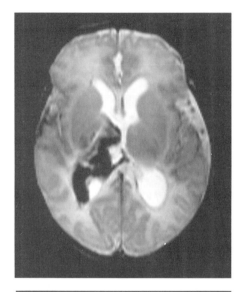

Figure 3K. On T2-weighted spin echo sequence (SE 2700/120), the hemorrhage is seen as predominantly low signal intensity.

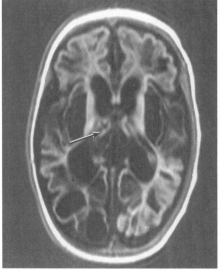

Figure 3L. Severe basal ganglia and white matter abnormalities. Inversion recovery sequence (IR 3800/30/950). Infant with stage II HIE, at 4 weeks of age. Atrophy and cystic breakdown throughout the basal ganglia and thalami (arrow) are apparent. There is cystic breakdown of the entire white matter.

infants who have died following severe basal ganglia and thalamic injury. There is however diffuse necrosis in these infants. Capillary proliferation occurs within hours of ischemic injury and this is probably responsible for the short T1 short T2 lesions seen on MRI.[40] In addition, the combination of very short T1 and very short T2 may result from neuronal mineralization, e.g., calcium deposition (Figure 3I). The bilateral abnormalities seen in term infants with severe HIE need to be distinguished from primary thalamic hemorrhage, which may rarely be bilateral (Figures 3J and 3K). Infants with primary thalamic hemorrhage may present with convulsions, but the clinical picture is not that of typical HIE.

Neurodevelopmental Outcome

Lesions within the basal ganglia and thalami can be scored. The severity of the score is directly related to the outcome of the infant.[14,22,24,25] Basal ganglia and thalamic lesions may be more simply graded as mild, moderate, and severe. Mild lesions are focal and are seen in the presence of normal signal intensity within the PLIC. They are typically inferior in position. Moderate lesions are also focal involving the posterior lentiform and lateral thalamus, but are accompanied by equivocal or abnormal signal intensity within the PLIC. Severe lesions are more widespread, involving all areas of the basal ganglia and thalami, and are always associated with abnormal signal intensity within the PLIC (Figure 3L).

All infants with persistent abnormal signal intensity within the basal ganglia have some neurodevelopmental impairment at follow-up. The outcome of mild lesions, with preservation of the signal from myelin in the PLIC, is not well documented. These infants may show mildly abnormal tone during the first year and develop a tremor in early childhood. More marked movement disorders may develop during adolescence if there was a history of mild birth asphyxia, but imaging data are not available for these cases.[41]

Moderate focal lesions that evolve into small cyst formation in the posterior part of the putamen (Figure 3F), and areas of increased T2 in the region of the ventrolateral nuclei of the thalami, are associated with the development of a fairly pure athetoid quadriplegia with intellectual preservation. These abnormalities may be very difficult to detect between 3 and 9 months of age. They then become more obvious, particularly with T2-weighted sequences. More extensive severe multifocal abnormalities are associated with a mixed spastic/athetoid quadriplegia with some intellectual deficit and, frequently, persistent convulsions.

Diffuse abnormalities resulting in severe atrophy throughout the basal ganglia and thalami are associated with the development of a spastic quadriplegia, severe intellectual deficit, and persistent convulsions, which are often difficult to control. There are additional marked feeding difficulties, which usually necessitate the insertion of a gastrostomy (Figures 3G and 3H). Imaging in these infants may show a loss of detail and a diffuse short T1, short T2 pattern throughout the midbrain extending into the mesencephalon (Figure 4A).

The Brainstem

Infants who develop Sarnat stage III HIE (see Chapter 12, Table 6) usually have severe basal ganglia lesions with extension into the midbrain (Figure 4B), pons, and medulla. These findings explain the clinical state of an unrousable infant with no gag reflex, no facial expression, and no normal eye movements. These infants are usually, but not always, unable to breathe independently. Brainstem lesions may also be seen as separate focal areas of low signal intensity on T1-weighted images and high signal intensity on T2-weighted images (Figures 4B and 4C). These features are consistent with infarction.

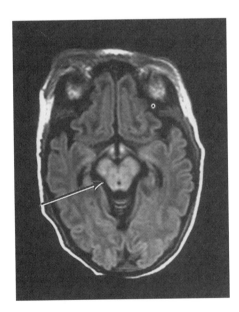

Figure 4A. Infant with stage III HIE, at age 12 days. There is a diffuse high signal within the mesencephalon bilaterally (arrow).

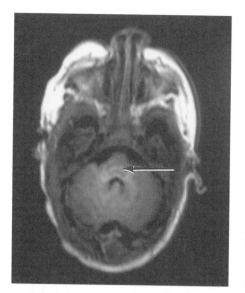

Figure 4B. Normal term infant. T1-weighted spin echo (SE 860/20) sequence. There is a small area of focal high signal intensity (arrow) consistent with myelin in the medial lemnisci. There is a thin low signal intensity region dorsal to the tracts.

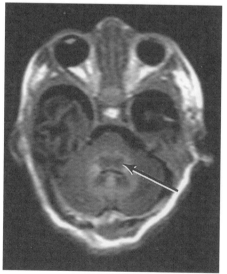

Figure 4C. Term infant with stage III HIE, T2-weighted spin echo sequence (SE 860/20). There are large bilateral abnormal low signal intensity lesions within the dorsal pons (arrow). Histology confirmed the presence of bilateral infarcts.

The Cortex

The newborn cortex has a relatively short T1 and T2 compared to adjacent white matter. This difference lasts for approximately 3 months.

Cortical Highlighting

Following perinatal asphyxia, areas of cortex may show abnormal highlighting with a shortening of both T1 and T2. This is most frequently seen around the central fissure, which can be the only abnormality on imaging in mild asphyxia (Figure 5A). The cortex around the interhemispheric fissure (Figure 5A) and the insula (Figure 5B) might also be involved, and in extreme cases almost the entire cortex may be abnormally highlighted (Figure 5B). The depths of the sulci are more frequently affected (Figures 5A and 5B). Infants with extensive cortical highlighting in the absence of basal ganglia abnormalities may have had a repetitive or chronic insult.

Evolution

An abnormal signal in the cortex may take several days to develop, then reach its maximum during the second week after the asphyxial insult, and last for several weeks. During the second week abnormal sig-

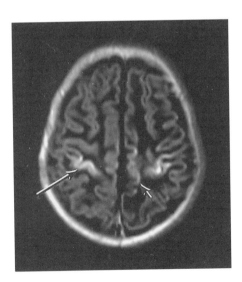

Figure 5A. Abnormal highlighting on the cortex. Inversion recovery sequence (IR 3800/30/950). Cortical highlighting around central fissure (long arrow). There is some highlighting at the depths of the sulci along the interhemispheric fissure (short arrow).

nal intensity may develop in the subcortical white matter adjacent to areas of highlighted cortex (Figure 5C). This is consistent with ischemic damage to the white matter, which then proceeds to break down and atrophy.

Barkovich described the appearances of "cortical edema" on proton density images in the first few days following delivery.[14] This finding is consistent with local areas of loss of gray/white matter differentiation from infarction (see below).

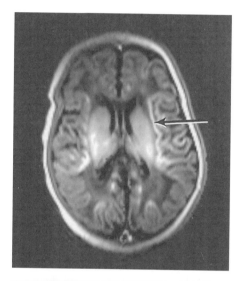

Figure 5B. Infant with stage II HIE whose mother had repeated episodes of vaginal bleeding in pregnancy. Delivery was precipitated by an acute severe antepartum hemorrhage. Widespread high lighting of the cortex. This is most marked along the insula (arrow).

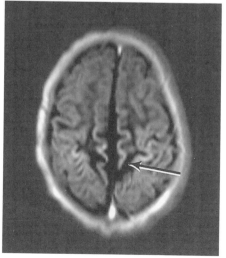

Figure 5C. Same infant as in Figure 5B. Level of the centrum semiovale. There is low signal intensity (arrow) developing in the subcortical white matter adjacent to areas of cortical highlighting.

Pathology

The abnormalities within the cortex on conventional imaging may represent ischemia of one or all cortical layers giving rise to laminar necrosis. The deep layers of the cortex are known to be more vulnerable to hypoxic-ischemic injury. It is unclear why necrosis of the cortex should give rise to a decrease in T1 and T2, but these changes probably reflect capillary proliferation at the cortex/white matter boundary. The subcortical white matter changes are probably secondary to infarction. This may occur from a direct insult to the white matter or may be secondary to the damage in the deep layers of the cortex. The low signal intensity takes at least 1 week to appear on conventional imaging.

Neurodevelopmental Outcome

Cortical highlighting is usually associated with other lesions in the brain and, therefore, it is difficult to identify specific neurodevelopmental sequelae. Minor degrees of highlighting may be associated with a normal outcome although long-term follow-up is necessary to identify more subtle cognitive deficits. Widespread highlighting has been associated with the development of a spastic diplegia, microcephaly, and moderate intellectual deficit, but without continuing convulsions. These clinical findings may be, in part, secondary to the associated white matter abnormalities (Figures 5B and 5C). Later imaging of the cortex is difficult although cortical structures clearly remain even after extensive highlighting. Abnormal signal intensity presumed to be secondary to laminar necrosis of the cortex has been reported in older children with cerebral palsy,[42] but it has not been possible to identify this level of detail with conventional imaging .

Gray/White Matter Differentiation

The normal term brain shows good differentiation between gray and white matter. This is apparent until the end of the first 3 months of life, by which time the T1 and T2 of the white matter have decreased and the T1 and T2 of the cortex have increased, and the differentiation is much less obvious.

Loss of Gray/White Matter Differentiation

Some loss of differentiation may be seen on T1-weighted spin echo images in the presence of brain swelling, but this may normalize to reveal an intact brain. If there is additional loss of differentiation on an inversion recovery sequence, this usually represents impending infarction (Figure 6A). These abnormalities may be seen in infants with focal infarction or with more widespread parasagittal injury effecting watershed areas in anterior and posterior subcortical and periventricular white matter.

T2-weighted imaging at the same time shows loss of differentiation with abnormal high signal in the cortex. This probably represents the same finding as Barkovich's sign of cortical edema on proton density images,[14] but it is unclear whether this is edema or actually represents infarction of some or all layers of the cortex. Regions with loss of differentiation may be easily identified with diffusion-weighted imaging, which shows a pattern consistent with restricted diffusion for the first week of life (Figure 6B). This becomes less obvious as conventional imaging becomes more abnormal (Figure 6C). During the second week, the gray/white matter differentiation returns but it is exaggerated because of a shortening of the T1 and T2 in the cortex, probably from capillary proliferation and an increase in T1 and T2 in the white matter (Figure 6D). White matter infarction is often found in infants with a more atypical course for HIE. There may be a history of antenatal problems that suggest a chronic or repetitive injury. In some infants a combination of widespread white matter infarction is seen in association with severe basal ganglia lesions (Figure 3L). This may result from a severe acute perinatal insult occurring after one or more chronic antenatal insults.

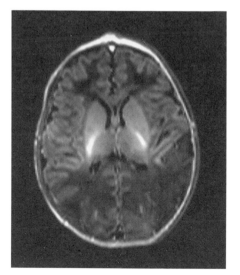

Figure 6A. Inversion recovery sequence (IR 3800/30/950). Loss of gray/white matter differentiation in the parietal, temporal and occipital lobes in an infant with stage II HIE, at age 5 days.

Pathology

The loss of differentiation is a result of cytotoxic edema resulting from severe ischemia, as seen in areas of focal infarction. Diffusion-weighted imaging confirms the presence of infarction.[42,43] The exaggeration of the cortical signal during the second week of life with a shortening of the T1 and T2 may also represent capillary proliferation.

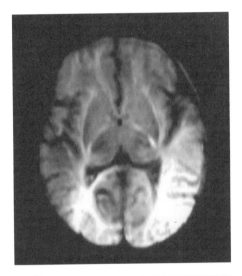

Figure 6B. Diffusion-weighted imaging in the same infant as in Figure 6A, also at 5 days of age. There are abnormal areas of high signal intensity consistent with restricted diffusion in the abnormal areas.

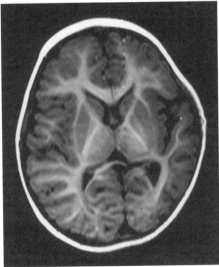

Figure 6C. Inversion recovery (IR 3600/30/70) sequence in the same infant at age 15 months. The areas of subsequent atrophy correspond to the abnormalities seen on early diffusion-weighted images. At the age of 5 years, this child was microcephalic with a global mild developmental delay and minimal asymmetry of tone.

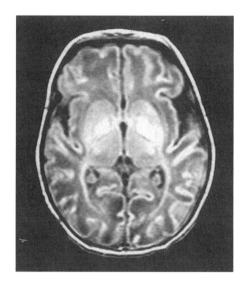

Figure 6D. Inversion recovery sequence (IR 3800/30/950). Term infant with stage II HIE, at age 10 days. Exaggerated gray/white matter differentiation, with low signal intensity in the entire white matter and abnormal high signal intensity within the cortex.

Neurodevelopmental Outcome

The clinical outcome in infants who show loss of gray/white matter differentiation proceeding infarction depends on the extent and site of the infarction and on the presence of other lesions. In the absence of basal ganglia lesions, the outcome may be surprisingly good even with extensive white matter loss and the development of a secondary microcephaly (Figure 6D).[44] The presence of hemorrhage is, however, associated with a worse outcome.

Intracranial Hemorrhage

As mentioned previously, infants with a clinical history of HIE occasionally develop major hemorrhagic lesions within the white matter (Figures 7A–7D). These are not common and occur in approximately 5% of cases, but may be more frequent in infants treated with hypothermia.[45] Underlying hemorrhagic or thrombotic conditions should be sought in these infants. Small hemorrhagic lesions are a frequent finding in infants who present with convulsions but not with a full encephalopathy.[46] Small subdural and subarachnoid hemorrhage may be seen in infants with HIE. Some subdural hemorrhage is a frequent finding in the posterior fossa. Large subdural hemorrhages may be associated with parenchymal infarction either of the cerebral or cerebellar

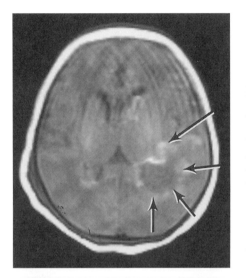

Figure 7A. Infant with stage II HIE, at 3 days of age, who also developed persistent hypoglycemia and neonatal hepatitis with prolonged conjugated jaundice. On T1-weighted spin echo (SE 860/20), there is a large hemorrhagic lesion in the left temporal region. This is slightly low signal intensity (short arrows) with a high signal rim (long arrow). The hemorrhage was seen as low signal intensity on T2-weighted spin echo (2700/120) sequence.

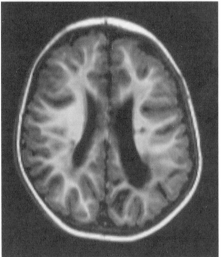

Figure 7B. Same infant as in Figure 7A. Inversion recovery sequence (IR 3600/30/700), at age 2 years. There is bilateral ventricular dilation with a paucity of myelin posteriorly.

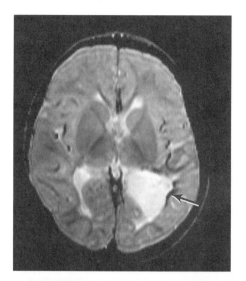

Figure 7C. T2-weighted spin echo (SE 2700/120), at age 2 years. Low ventricular level. There is left ventricular dilation and residual low signal intensity at the site of the neonatal hemorrhage (arrow). This is consistent with the presence of hemosiderin.

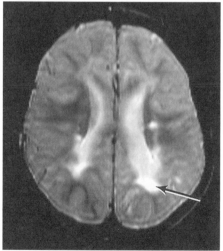

Figure 7D. There is abnormal high signal in the periventricular white matter most marked posteriorly (arrow). This is consistent with glial tissue and is more prominent on the fluid attenuated inversion recovery sequence (FLAIR). The abnormalities that develop following perinatal white matter injury at term are reminiscent of those found in more classic periventricular leukomalacia occurring in the preterm infant.

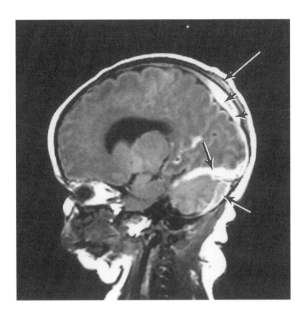

Figure 8. Subdural hemorrhage in an infant with stage II HIE, delivered by vacuum extractor following a failed attempt with forceps. T1-weighted spin echo sequence (SE 2700/120), sagittal plane. There is abnormal high signal intensity consistent with hemorrhage in the subdural space over the parietal lobe (arrowheads). An additional collection at the site of the vacuum application is apparent, consistent with a cephalhematoma (long arrow). There is hemorrhage in the posterior fossa behind the cerebellum and around the tentorium (short arrows).

hemispheres. Larger extracerebral hemorrhages in HIE are usually associated with a traumatic delivery (Figure 8).

The Cerebellum

The cerebellum is relatively resistant to hypoxic-ischemic damage. In infants with widespread destruction of all other areas of the brain, the cerebellum often remains intact and looks relatively normal. Certain regions of the cerebellum (e.g., the dentate nucleus) are reported as being sensitive to asphyxial damage in animal studies. Changes in the dentate nucleus are difficult to identify with MRI. The visualization of these structures is angle-dependent in the transverse plane. Abnormalities probably represent an exaggeration of the normal low and high signal intensity, which are difficult to assess. In a study comparing MRI to histologic appearances following severe birth asphyxia, we were unable to detect any abnormal signal intensity within the dentate nucleus although at histology the dentate was classified as abnormal in every infant.[36]

Prediction of Outcome: Pattern Recognition and Grading Systems

Several authors have described scoring systems for the pattern of injury detected on early MRI following birth asphyxia. These scoring systems are useful for classifying lesions for research studies.[1,14,21,22,25] However, many of them are too complicated for routine clinical use. An ideal imaging sign for prediction of neurodevelopmental outcome is one where the signal intensity within a structure is either lost or reversed from normal, as is found in the PLIC.[25] Exaggerations of the normal signal intensity are very subjective and influenced by the windowing applied before processing the images. Magnetic resonance imaging has a vital role in the prediction of outcome, but correct interpretation of imaging findings may be difficult. Thus, MRI should not be used as the sole technique for the prediction of outcome and/or for decisions to alter clinical management. Some abnormal outcomes may not be severe enough to warrant the possible complications inherent in some interventions (e.g., hypothermia), as these become more widely available.[45] Magnetic resonance imaging provides invaluable information on the patterns and evolution of injury following HIE. This information will prove vital for monitoring both the beneficial and deleterious effects of any future interventions.

Insults Prior to Term

The pattern of injury seen in the preterm fetal brain, as in the term brain, depends on the nature of the insult and, to a lesser extent, the gestational age of the fetus or infant. Severe acute insults, which may correspond to a documented clinical event (e.g., attempted maternal suicide), result in injury to the basal ganglia and thalami (Figures 9A and 9B). Infants subjected to these insults may be born by normal delivery at term but present with arthrogryposis.[47] The specific regions within the basal ganglia and thalami may be different from the asphyxiated term brain.[18] These severe events may occur in preterm infants following delivery (Figures 3H and 3I), but with appropriate neonatal intensive care, they are relatively rare. The more common injury seen in the preterm brain is to white matter. This is probably because of the type of insult to which preterm infants are usually exposed (e.g., sepsis and chronic hypoxia)[48] and because the white matter is particularly vulnerable.

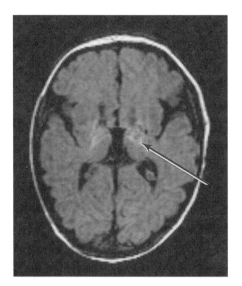

Figure 9A. Infant born at 27 weeks with arthrogryposis. There was a failed attempt at maternal suicide during the pregnancy. Inversion recovery sequence (IR FSE 3500/30/950), at age 5 days. Atrophy of the basal ganglia and thalami and abnormal high signal intensity within the thalamus (arrow).

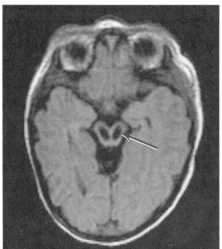

Figure 9B. Same infant as in Figure A. Bilateral low signal intensity (arrow) consistent with infarction in the mesencephalon.

Timing of Brain Injury

Currently, many infants and children are imaged primarily for medico-legal reasons. The interpretation of scans acquired later in childhood is very difficult. Imaging older children with neurodevelopmental problems is problematic, as few are able to remain motionless enough for the duration of the examination. This results in motion-artifacted images, which are difficult to interpret, as well as a more limited acquisition. A thorough examination may be possible only with the use of general anesthesia.

It is important to note that the imaging changes relate to the type of insult and not necessarily the time of injury (Table 2). The infant's brain, damaged or not, grows and develops with time, which means that the original pattern of lesions may be difficult to identify. It may be easier to detect abnormal signal intensity within the brain than to notice that tissue is missing or atrophic. Subtle degrees of atrophy within a brain structure may not be detectable from visual analysis alone. Not all abnormalities detected later in life may be attributable to the documented perinatal insult. Additional white matter lesions may have been acquired since birth as the result of viral infections and other etiologies. Interpretation of late scans needs to be done with full knowledge of the history and clinical status of the child. This will be of particular value in identifying any major discrepancies between the neonatal signs, the current clinical state of the child, and the imaging findings. A full knowl-

Table 2

Summary of Neuroimaging

- MRI and cranial ultrasound provide the best approach for assessment of the neonatal brain in HIE.
- Most commercial MRI scanners need adaptations to coils and sequences for optimal imaging of the newborn.
- Specific patterns of injury are associated with HIE, which are often bilateral and symmetrical, but may also be quite subtle.
- Lesions of the basal ganglia and thalamus have a worse prognosis than isolated lesions of the white matter, even if the latter are extensive.
- Knowledge of the normal neonatal appearances with different sequences is essential.
- Determination of the time of insult and the prediction of outcome are often possible using MRI; however, images must be assessed in conjunction with historical and clinical findings.
- The site or pattern of brain injury is related to the type of insult and not always to gestational age.
- Late images must be interpreted with great care. Lesions acquired in the perinatal period evolve rapidly but predictably. They may also "disappear" on certain sequences as they evolve.

MRI = magnetic resonance imaging; HIE = hypoxic-ischemic encephalopathy.

edge in all three areas is needed when attempting to ascertain the timing and the likely cause of a child's neurodevelopmental problems.

It is likely that the population of young children with cerebral lesions and disabilities who survive into adolescence and adulthood will increase. Thus, it is important that we understand the *evolution* of cerebral lesions, especially as new modalities, including functional imaging, are introduced. Indeed, the normal life expectancy of many children with milder disabilities as a result of brain lesions means that they will eventually become exposed to ischemic and hemorrhagic brain lesions that normally accompany the aging process. One challenge is to collect serial imaging information so that we can better understand the effects of cerebral lesions acquired before or around the time of birth on brain growth and maturation. This may, in turn, enable potential interventional strategies to improve long-term outcomes.

References

1. Rutherford MA, Pennock JM, Dubowitz LMS: Cranial ultrasound and magnetic resonance imaging in hypoxic-ischemic encephalopathy: a comparison with outcome. Dev Med Child Neurol 1994;36:813–825.
2. Eken P, Jansen GH, Groenendaal F, et al: Intracranial lesions in the full-term infant with hypoxic-ischemic encephalopathy: ultrasound and autopsy correlation. Neuropediatrics 1994;25:301–307.
3. Goevart P, De Vries L: *An Atlas of Neonatal Brain Sonography.* MacKeith Press, Cambridge, England, 1997.
4. DeVries LS, Eken P, Beek E, et al: The posterior fontanelle: a neglected acoustic window. Neuropediatrics 1996;27:101–104.
5. Archer LN, Levene MI, Evans DH: Cerebral artery Doppler ultrasonography for prediction of outcome after perinatal asphyxia. Lancet 1986;ii: 1116–1118.
6. Adsett DB, Fitz CR, Hill A: Hypoxic-ischemic cerebral injury in the term newborn: correlation of CT findings with neurological outcome. Dev Med Child Neurol 1985;27:155–160.
7. Cullen A, Donoghue V, King MD: High attenuation gyri CT in postasphyxial encephalopathy. Irish J Med Sci 1998;167:193–195.
8. Mitchell DG: *MRI Principles.* Philadelphia, W.B. Saunders, 1999.
9. Westbrook C, Kaut C: *MRI in Practice.* 2nd ed. Oxford, Blackwell Science, England, 1988.
10. Barkovich AJ, Latal-Hajnal B, Partridge JC, et al: MR contrast enhancement of the normal neonatal brain. Am J Neuroradiol 1997;18:1713–1717.
11. Noguchi K, Ogawa T, Seto H, et al: Subacute and chronic subarachnoid hemorrhage: diagnosis with fluid-attenuated inversion recovery MR imaging. Radiology 1997;203:257–262.
12. Bakshi R, Caruthers SD, Janardhan V, Wasay M: Intraventricular CSF pulsation artifact on fast fluid-attenuation inversion recovery MR images: analysis of 100 consecutive normal studies. Am J Neuroradiol 2000;21: 503–508.

13. Okuda T, Korogi Y Ikushima I, et al: Use of fluid-attenuated inversion recovery (FLAIR) pulse sequences in perinatal hypoxic-ischemic encephalopathy. Br J Radiol 1998;71:282–290.
14. Barkovich AJ, Hajnal BL, Vigneron D, et al: Prediction of neuromotor outcome in perinatal asphyxia: evaluation of MR scoring systems. Am J Neuroradiol 1998; 19:143–149.
15. Sarnat HB, Sarnat MS: Neonatal encephalopathy following fetal distress: a clinical and electrophysiological study. Arch Neurol 1976;33:696–705.
16. Barkovich AJ, Truwit CL: Brain damage from perinatal asphyxia: correlation of MR findings with gestational age. Am J Neuroradiol 1990;11:1087–1096.
17. Barkovich AJ: MR and CT evaluation of profound neonatal and infantile asphyxia. Am J Neuroradiol 1992;13:959–972.
18. Barkovich AJ, Sargent SK: Profound asphyxia in the premature infant: imaging findings. Am J Neuroradiol 1995;16:1837–1846.
19. Byrne P, Welch R, Johnson MA, et al: Serial magnetic resonance imaging in neonatal hypoxic-ischemic encephalopathy. J Pediatr 1990;117:694–700.
20. Keeney SE, Adcock EW, McArdle CB: Prospective observations of 100 high risk newborns by high-field (1.5 Tesla) magnetic resonance imaging of the central nervous system. II. Lesions associated with hypoxic-ischemic encephalopathy. Pediatrics 1991;87:431–438.
21. Kuenzle C, Baenziger O, Martin E, et al: Prognostic value of early MR imaging in term infants with severe perinatal asphyxia. Neuropediatrics 1994;4:191–200.
22. Rutherford MA, Pennock JM, Murdoch-Eaton DM, et al: Athetoid cerebral palsy and cysts in the putamen after hypoxic-ischemic encephalopathy. Arch Dis Child 1992;67:846–850.
23. Rutherford MA, Pennock JM, Schwieso JE, et al: Hypoxic-ischemic encephalopathy: early magnetic resonance imaging findings and their evolution. Neuropediatrics 1995;26:183–191.
24. Rutherford MA, Pennock JM, Schwieso JE, et al: Hypoxic-ischemic encephalopathy: early and late MRI findings and clinical outcome. Arch Dis Child 1996;75:141–151.
25. Rutherford MA, Pennock J, Counsell S, et al: Abnormal magnetic resonance signal in the internal capsule predicts poor developmental outcome in infants with hypoxic-ischemic encephalopathy. Pediatrics 1998;102: 323–328.
26. Pasternak JF, Predey TA, Mikhael MA: Neonatal asphyxia: vulnerability of basal ganglia, thalamus and brainstem. Pediatr Neurol 1991;7:147–149.
27. Pasternak JF, Goery MT: The syndrome of acute near-total intrauterine asphyxia in the term infant. Pediatr Neurol 1998;18:391–398.
28. Roland EH, Hill A, Norman MG, et al: Selective brainstem injury in an asphyxiated newborn. Ann Neurol 1988;23:89–92.
29. Leech RW, Alvord EC: Anoxic-ischemic encephalopathy in the human neonatal period: the significance of brain stem involvement. Arch Neurol 1977;34:109–113.
30. Rademakers RP, van der Knaap MS, Verbeeten B, et al: Central corticosubcortical involvement: a distinct pattern of brain damage caused by perinatal and postnatal asphyxia in term infants. J Comput Assist Tomogr 1995;19:252–263.
31. Volpe JJ, Herscovitch P, Perlman JM, et al: Positron emission tomography

in the asphyxiated term newborn: parasagittal impairment of cerebral blood flow. Ann Neurol 1985;17:287–296.

32. Traill Z, Squier M, Anslow P: Brain imaging in neonatal hypoglycemia. Arch Dis Child 1998;79:F145-F147.

33. Barkovich AJ, Ali FA, Rowley HA, Bass N: Imaging patterns of neonatal hypoglycemia. Am J Neuroradiol 1998;19:523–528.

34. Yokochi K: Clinical profiles of subjects with subcortical leucomalacia and border-zone infarction revealed by MR. Acta Pediatr 1998;87:879–883.

35. Kinnala A, Rikalainen H, Lapinleimu H, et al: Cerebral magnetic resonance imaging and ultrasonography findings after neonatal hypoglycemia. Pediatrics 1999;103:724–729.

36. Jouvet P, Cowan FM, Cox P, et al: Reproducibility and accuracy of MR imaging of the brain after severe birth asphyxia. Am J Neuroradiol 1999; 20:1343–1348.

37. Willis TA, Davidson J, Gray R, et al: Cytochrome oxidase deficiency presenting as birth asphyxia. Dev Med Child Neurol 2000;42:414–417.

38. Chugani HT, Phelps ME: Maturational changes in cerebral function in infants determined by 18FDG positron emission tomography. Science 1986;231:840–843.

39. Malamud N: Status marmoratus: a form of cerebral palsy following birth injury or inflammation of the central nervous system. J Pediatr 1950;37:610.

40. Shewmon DA, Fine M, Masdeu JC, Palacios E: Postischemic hypervascularity of infancy: a stage in the evolution of ischemic brain damage with characteristic CT scan. Ann Neurol 1981;9:358–365.

41. Saint-Hilaire MH, Burke RE, Bressman SB, et al: Delayed-onset dystonia due to perinatal or early childhood asphyxia. Neurology 1991;41:216–222.

42. Van der Knaap MS, Smit LS, Nauta JP, et al: Cortical laminar abnormalities: occurrence and clinical significance. Neuropediatrics 1993;24:143–148.

43. Cowan FM, Pennock JM, Hanrahan JD, et al: Early detection of cerebral infarction and hypoxic ischemic encephalopathy in newborns using diffusion weighted magnetic resonance imaging. Neuropediatrics 1994;25:172–175.

44. Mercuri E, Ricci D, Cowan F, et al: Head growth in infants with hypoxic-ischemic encephalopathy: correlation with neonatal magnetic resonance imaging. Pediatrics 2000;106:235–243.

45. Azzopardi D, Robertson N, Cowan F, et al: Pilot study of treatment with whole body hypothermia for neonatal encephalopathy. Pediatrics 2000; 106:684–694.

46. Mercuri E, Cowan F, Rutherford M, et al: Ischemic and haemorrhagic brain lesions in newborns with seizures and normal Apgar scores. Arch Dis Child 1995;73:F67-F74.

47. Maalouf E, Battin M, Counsell S, et al: Arthrogryposis multiplex congenita and bilateral mid-brain infarction following maternal overdose of co-proxamol. Eur J Paediatr Neurol 1997;1:183–186.

48. Dammann O, Leviton A: Maternal intrauterine infection, cytokines, and brain damage in the preterm newborn. Pediatr Res 1997;42:1–8.

CHAPTER 14

Thermal Influence on the Asphyxiated Newborn

Marianne Thoresen

Introduction

The main mechanisms of defense against asphyxia are similar among reptiles, birds, and mammals. An important response to decreased oxygen/glucose availability is to reduce metabolic demand. This can be achieved in several ways. One is by lowering the temperature (endogenous cooling), which is accomplished in small homeotherms through both autonomic and behavioral heat-dissipating responses.[1–3] The mildly asphyxiated newborn infant was shown to be 2°C colder than healthy newborns for the first 20 hours after birth.[4] Even the adult human has a reduced threshold for shivering during hypoxia, leading to a reduction in body temperature.[5] The second mechanism of decreasing metabolic demand is achieved by decreasing neuronal activity by an increase in inhibitory neuromodulators like gamma-aminobutyric acid (GABA)[6] and adenosine.[7] GABA or GABA agonists are also shown to induce hypothermia by reducing the temperature sensitivity of hypothalamic neurons.[8]

Studies involving the cooling of newborn[9–11] and adult[12] animals by 2–6°C after hypoxia-ischemia have shown promising results. Clinical trials are now in progress to investigate whether cooling initiated soon after the insult offers long-term neuroprotection.[13–17] Anecdotal experience derived from the work of Miller and Westin,[18,19] and others,[20,21] suggests confirmation of the hypothesis that hypothermia will improve the survival of asphyxiated newborns.

In 1973, Swan reviewed the historical use of *therapeutic hypothermia*.[22] The Hippocratic School on Cos, Greece (500 B.C.), used cold water and ice for sprains, fractures, gouty swellings, hemor-

This work was supported by The Norwegian Research Council, the Laerdal Foundation for Acute Medicine, and The Wellcome Trust.
From Donn SM, Sinha SK, Chiswick ML (eds): *Birth Asphyxia and the Brain: Basic Science and Clinical Implications.* © 2002, Futura Publishing Co., Inc., Armonk, NY.

rhages, tetanus, and febrile convulsions. Hypothermia and alcohol ingestion were the only anesthetic agents for amputations until chloroform was first used in the 19th century. Fay observed that cooling not only relieved pain but also decreased the growth of tumors.[23] To treat cerebral metastasis, he implemented selective brain cooling by inserting capsules perfused with cold liquid into the brain.[23]

The use of induced hypothermia to prevent hypoxic-ischemic brain damage (cooling *during* the insult, or intra-ischemic hypothermia) was first investigated by Miller.[24] He showed that the colder the newborn animals were, the longer the time period they were able to tolerate anoxia. Moreover, the more immature the species, the more prominent the effect. Anoxic tolerance for rats was 45 minutes, and for guinea pigs, who have a more mature and myelinated brain, only 6 minutes. A major breakthrough for cardiac surgery was achieved in 1950, when Bigelow et al. demonstrated that the heart could be isolated from the rest of the circulation during deep hypothermia (15–20°C).[25]

There is ample experimental evidence that low temperature *during* a hypoxic-ischemic insult ameliorates the damaging processes initiated by hypoxia.[26,27] The therapeutic benefit of cooling *after the insult* to prevent the development of brain damage has been more difficult to prove. The first study of post-insult hypothermia in adults was reported in 1958; four patients were cooled to 30–34°C for 72 hours after cardiac arrest with better outcome than historical controls.[28] Early in the 20th century, it was common practice to stimulate unresponsive newborns with cold water. (Many related anecdotes exist. Allegedly, the singer and actor, Frank Sinatra, was left for dead after a difficult breech delivery when his grandmother put him under cold water and revived him.)

Westin and Miller immersed newborn infants who did not breathe by 5 minutes in cold water until respiration ensued, which occurred in 2–14 minutes. The infants had rectal temperatures of 25–33°C.[29] They were then dried and allowed to re-warm slowly to 37°C by the rate of their own metabolism, which took up to 24 hours. Neurologic outcome was reported to be better than for those who received standard care at the time.[30] No randomized trials were undertaken and a total of 288 infants were cooled among several series.[29,31–35] The mortality rate was 12–15% in all the series, similar to that after standard care.[30] Russian investigators modified the technique and cooled the body to a rectal temperature of 30°C, selectively cooling the head by flushing ice cold water through a cap made of circular rubber tubing.[36] Tympanic membrane temperature was, on average, 1.5°C lower than rectal temperature.[37] (It must be noted, however, that tympanic temperature is not thought to be a good surrogate for brain temperature). After reaching target temperature, cooling was discontinued and the infants were allowed to passively re-warm by their own metabolism over the next 24 hours. When it was shown by Glass, Day, and Silverman et al,[20,21,38] in randomized controlled trials, that a long-term cold environment impaired growth and increased mortality in premature infants, all forms of cooling were thought to be unsafe. Subsequently, cooling as a resuscitative measure was abandoned for many years. The clinical use of hypothermia as a post-insult intervention did not develop further until basic research documented its beneficial effect in many experimental studies.[26,27,39,40]

Brain Metabolism and Energy Failure

At least 50% of brain metabolism is used to maintain ion gradients in neurons. During anoxia, adenosine triphosphate (ATP) must fall to less than 25% of normal levels before neurons start to exhibit signs of injury. However, at 0–10% of normal ATP concentrations, irreversible neuronal death occurs. These critical levels are similar across all species and ages. Brain maturity determines the time it takes until critical energy depletion and depolarization occur. Immature brains have smaller neurons with fewer ion channels and are more resistant to hypoxia.[41–44] Some neurons are irreversibly damaged, suffering the so-called primary injury. There are multiple factors, however, that determine the fate of neurons that are *reversibly* injured. Thus, there may be windows of opportunity to reduce, and possibly cease, the neurotoxic cascade, thereby rescuing reversibly injured neurons after the acute insult.

Physiology of Hypothermia

Metabolism in mammals is strongly related to temperature. For every 1°C reduction in body temperature, there is a 6–8% drop in metabolism. In the piglet brain, magnetic resonance spectroscopy (MRS) demonstrated a 5.3% reduction in cerebral metabolic rate per degree of temperature decrease.[45] Heart rate drops linearly with temperature. Mild hypothermia has been shown either to decrease[46] or increase cardiac output.[47] Low temperature increases vascular resistance in the pulmonary circulation,[48,49] and the development of persistent pulmonary hypertension is of significant concern as an adverse effect of hypothermia in the newborn. Hypothermia induces a leftward shift of the oxygen-hemoglobin dissociation curve,[50] as does fetal hemoglobin. Thus, oxygen is even more tightly bound to hemoglobin. Also, blood viscosity increases by 2–4% per degree of temperature decrease, which may be clinically important in newborns with a high hematocrit. Therefore, tissues could effectively be hypoxic even at sufficient oxygen saturation. Per degree decrease in temperature, PaO_2 is typically reduced by 4–7 mmHg and $PaCO_2$ is reduced by about 4.5%. Lower $PaCO_2$ will also shift the dissociation curve to the left, making it even more difficult to release oxygen to the tissue.[50] Low $PaCO_2$ (as with inadvertent overventilation) during hypothermia might therefore be particularly undesirable. An experiment on newborn piglets studied two different CO_2 strategies during hypothermic extracorporal circulation and cardiac arrest. Those with high $PaCO_2$ had a more uniform cerebral perfusion and less brain damage than those with lower $PaCO_2$. During re-warming there is a mismatch between metabolism and oxygen delivery,[51] and a study in which patients were kept hypercapnic during re-warming reported the avoidance of jugular venous desaturation.[52]

Fluid management requires particular attention during hypothermia. Hypothermia inhibits antidiuretic hormone production and increases diuresis ("cold diuresis"). Also, tubular reabsorption of sodium is reduced, and thus serum sodium needs to be followed closely in hypothermic patients.[53] There is also a trend for fluid to shift into tissues, depleting intravascular volume and risking hypotension. Measurement of central venous pressure and echocardiographic assessment of atrial filling are useful in the determination of intravascular volume.

Enzymes have differing sensitivities to changes in temperature; some effects may be beneficial and some deleterious.[54] Blood coagulation reactions are enzymatic and are dependent on temperature. In adult humans, prothrombin time and partial thromboplastin time increase by 25% at 31°C compared to 37°C. In a group of accidentally cooled newborn infants, thrombin clotting time was 80% longer in infants with rectal temperatures of 34°C or less, compared to controls at 37°C.[55] Bleeding time reflects the *in vivo* interactions of platelets, several clotting factors, and the vessel wall. In monkeys, who have a similar clotting cascade to humans, skin bleeding time was 125% longer at skin temperature of 28°C compared to 34°C.[56] In these studies, clotting was examined at actual temperature. Since standard clotting assays are performed at 37°C, significant hypothermic coagulopathy may be missed. However, clotting times are more severely prolonged when hypothermic temperatures are encountered during laboratory testing than when body temperatures are hypothermic.[57]

In the 1960s, severe hypothermia in newborns who were born at home was not uncommon. Uncontrolled observations report that these children had an increased risk of pulmonary and cerebral hemorrhages.[55,58] The implication for newborns kept hypothermic for several days as a neuroprotective strategy is that coagulopathy may be a significant concern.

There is conflicting evidence as to whether mild hypothermia increases the susceptibility to infection. Hypothermia reduces the number of circulating white blood cells, particularly neutrophils, and this effect is reversed on re-warming.[59] Adult studies have shown reduced phagocytic and chemotactic activity during cooling. In a study of brain trauma patients who were treated with a combination of barbiturates and hypothermia, and who developed pneumonia, granulocyte colony-stimulating factor was effective in increasing the white cell count.[60] In another study of 10 patients who were cooled for 24 hours after trauma, eight developed increased serum lipase activity, four of whom had clinical pancreatitis; all normalized with re-warming.[61] In a randomized study of 24 hours of hypothermia and 3 days survival in 36 newborn piglets, no infections were documented, although the white blood cell count was reduced by 50% during hypothermia (Thoresen, unpublished data).

Experimental Models: Cooling After Injury

Three questions are of critical importance in inducing hypothermia after brain injury: (1) How much should the temperature be decreased? (2) How long should cooling be continued? (3) How much time can elapse before cooling is started after the insult in order for it to have a neuroprotective effect? In adult rats and gerbils, the shorter the delay until initiation of cooling, the stronger the effect; the protection was lost after a 3–12 hour delay in other studies.[12] A major concern is that most adult animal studies did not demonstrate long-term protection. Hypothermia merely postponed the development of damage. However, Colbourne et al reported that cooling begun after 6–12 hours, and continued for 48 hours, resulted in significant long-lasting protection.[62,63] It appears that a longer cooling period can partially compensate for a delayed start.

A randomized study of newborn animals, using the 7-day-old rat model, first showed that cooling initiated *after* the injury uniformly protected all areas of the brain.[14] Pups were cooled from 38°C to 32°C for 3 hours, reaching the target temperature within 15 minutes. Histologic injury evaluated after 1 week of survival showed more than 50% protection. Trescher et al used the same model and found that cooling by 4°C afforded similar protection after 1 week, but no protection after 4 weeks of survival.[64] In a repeat study using cooling by 5°C for 6 hours and randomizing animals to survive for either 1 or 6 weeks, both groups showed significant protection compared with normothermic controls.[65] It appears that there is a threshold for the "cooling dose," by depth or duration, to achieve long-term protection. The rat pup is small (10–12 g) and continuous cardiovascular monitoring and blood sampling is not possible. For such studies, larger models such as the fetal sheep and newborn pig are used. In a model of global hypoxia-ischemia, a 4°C reduction in temperature lasting 3 hours was protective for milder insults,[66] but not protective for severe insults when the animals developed post-hypoxic seizures.[15]

Mechanisms of Hypothermic Neuroprotection

Although the specific mechanisms of protection by hypothermia are not known, it appears that hypothermia may intervene at several stages in the sequence of events between metabolic inhibition and neuronal death. In addition, the current knowledge is derived mostly from adult animal models and from intra-ischemic, rather than post-ischemic, hypothermia.

The largest neuroprotective effect of low temperature is exemplified in ectoderms such as the turtle. Turtles survive in an anoxic environment for weeks or months; the lower the temperature, the longer the duration of survival.[67] Miller showed that warm-blooded animals that are immature at birth, such as the rat or dog pup and kitten, increased their anoxic tolerance eightfold between 37°C and 15°C.[24,68] However, guinea pigs, which are even more mature at birth than human newborns,[69] show an increase of anoxic tolerance during moderate hypothermia of only 5–9 minutes.[24]

A widespread defense strategy used by hypoxia-tolerant animals is metabolic depression. Sodium channel density is downregulated during anoxia.[70] There are increased levels of inhibitory neurotransmitters/neuromodulators such as glycine, taurine, GABA, and adenosine during anoxia[6] that decrease synaptic excitability and, thus, brain activity and energy consumption. Adenosine added to hippocampal slices after chemical anoxia (no oxygen or glucose) increases the critical survival period of the slice from 10 to 15–20 minutes. In theory, drugs such as profentophyllin (re-uptake inhibitor) or allopurinol (xanthine oxidase inhibitor) that increase adenosine levels might be neuroprotective. Accordingly, adenosine antagonists, such as theophylline, might not be beneficial.

Low temperature reduces ATP consumption and delays depolarization when ATP production stops.[71] In the newborn, the neurons are smaller, the membrane contains fewer ion channels, and there are far fewer synaptic connections – all of which are factors that reduce the energy demand and increase tolerance to anoxia. Zeevalk and Nicklas showed that hypothermia reduced the rate of ion leakage in the chick retina.[72] Major reductions in brain injury that result from even mild reductions in brain temperature suggest that the mechanism is not only decreased metabolic rate.[26] When cerebral metabolic rate is reduced correspondingly by drugs, the neuroprotection that is achieved is not the same as with hypothermia.[73]

During intra-ischemic hypothermia, extracellular glutamate release is reduced[74] and expression of early genes occurs even faster.[75,76] Increased intracranial pressure is rarely a problem in the newborn who has an open fontanel. In children and adults, reduction of intracranial pressure is an important beneficial effect of hypothermia when applied after brain trauma.[77,78]

The development of brain damage is also thought to be mediated by the neurotoxic cascade of inflammatory processes (see Chapters 3 and 4).[79] A study in rats using hypothermia and interleukin-10 (IL-10, anti-inflammatory cytokine) showed long-lasting protection which was not achieved by hypothermia alone.[80] A combination of hypothermia and an anti-inflammatory drug which reduced the core temperature by 1°C for 1 week also provided effective long-term neuroprotection.[81] In brain trauma studies in which hypothermia was neuroprotective, there was a reduction in plasma IL-6[82] and intraventricular IL-1β.[83]

Few experimental studies have been carried out in newborns to investigate mechanisms of post-hypoxic hypothermic neuroprotection. Cerebral energy metabolism in human infants who are severely depressed after birth can be assessed by phosphorus magnetic resonance spectroscopy (^{31}P MRS) and is usually normal on the first day of life. After 24 hours, impairment of cerebral metabolism develops, as shown by falling phosphocreatine/inorganic phosphorus (PCr/Pi) and ATP.[84,85] The severity of this secondary energy failure is closely related to the risk of death or severe long-term neurodevelopmental disability[86] (see Chapter 6).

The piglet carotid occlusion model develops secondary energy failure with a similar time course as asphyxiated infants.[87] In newborn pigs subjected to transient bilateral carotid occlusion severe enough to deplete ATP by 75–90%, it was shown that 12 hours of post-hypoxic cooling of 4°C ameliorated secondary energy failure[13] and the late rise in lactate.[88] The animals survived for only 3 days, and thus it is unknown whether the impressive improvement in metabolic state was long-lasting. In adult models of trauma and infection, the blood-brain barrier has been shown to be less permeable during hypothermia.[89,90] There are no studies examining post-hypoxic hypothermia on the neonatal blood-brain barrier.

Apoptosis and Necrosis

It has been suggested that hypothermia exerts its protection primarily by inhibiting apoptotic cell death.[91] In the immature brain, more cells have the fate of apoptotic cell death than in the mature brain. Also, glutamate toxicity is different. Blockade of N-methyl-D-aspartate (NMDA) glutamate receptors for only a few hours during late fetal or early neonatal life triggers widespread apoptotic neurodegeneration in the developing brain.[92] Determination of apoptotic versus necrotic cell death is not straightforward. The frequently used DNA fragmentation analysis has been found to be of little value, because only ultrastructural analysis has the capability of distinguishing between excitotoxic and apoptotic neurodegeneration.[93] (See also Chapter 7.)

In a global model of asphyxia, collection of extracellular fluid from the brain using microdialysis for 6 hours post-insult, during hypothermia or normothermia, revealed that the concentration of excitatory amino acids and the citrulline/arginine ratio (a measure of nitric oxide) was significantly reduced during post-hypoxic cooling.[94]

Deleterious Effects of Hyperthermia

Hyperthermia during ischemia is deleterious. A 2°C increase in core temperature results in a 40% increase in neuronal loss in an adult rat model of brain ischemia.[95] High temperature after stroke was predictive of neurologic impairment in a prospective Danish study.[96] Fever is the hallmark of inflammation, and it is suggested that the severity of the ischemic insult determines the release of factors such as cytokines, which induce hyperthermia as well as aggravate brain injury.[79] Clifton et al suggested that the clinical studies that showed neuroprotection by hypothermia in fact did so by the detrimental effect of actively warming the normothermic group.[97]

Fetal Temperature

The damaging effect of hyperthermia is particularly relevant to the fetus. Grether and Nelson showed that maternal pyrexia had the highest odds ratio of all single risk factors for the development of cerebral palsy in offspring.[98] *In utero,* the fetus is always warmer than the mother and the placental circulation drains the excess heat from the fetus. In the fetal sheep, neuroprotection was achieved only if the brain temperature was less than 34°C.[99]

Adult Human Studies on Cooling After Injury

A pilot study of 48 hours of cooling after severe stroke has shown promising results.[78] Target temperature of 33°C was reached as late as 14 hours after the insult and continued for 48–72 hours.[100] Hypothermia was effective in reducing intracranial pressure. One randomized, single center study in adult humans with closed head trauma used whole body cooling to 33.5°C for 24 hours and found improved outcome at 6 months in those with mild or moderate insults.[77] In a recent larger study,[97] 392 patients with coma after head injury were randomly assigned to be cooled within 6 hours to 33°C, which continued for the first 48 hours after injury. Functional status after 6 months showed no difference in outcome in the two groups (57% suffered severe disability or death). Subgroup analysis showed that the rate of poor outcome was significantly higher in cooled patients older than 45 years of age, as was the occurrence of complications. However, in 81 patients younger than or equal to 45 years of age who had had a core temperature less than 35°C on admission, 52% in the hypothermia group versus 76% in the normothermia group had a poor outcome (p=0.02). This suggests protection in a subgroup of younger individuals.

Systemic Adverse Effects of Mild and Moderate Hypothermia

Animal cerebral ischemia models are not appropriate for studies of the adverse systemic effect of hypothermia, because only the brain, and not the rest of the body, is subjected to hypoxic-ischemia. In piglet survival studies after global hypoxia-ischemia with post-hypoxic hypothermia, investigators found no increase in complications in the hypothermia group, although there was a transiently higher need for oxygen supplementation during hypothermia.[15] Some human brain trauma or stroke trials report no serious adverse effects such as hypotension, arrhythmia, infection, bleeding, or requirement for ventilatory support,[61,83] although pneumonia[78] and pancreatitis[61] occurred more frequently in the hypothermia group. In a recent large 48-hour hypothermia trial,[97] the hypothermia group had more hospital days with complications than the patients in the normothermia group. However, it was also reported that fewer hypothermic patients had elevated intracranial pressure. In the dog, mild (34°C) whole body hypothermia after cardiac arrest gave better overall outcomes than moderate (28–32°C) or severe (15–25°C) hypothermia. The investigators suggested that this resulted from fewer systemic adverse effects of mild hypothermia.[102]

Hypothermia is reported to increase the susceptibility to infection in adults; however, there are no data available for the effect of prolonged mild hypothermia. *In vitro* experiments with human granulocytes have shown reduced phagocytosis outside the range of 32–39°C.[103] In adult patients treated with hypothermia who developed severe infections, treatment with granulocyte colony-stimulating factor was effective.[60] In newborn infants, coagulation disturbances are seen with temperatures below 33°C.[55] Hypothermia increases viscosity, with a 2–4% increase per 1°C,[54] which might impair perfusion and possibly oxygenation if the hematocrit is already high.

Another clinically important aspect of hypothermia is its effect on drug metabolism.[104] In a pilot study of total body cooling, two infants who had repeated post-hypoxic seizures received 40 mg/kg of phenobarbital within 6 hours. Plasma levels were checked for 5 days and a half-life of greater than 450 hours was found compared to 150 hours in normothermic, asphyxiated infants (Thoresen, unpublished data). The half-life of gentamicin, which is mainly handled by the kidneys, was not affected by 24 hours of hypothermia in a piglet model of hypoxia-ischemia.[105]

Cooling and Stress

The physiologic response to cooling in healthy individuals is an increased metabolic rate, to counteract the cooling. Adults shiver while cooled, which increases metabolism by up to 600%. However, newborns do not have the motor maturity to shiver, and instead metabolize brown fat.[106] Hypoxic newborn animals do not mount a metabolic response to cold. This may be a teleologic adaptation to prevent survival with severe impairment.

A frequently used standardized stress intervention in animals is restraint from free movement. In rats, hypothermia was applied with and without additional restraint stress. In the group that was restrained from moving freely, the protective effect of hypothermia was lost.[107] This supports the study by Yager et al in 1993 that demonstrated no effect of 3 hours of 3°C or 6°C post-hypoxic hypothermia, using the same model when all animals were restrained.[108] Miller and Miller showed in 1962 that the tolerance to anoxia during hypothermia was increased if the animals were sedated.[109] In a study of 24 hours of cooling after a global insult, the hypothermic animals were not sedated or anesthetized during cooling.[101] Contrary to results of previous studies,[13,15] no protection from hypothermia was observed. It was speculated that this was associated with the stress of being cooled, as the hypothermic animals had a threefold increase in cortisol levels compared with those who were kept normothermic.[101,110]

There are no data regarding newborn infants and the effect of stress or metabolism on the degree of injury. Experimental work indicates that stress, as measured by increased cortisol, increases brain damage and, particularly, apoptosis in the hippocampus. Reducing cortisol by pharmacologic blockade or adrenalectomy reduces the brain damage.[111] Newborns in intensive care units are subjected to many stressful and painful procedures. There is no consensus as to when and how one should give analgesia and sedation. A recent pilot trial on ventilated preterm infants investigated three different regimens of analgesia and sedation, with morphine and midazolam. In the group receiving morphine, a poor outcome was found in 4% of the infants, compared to 34% in the midazolam group, and 33% in the placebo group.[112] Until further knowledge is available, it is advisable to give sufficient sedation to infants subjected to hypothermia because the implications of stress are as yet unknown.

Head Versus Body Cooling

No valid noninvasive method is available for measuring the cerebral temperature in newborn infants. In adults, the brain is 0.5°C warmer than core temperature. Temperature gradients also exist within the brain. In an MRS study of healthy adult humans, the thalamus was 37.7°C and the frontal cortex was 37.2°C.[113] In adult neurosurgical and stroke patients with brain injury, brain temperature was found to be 1–3°C higher than core temperature[100,114] and, during body cooling, this gradient was reduced to 0.3°C.[100] One mechanism for higher brain temperature in trauma patients is "thermopooling" secondary to low perfusion. When the perfusion pressure was increased by elevating the arterial blood pressure, more heat could be transported from the brain via improved blood flow.[115] Similar measurements are not available for newborns, and it is unknown whether the asphyxiated brain is actually warmer than the healthy brain.

Selective brain cooling is a natural mechanism that enables mammals to maintain their brain temperature below the temperature of the rest of the body during conditions of hyperthermia.[116,117] Those mammals with rete mirabilis (in which the inflowing artery divides into a network of vessels intermingled with venous plexuses at the base of the brain, receiving blood from cooler mucosal or cutaneous areas) have the ability to cool cerebral blood on its arrival into the brain. It is postulated that humans, who lack a cerebral rete, cool inflowing arterial blood via the veins in close proximity, the plexus caroticus, and the venous plexuses in the spinal canal surrounding the vertebral arteries.[118] Anatomically, there are connections between extra- and intracranial venous plexuses. In theory, cooling the scalp should also cool the venous blood. The extent to which the brain itself is cooled, and the depth from the brain surface at which cooling is effective, are not known. In adults with a thick skull, a cooling cap perfused with water of 10°C did not lower the brain temperature even at very superficial levels.[119]

Mellergård found in neurosurgical patients who were body-cooled that the epidural, intraventricular, and rectal temperatures responded similarly during cooling. When a cooling cap was added for 8 hours, the epidural temperature fell by 1°C; however, rectal and intraventricular (brain) temperatures were unaffected. This suggests that a cooling cap has no selective effect on brain temperature in adults.[120]

When cold water is circulated in a cooling cap, a temperature gradient from the cold surface under the cap and into the brain is thought to occur. Fetal lamb studies with a cooling coil around the head support the assumption that the neuroprotection is far better in the superficial cortex compared to the deeper basal ganglia.[17] Since basal ganglia damage is one of the significant pathologic features of severe intrapartum asphyxia, the aim should also be to cool the core of the brain. In 2-week-old piglets, Gelman et al were able to cool the basal ganglia using a cap perfused with ethylene glycol at a temperature of $-30°C$ for 45 minutes.[121] The author and co-investigators have applied selective head cooling to newborn piglets after global hypoxia-ischemia while monitoring brain and body temperature. In this small brain, it was possible to maintain deep brain temperature at 5°C lower than core temperature by circulating water at about 10°C around the head.[122]

It is likely that the degree of systemic hypothermia is particularly important in the cooling of the basal ganglia. With head cooling, the additional protection of the cortex might be encountered. Our data suggest that, at least in a small brain, selective head cooling can also cool the deeper parts of the brain.[122] Cooling the head is also effective as a means of body cooling in newborns, in whom the head represents a large surface area; unlike other skin surfaces, the scalp does not undergo vasoconstriction,[123] increasing the effectiveness of heat transfer.

Safety Studies of Mild Neonatal Hypothermia

In 1998, Gunn et al reported a pilot study of selective head cooling and mild hypothermia in six asphyxiated infants who were cooled to a rectal temperature of $36.3 \pm 0.2°C$, and six asphyxiated infants cooled to $35.7 \pm 0.2°C$.[124] None of the infants developed arrhythmias or hypotension (mean arterial pressure < 40 mmHg) during cooling. One infant, whose rectal temperature inadvertently fell to 34.2°C, developed an increase in oxygen requirement to 40% and the pH fell to 7.29, but both of these changes reversed when the rectal temperature was raised to 35.5°C.

Another pilot study of selective head cooling reported the cardiovascular effects of therapeutic hypothermia.[125] The study recruited sicker patients than Gunn et al, including Apgar scores at 10 minutes that were less than or equal to 5, pH less than 7.0, and significant amplitude-integrated electroencephalographic (EEG) abnormalities (shown to predict poor outcome[126]). In the pilot study of 72 hours of mild hypothermia, the target core temperature was 33–34°C in three total body-cooled infants and 34–35°C in six selectively head-cooled infants. During cooling, the blood pressure rose slightly and the pulse rate fell. In two infants, there was worsening of pulmonary gas exchange during cooling consistent with persistent pulmonary hypertension, which normalized during re-warming. Avoidance of overcooling required experience, particularly when drugs were given that inhibited movements or heat production, such as sedatives, anticonvulsants, and skeletal muscle relaxants. It was necessary that re-warming be accomplished slowly, with special attention to hypotension, the need for volume replacement, and oxygenation. (During cardiopulmonary bypass in rabbits, rapid re-warming caused an increase in cerebral oxygen consumption that was temporarily unmatched by cerebral blood flow.[51]) Cerebral fractional oxygen extraction, monitored with near-infrared spectroscopy, was reduced in children during re-warming after hypothermic cardiopulmonary bypass.[127] The patients experienced no serious complications that could not be corrected with careful monitoring. Significant subdural hematomas were found in two children and a small intraventricular hemorrhage was found in one. Both subdural bleeds resolved by 2 months and there was no parenchymal damage. Subdural hematomas may be present in children after instrument-assisted deliveries, and therefore might not be associated with cooling in this small pilot study.

A large international 26-center, randomized, controlled trial of selective brain cooling in the treatment of hypoxic-ischemic encephalopathy completed recruitment of 235 patients by January 2002. This study, which utilized the Cool Care® cold water recirculating cap (Olympic Medical, Seattle, WA, USA), will examine neurologic status at 18 months of age. Other current multicenter studies are investigating the neuroprotective benefits of total body cooling on asphyxiated newborns.

Conclusions

In terms of its implications for clinical use, following intrapartum asphyxia, hypothermia is a highly experimental intervention which has not yet been proven to be effective in randomized trials. The asphyxiated infant is best managed according to current guidelines.[128,129] Also, perinatal hyperthermia, both maternal and neonatal, should be avoided, since hyperthermia increases neurologic damage.[26,97] A child who becomes hypothermic after resuscitation should be re-warmed slowly and attention should be paid to volume replacement in order to avoid hypotension.

It is plausible that future neuroprotective treatment will consist of hypothermia in combination with a "cocktail" of drugs, each specifically inhibiting a different point of the neurotoxic cascade, or facilitating repair.[80] As with any other therapeutic measure, hypothermia must be administered with an understanding of the extensive physiologic effects. The promising aspects of hypothermia lie in its ability to intercept the neurotoxic cascade at multiple levels.

References

1. Gordon C, Fogelson L: Comparative effects of hypoxia on behavioral thermoregulation in rats, hamsters and mice. Am J Physiol 1991;260: R120–R125.
2. Gordon CJ: Homeothermy: does it impede the response to cellular injury? J Therm Biol 1996;21:29–36.
3. Dawkins MJR, Hull D: Brown adipose tissue and the response of newborn rabbits to cold. J Physiol 1964;172:216–238.
4. Burnard ED, Cross KW: Rectal temperature in the newborn after birth asphyxia. Br Med J 1958;1197–1199.
5. Johnston CE, White MD, Wu M, et al: Eucapnic hypoxia lowers human cold thermoregulatory response thresholds and accelerates core cooling. J Appl Physiol 1996;80:422–429.
6. Nilsson GE, Lutz PL: Release of inhibitory neurotransmitters in response to anoxia in turtle brain. Am J Physiol 1991;261:R32–R33.
7. Perez-Pinzon MA, Lutz PL, Sick TJ, Rosenthal M: Adenosine, a "retaliatory" metabolite, promotes anoxia tolerance in turtle brain. J Cereb Blood Flow Metab 1993;13:728–732.
8. Yakimova K, Sann H, Schmid H, Pierau F-K: Effects of GABA agonists and antagonists on temperature sensitive neurones in the rat hypothalamus. J Physiol 1996;494:217–230.
9. Thoresen M, Wyatt J: Keeping a cool head, post-hypoxic hypothermia—an old idea revisited. Acta Paediatr Scand 1997;86:1029–1033.
10. Wagner CL, Eicher DJ, Katikanemi LD, et al: The use of hypothermia: a role in the treatment of neonatal asphyxia. Pediatr Neurol 1999;21: 429–443.
11. Gunn AJ, Gunn TR: The "pharmacology" of neuronal rescue with cerebral hypothermia. Early Human Dev 1998;53:19–35.
12. Colbourne F, Sutherland G, Corbett D: Postischemic hypothermia: a critical appraisal with implications for clinical treatment. Mol Neurobiol 1997;14:171–201.
13. Thoresen M, Penrice J, Lorek A, et al: Mild hypothermia following severe transient hypoxia-ischemia ameliorates delayed ("secondary") cerebral energy failure in the newborn piglet. Pediatr Res 1995;5:667–670.
14. Thoresen M, Bågenholm R, Løberg EM, et al: Post-hypoxic cooling of neonatal rats provides protection against brain injury. Arch Dis Child 1996;74:F3–F9.
15. Haaland K, Løberg EM, Steen PA, Thoresen M: Post-hypoxic hypothermia in newborn piglets. Pediatr Res 1997;41:505–512.
16. Sirimanne ES, Blumberg RM, Bossano D, et al: The effect of prolonged modification of cerebral temperature on the outcome after hypoxic-ischemic brain injury in the infant rat. Pediatr Res 1996;39:591–597.
17. Gunn AJ, Gunn TR, deHaan HH, et al: Dramatic neuronal rescue with prolonged selective head cooling after ischemia in fetal lambs. J Clin Invest 1997;99:248–256.
18. Silverman W: Cooling the asphyxiated newborn—responsibly. Pediatrics 1998;101:697–698.
19. Westin B, Nyberg R, Miller JA, Wedenberg E: Hypothermia and transfu-

sion with oxygenated blood in the treatment of asphyxia neonatorum. Acta Paediatr Scand 1962;51:1–80.

20. Glass L, Silverman WA, Sinclair JC: Effect of the thermal environment on cold resistance and growth of small infants after the first week of life. Pediatrics 1968;41:1033–1046.

21. Day RL, Caliquiri L, Kamenski C: Body temperature and survival of premature infants. Pediatrics 1964;34:163–167.

22. Swan H: Clinical hypothermia: a lady with a past and some promise for the future. Surgery 1973;73:736–758.

23. Fay T: Early experiences with local and generalized refrigeration of the human brain. J Neurosurg 1959;16:239–260.

24. Miller JA: Factors in neonatal resistance to anoxia. I. Temperature and survival of newborn guinea pigs under anoxia. Science 1949;110:113–114.

25. Bigelow WG, Callaghan JC, Hopps JA: General hypothermia for experimental intracardiac surgery. Ann Surg 1950;132:531–539.

26. Busto R, Dietrich WD, Globus MYT, et al: Small differences in intra-ischemic brain temperature critically determine the extent of ischemic neuronal injury. J Cereb Blood Flow Metab 1987;7:729–738.

27. Dietrich WD: The importance of brain temperature in cerebral injury. J Neurotrauma 1992;9:S475–S445.

28. William GR, Spencer FC: The clinical use of hypothermia following cardiac arrest. Ann Surg 1958;148:462–466.

29. Westin B: Infant resuscitation and prevention of mental retardation. Am J Obstet Gynecol 1971;110:1134–1138.

30. Drage JS, Berendes H: Apgar scores and the outcome of the newborn. Pediatr Clin N Am 1966;13:635–643.

31. Dunn JM, Miller JMJ: Hypothermia combined with positive pressure ventilation in resuscitation of the asphyxiated neonate. Am J Obstet Gynecol 1969;104:58–67.

32. Ehrström J, Hirvensalo M, Donner M, Hietalathi J: Hypothermia in the resuscitation of severely asphyctic newborn infants. Ann Clin Res 1969;1:40–49.

33. Krokfors E, Pitkänen H, Hirvensalo M, Rhen K: The use of hypothermia in severe neonatal asphyxia. Finlands Läkartidning 1961;17:987–989.

34. Miller JA, Miller FS, Westin B: Hypothermia in the treatment of asphyxia neonatorum. Biol Neonat 1964;6:148–163.

35. Westin B, Miller JA, Nyberg R, Wedenberg E: Neonatal asphyxia pallida treated with hypothermia alone or with hypothermia and transfusion of oxygenated blood. Surgery 1959;45:868–879.

36. Kopchev SN. Cranio-cerebral hypothermia. In *Obstetrics*. Medicina, Moscow, 1985, pp 1–112.

37. Shiraki K, Sagawa S, Tajima F, et al: Independence of brain and tympanic temperatures in an unanesthetized human. J Appl Physiol 1988;65: 482–486.

38. Silverman WA, Fertig JW, Berger AP: The influence of the thermal environment upon the survival of newly born premature infants. Pediatrics 1958;22:876–886.

39. Busto R, Dietrich WD, Globus MYT, Ginsberg MD: Postischemic moderate hypothermia inhibits CA1 hippocampal ischemic neuronal injury. Neurosci Lett 1989;101:299–304.

40. Dietrich WD: Effect of mild hypothermia on cerebral energy metabolism during the evolution of hypoxic-ischemic brain damage in the immature rat. Stroke 1996;27:926.

41. Friedman JE, Haddad GG: Major differences in Ca_I^{2+} response to anoxia between neonatal and adult rat CA1 neurons: role of Ca_O^{2+} and Na_O^+. J Neurosci 1993;13:63–72.

42. Haddad GG, Donnelly DF: O_2 deprivation induces a major depolarization in brain stem neurons in the adult but not in the neonatal rat. J Physiol 1990;429:411–428.

43. Jiang C, Xia Y, Haddad GG: Role of ATP-sensitive K^+ channels during anoxia: major differences between rat (newborn and adult) and turtle neurons. J Physiol 1992;448:599–612.

44. Xia Y, Jiang C, Haddad GG: Oxidative and glycolytic pathways in rat (newborn and adult) and turtle brain: role during anoxia. Am J Physiol 1992;262:R595–R603.

45. Laptook AR, Corbett RJT, Sterett R, et al: Quantitative relationship between brain temperature and energy utilization rate measured in vivo using ^{31}P and ^1H magnetic resonance spectroscopy. Pediatr Res 1995;38:919–925.

46. Dudgeon DL, Randall PA, Hill RB, McAfee JG: Mild hypothermia: its effect on cardiac output and regional perfusion in the neonatal piglet. J Pediatr Surg 1980;15:805–810.

47. Ohta S, Yukioka T, Wada T, et al: Effect of mild hypothermia on the coefficient of oxygen delivery in hypoxemic dogs. J Appl Physiol 1995;78:2095–2099.

48. Benumof JL, Wahrenbrock EA: Dependency of hypoxic pulmonary vasoconstriction on temperature. J Appl Physiol 1977;42:56–58.

49. Stern S, Braun K: Pulmonary arterial and venous response to cooling: role of alpha adrenergic receptors. Am J Physiol 1970;219:982–985.

50. Dill D: Respiratory and metabolic effects of hypothermia. Am J Physiol 1941;132:685.

51. Enomoto S, Hindman BJ, Dexter F, et al: Rapid re-warming causes an increase in the cerebral metabolic rate for oxygen that is temporarily unmatched by cerebral blood flow: a study during cardiopulmonary bypass in rabbits. Anesthesiology 1996;84:1392–1400.

52. Hänel F, Knoblesdorff GV, Werner C, et al: Hypercapnia prevents jugular bulb desaturation during re-warming from hypothermia cardiopulmonary bypass. Anesthesiology 1998;89:19–23.

53. Moyer JH, Morris G, DeBakey ME: Hypothermia. I. Effect on renal hemodynamics and on excretion of water and electrolytes in dog and man. Ann Surg 1957;145:26–40.

54. Schubert A: Side effect of mild hypothermia. J Neurosurg Anesthesiol 1995;7:139–147.

55. Chadd MA, Gray OP: Hypothermia and coagulation defects in the newborn. Arch Dis Child 1972;41:819–821.

56. Valeri CR, Feingold H, Cassidy G, et al: Hypothermia-induced reversible platelet dysfunction. Ann Surg 1986;205:175–181.

57. Reed RL, Johnston TD, Hudson JD: The disparity between hypothermic coagulopathy and clotting studies. J Neurotrauma 1992;33:465–468.

58. Mann TP, Elliott RIK: Neonatal cold injury due to accidental exposure to cold. Lancet 1957;i:229–234.
59. Shenaq SA, Yawn DH, Saleem A, et al: Effect of profound hypothermia on leukocytes and platelets. Ann Clin Lab Sci 1986;16:130–133.
60. Ishikawa K, Tanaka T, Takaoka M, et al: Granulocyte colony-stimulating factor ameliorates life-threatening infections after combined therapy with barbiturates and mild hypothermia in patients with severe head injury. J Trauma 1999; 46:999–1007.
61. Metz C, Holzschuh M, Bein T, et al: Moderate hypothermia in patients with severe head injury: cerebral and extracerebral effects. J Neurosurg 1996;85:533–541.
62. Colbourne F, Sutherland GR, Auer RN: Electron microscopic evidence against apoptosis as the mechanisms of neuronal death in global ischemia. J Neurosci 1999;19:4200–4210.
63. Colbourne F, Li H, Bucham AM: Indefatigable CA1 sector neuroprotection with mild hypothermia induced 6 hours after severe forebrain ischemia in rats. J Cereb Blood Flow Metab 1999;19:742–749.
64. Trescher WH, Ishiwa S, Johnston MV: Brief post-hypoxic-ischemic hypothermia markedly delays neonatal brain injury. Brain Dev 1997;19: 326–338.
65. Bona E, Løberg EM, Bågenholm R, Kjellmer I, et al: Protective effects of moderate hypothermia after neonatal hypoxia-ischemia: short and long-term outcome. Pediatr Res 1998;40:738–748.
66. Thoresen M, Haaland K, Løberg EM, et al: A piglet survival model for post-hypoxic encephalopathy. Pediatr Res 1996;40:738–748.
67. Belkin DA: Anoxia: tolerance in reptiles. Science 1963;139:492–493.
68. Miller FS, Miller JA: Body temperature and tolerance of asphyxia in newborn kittens. Bull Tulane Med Faculty 1967;24:197–209.
69. Dobbing J, Sands J: Comparative aspect of the brain growth spurt. Early Hum Dev 1979;3:79–83.
70. Perez-Pinson MA, Rosenthal M, Sick TJ, et al: Downregulation of sodium channels during anoxia: a putative survival strategy of turtle brain. Am J Physiol 1992;262.
71. Bart RD, Takaoka S, Pearlstein RD, et al: Interactions between hypothermia and the latency to ischemic depolarization. Anesthesiology 1998;88: 1266–1273.
72. Zeevalk GD, Nicklas WJ: Hypothermia, metabolic stress, and NMDA-mediated excitotoxicity. J Neurochem 1993;61:1445–1453.
73. Nakashima K, Todd M, Warner D: The relationship between cerebral metabolic rate and ischemic depolarization: a comparison of the effects of hypothermia, pentobarbital and isoflurane. Anesthesiology 1995;82: 1199–1208.
74. Busto R, Globus MYT, Dietrich WD, et al: Effect of mild hypothermia on ischemia-induced release of neurotransmitters and free fatty acids. Stroke 1989;20:904–910.
75. Kumar K, Wu XL, Evans AT: Expression of c-fos and fos-B proteins following transient forebrain ischemia: effect of hypothermia. Mol Brain Res 1996;42:337–343.
76. Kamme F, Wieloch T: Induction of junD mRNA after transient forebrain ischemia in the rat: effect of hypothermia. Mol Brain Res 1996;43:51–56.

77. Shiozaki T, Sugimoto H, Taneda M, et al: Effect of mild hypothermia on uncontrollable intracranial hypertension after severe head injury. J Neurosurg 1993;79:363–368.
78. Schwab S, Schwarz S, Spranger M, et al: Moderate hypothermia in the treatment of patients with severe middle cerebral artery infarction. Stroke 1998;29:2461–2466.
79. Arvin B, Neville LF, Barone FC, Feuerstein GZ: The role of inflammation and cytokines in brain injury. Neurosci Biobehav Rev 1996;20:445–452.
80. Dietrich WD, Busto R, Bethea JR: Postischemic hypothermia and IL-10 treatment provide long-lasting neuroprotection of CA1 hippocampus following transient global ischemia in rats. Exp Neurol 1999;158: 444–450.
81. Coimbra C, Drake M, Borismoller F, Wieloch T: Long-lasting neuroprotective effect of postischemic hypothermia and treatment with an anti-inflammatory/antipyretic drug: evidence for chronic encephalopathic processes following ischemia. Stroke 1996;27:1578–1585.
82. Aibiki M, Maekawa S, Ogura S, et al: Effect of moderate hypothermia on systemic and internal jugular plasma IL-6 levels after traumatic brain injury in humans. J Neurotrauma 1999;16:225–232.
83. Marion DW, Penrod LE, Kelsey ST, et al: Treatment of traumatic brain injury with moderate hypothermia. N Engl J Med 1997;336:540–546.
84. Hope PL, Cady EB, Delpy DT, et al: Brain metabolism and intracellular pH during ischaemia and hypoxia: an in vivo ^{31}P and ^1H nuclear magnetic resonance study in the lamb. J Neurochem 1987;49:75–82.
85. Azzopardi D, Wyatt S, Cady EB, et al: Prognosis of newborn infants with hypoxic-ischemic brain injury assessed by phosphorus magnetic resonance spectroscopy. Pediatr Res 1989;25:445–451.
86. Roth SC, Edwards AD, Cady EB, et al: Relation between cerebral oxidative metabolism following birth asphyxia, and neurodevelopmental outcome and brain growth at one year. Devel Med Child Neurol 1992;34: 285–295.
87. Lorek A, Takei Y, Cady EB, et al: Delayed ("secondary") cerebral energy failure after acute hypoxia-ischemia in the newborn piglet: continuous 48-hour studies by phosphorus magnetic resonance spectroscopy. Pediatr Res 1994;36:699–706.
88. Amess PN, Penrice J, Lorek A, et al: Mild hypothermia after severe transient hypoxia-ischemia reduces the delayed rise in cerebral lactate in the piglet. Pediatr Res 1997;41:803–808.
89. Dietrich WD, Busto R, Halley M, Valdes I: The importance of brain temperature in alterations of the blood-brain barrier following cerebral ischemia. J Neuropathol Exp Neurol 1990;49:486–497.
90. Huang ZG, Xue D, Preston E, et al: Biphasic opening of the blood-brain barrier following transient focal ischemia: effects of hypothermia. Can J Neurol Sci 1999;26:298–304.
91. Edwards AD, Yue X, Squier MV, et al: Specific inhibition of apoptosis after cerebral hypoxia-ischemia by moderate post-insult hypothermia. Biochem Biophys Res Comm 1995;217:1193–1199.
92. Ikonomodou CEA: Blockade of NMDA receptors and apoptotic neurodegeneration in the developing brain. Science 1999;283:70–74.
93. Ishimaru MJ, Ikonomodou C, Tenkova TI, et al: Distinguishing excitotoxic

from apoptotic neurodegeneration in the developing rat brain. J Comp Neurol 1999;408:461–476.

94. Thoresen M, Satas S, Puka-Sundvall M, et al: Post-hypoxic hypothermia reduces cerebrocortical release of NO and excitotoxins. Neuroreport 1997;8:3359–3362.

95. Miyazawa T, Bonnekoh P, Widmann R, Hossmann K-A: Heating of the brain to maintain normothermia during ischemia aggravates brain injury in the rat. Acta Neuropathol 1993;85:488–494.

96. Reith J, Jørgensen HS, Pedersen PM, et al: Body temperature in acute stroke: relation to stroke severity, infarct size, mortality and outcome. Lancet 1996;347:422–425.

97. Clifton GL, Miller ER, Sung RN, et al: Lack of effect of induction of hypothermia after acute brain injury. N Engl J Med 2001;344:556–563.

98. Grether JK, Nelson KB: Maternal infection and cerebral palsy in infants of normal birthweight. JAMA 1997;278:207–211.

99. Gunn TR, Gunn AJ, Gluckman PD: Substantial neuronal rescue with prolonged selective head cooling begun 5.5h after cerebral ischemia in the fetal sheep. Pediatr Res 1997;41:152A.

100. Schwab S, Spranger M, Aschoff A, et al: Brain temperature monitoring and modulation in patients with severe MCA infarction. Neurology 1997; 48:762–767.

101. Thoresen M, Satas S, Løberg EM, et al: Twenty-four hours of mild hypothermia in unsedated newborn pigs starting after a severe global hypoxic-ischemic insult is not neuroprotective. Pediatr Res 2001;50: 405–411.

102. Leonov Y, Sterz F, Safar P, et al: Mild cerebral hypothermia during and after cardiac arrest improves neurologic outcome in dogs. J Cereb Blood Flow Metab 1990;10:57–70.

103. Leijh PCJ, van den Barselar MT, Zwet TLV, et al: Kinetics of phagocytosis of Staphylococcus aureus and Escherichia coli by human granulocytes. Immunology 1979;37:453–465.

104. Heier T, Caldwell JE, Sessler DI, Miller RD: Mild intraoperative hypothermia increases duration of action and spontaneous recovery of vecuronium blockade during nitrous oxide-isoflurane anesthesia in humans. Anesthesiology 1991;74:815–819.

105. Satas S, Hoem N, Melby K, et al: Influence of mild hypothermia after hypoxia-ischemia on the pharmacokinetics of gentamicin in newborn pigs. Biol Neonate 2000;77:50–57.

106. Dawkins MJR, Hull D: The production of heat by fat. Sci Am 1965;62–67.

107. Thoresen M, Apricena F, Løberg EM, et al: Post-hypoxic-ischemic hypothermia reduces necrosis and apoptosis correspondingly in the newborn rat, however restraint stress ameliorates neuroprotection. Pediatr Res 1998;44:421. Abstract.

108. Yager J, Towfighi J, Vannucci RC: Influence of mild hypothermia on hypoxic-ischemic brain damage in the immature rat. Pediatr Res 1993; 34:525–529.

109. Miller JA, Miller FS: Factors in neonatal resistance to anoxia. III. Potentiation by narcosis of the effect of hypothermia in the newborn guinea pig. Am J Obstet Gynecol 1962;84:44–56.

110. Becker BA, Nienaber JA, Christenson RK, et al: Peripheral concentrations of cortisol as an indicator of stress in the pig: a reevaluation. Am J Veterin Res 1985;46:1034–1040.

111. Johnson EO, Kamilaris TC, Chrousos GP: Mechanisms of stress: a dynamic overview of hormonal and behavioral homeostasis. Neurosci Biobehav Rev 1992;16:115–130.

112. Anand KJ, McIntosh N, Lagercrantz H, et al: Analgesia and sedation in preterm neonates who require ventilatory support: results from the NOPAIN trial: Neonatal Outcome and Prolonged Analgesia in Neonates. Arch Pediatr Adol Med 1999;153:331–338.

113. Corbett R, Laptook A, Weatherall P: Noninvasive measurements of human brain temperature using volume-localized proton magnetic resonance spectroscopy. J Cereb Blood Flow Metab 1997;17:363–369.

114. Mellergård P, Nordstrøm C-H: Intracerebral temperature in neurosurgical patients. Neurosurgery 1991;28:709–713.

115. Hayashi N, Hirayama T, Udagawa A, et al: Systemic management of cerebral edema based on a new concept in severe head injury patients. Acta Neurochirurgica Suppl 1994;60:541–543.

116. Baker MA: Brain cooling in endotherms in heat and exercise. Ann Rev Physiol 1982;44:85–96.

117. Cabanac M, Caputa M: Natural selective cooling of the human brain: evidence of its occurrence and magnitude. J Physiol 1979;286:255–264.

118. du Boulay GH, Lawton M, Wallis A: The story of the internal carotid artery of mammals: from Galen to sudden infant death syndrome. Neuroradiology 1998;40:697–703.

119. Corbett R, Laptook AR: Failure of localized head cooling to reduce brain temperature in adult humans. Neuroreport 1998;9:2721–2725.

120. Mellergård P: Changes in human intracerebral temperature in response to different methods of brain cooling. Neurosurgery 1992;31:671–677.

121. Gelman B, Schleien CL, Lohe A, Kuluz JW: Selective brain cooling in infant piglets after cardiac arrest and resuscitation. Crit Care Med 1996;24:1009–1017.

122. Thoresen M, Simmonds M, Satas S, et al: Effective selective head cooling during posthypoxic hypothermia in newborn piglets. Pediatr Res 2001; 49:594–599.

123. Froese G, Burton A: Heat losses from the human head. J Appl Physiol 1957;10:235–241.

124. Gunn AJ, Gluckman PD, Gunn TR: Selective head cooling in newborn infants after perinatal asphyxia: a safety study. Pediatrics 1998;102: 885–892.

125. Thoresen M, Whitelaw A: Cardiovascular changes during mild therapeutic hypothermia and rewarming in infants with hypoxic-ischemic encephalopathy. Pediatrics 2000;106:92–99.

126. Hellström Westaas L, Rosén I, Svenningsen NW: Predictive value of early continuous amplitude integrated EEG recordings on outcome after severe birth asphyxia in full term infants. Arch Dis Child 1995;72: F34–F38.

127. Wardle SP, Yoxall CW, Wendling AM: Cerebral oxygenation during cardiopulmonary bypass. Arch Dis Child 1998;78:26–32.

128. Levene MI: Management of the asphyxiated full term infant. Arch Dis Child 1993;68:612–616.
129. Kattwinkel J, Niermeyer S, Nadkarni V, et al: Resuscitation of the newly born infant: an advisory statement from the Pediatric Working Group of the International Liaison Committee on Resuscitation. Resuscitation 1999;40:71–88.

PART IV

Medico-Legal Aspects

CHAPTER 15

Medico-Legal Implications of Hypoxic-Ischemic Brain Injury

Steven M. Donn, Malcolm L. Chiswick, Paula Whittell, Susan Anderson

Introduction

In 2000, there were more than 15,600 reports of medical malpractice payments by physicians in the United States. The mean payment was nearly $250,000 resulting in a total of almost 4 billion dollars in verdicts or settlements (2000 Annual Report, National Practitioner Data Bank). In England and Wales, at the end of March 2001, there were 23,000 claims outstanding. In the fiscal year 1999/2000 alone, there were 10,000 new claims filed. The outlay in damages as a result of medical negligence claims in 1999/2000 was £373,000,000, according to the National Audit Commission, partly as a result of changes in the law covering the quantification of future losses. In the United Kingdom, between 1992 and 1998, new claims per thousand consultant contacts (all specialties) increased by 72%.

Many of these claims involved allegations of medical negligence that led to fetal or neonatal hypoxic-ischemic brain injury. It has been estimated that approximately 30% of the members of the American Academy of Pediatrics, and more than 75% of the members of the American College of Obstetricians and Gynecologists, have been sued for medical malpractice at least once. The average obstetrician-gynecologist in the United States can expect to be sued for medical malpractice two or three times in his or her career. Obstetrical claims have an average damage award of $417,181. The vulnerability of obstetricians and pediatricians results from the high costs associated with lifelong medical disabilities, a long statute of limitations, and the emotional tragedy of unfulfilled potential.

Many of the reasons that prompt parents to take medico-legal action are related to unsatisfactory interactions with health care pro-

From Donn SM, Sinha SK, Chiswick ML (eds): *Birth Asphyxia and the Brain: Basic Science and Clinical Implications.* © 2002, Futura Publishing Co., Inc., Armonk, NY.

fessionals, and/or to unreasonable expectations that inevitably were not met. For some parents, seeking legal action is a way of coping with grief; for others it is driven by anger, a desire for retribution, and sometimes guilt. Moreover, in the United States, plaintiff attorneys frequently advertise their services in such a way that leads parents to mistakenly believe that all cerebral palsy, for example, results from obstetrical or pediatric negligence and that litigation is the means to financial security for the child.

In England and Wales, the socialized health care system formerly provided fully for the disabled, but this funding system has been eroded by successive governments – partly as a result of the rising costs of providing the National Health Service in the face of medical advances during the past 30 years. Parents who previously never would have considered claiming damages on behalf of their children are now motivated by financial need. As in the United States, parents often have unreasonable expectations, but this may be partially the fault of midwives and medical professionals themselves. Some professionals may inadvertently lead pregnant women to believe that different styles of childbirth are largely a matter of choice; as a result, parents have high expectations of a controlled labor, culminating in a smooth delivery in which the mother is in control and participates in all decisions. The shock of losing control of the delivery and the possibility of the baby being injured at birth is something for which they are not prepared.

Medical malpractice litigation is governed by civil law. In order to claim damages, a plaintiff (in the U.K., claimant) must: (1) establish that there was a duty on the part of the defendant health care provider or institution to the plaintiff; (2) show that the defendant breached the applicable standards of care in the performance of that duty; (3) prove that the negligent care was the proximate cause of the injury or disability – in other words, "but for" the negligent care, the injury or disability would not have occurred; and (4) prove the existence of an injury. Damages are not awarded for negligence unless the injury is also proved. Each of the four elements must be proved for the defendant to be found negligent. The plaintiff need only prove his or her case "on the balance of probability," or "more likely than not" (i.e., with more than 50% probability). This is a lesser degree of proof than is required in medical research, which is conventionally a probability of 95% or more ($p < 0.05$).

If a malpractice verdict is rendered, monetary damages must be paid to the plaintiff. The valuation of a birth-injured child is complex and time consuming, but the underlying principle is that damage awards should restore the plaintiff to the position they would have been in, had the negligence not happened. Obviously, this is arbitrary, since health cannot be quantified in monetary terms.

The settlement represents the cost caused by the negligence, and includes calculable damages, such as the loss of future earnings, and noncalculable damages, such as pain, suffering, and loss of amenity. Thus, the amount of damages is strongly influenced by the plaintiff's life expectancy, which is decided by the Court and is based on the opinions of experts. In England and Wales, as in the United States, a structured settlement is attractive to many parents. The settlement sum provides for the child throughout his/her life, however long or short the expected life span, and is funded by a series of annuities.

Genesis of a Medical Malpractice Lawsuit in the United States

Most, but not all, medical malpractice cases that proceed to trial in the United States are decided by the jury system. Occasionally, in some jurisdictions, there may be a bench trial, where the verdict is decided solely by a judge. Most civil law involving medical malpractice is determined at the state or county level; cases involving two or more states or a federal government entity may be tried in a federal court and are then subject to federal law.

Although the process varies slightly among the states, the general principles are similar. Most lawsuits begin with the plaintiff filing a Notice of Intent, whereby the plaintiff notifies the defendant(s) that a malpractice suit will be filed, and the act(s) of negligence are broadly specified. Within a short period of time, a complaint is filed with the Court, listing the specific allegations of medical malpractice and the way(s) in which they resulted in injury. In some jurisdictions, a specific demand for damages may be included.

The next phase involves discovery, or fact-finding. Health care providers who were involved in the care of the patient will be interviewed under oath by the attorneys, to ascertain their roles in the care of the patient and elements of fact. The plaintiffs (parents) may also be questioned by the defendants' attorney(s) to explore other possible explanations for the poor outcome, such as genetic diseases, possible exposure to teratogens, and/or other health problems, and also to determine the child's present condition and ongoing treatments.

After discovery of fact has been completed, expert witnesses are retained by each side to review the medical records and discovery transcripts, and to render their opinions in the case (see "Role of the Expert Witness"). In some states, expert witnesses are deposed (questioned under oath) by the opposing side to uncover the opinions they will express at trial. In other states, experts prepare written reports that are exchanged prior to trial. In some jurisdictions, there is no pretrial discovery of expert opinions and the experts are not even identified until they appear at trial.

After the period of discovery closes, there may be attempts to get the opposing parties to settle the case before trial. Settlement conferences may be mandated, during which the parties try to arrive at a compromise position. Some states use a panel system, in which physicians, attorneys, or others hear the case and make a nonbinding recommendation. Other states use nonbinding mediation, which is similar, or binding arbitration, in which the decision is final. The aim of all of these processes is to avoid a costly and time-consuming trial.

If the two parties fail to reach an agreement, the case proceeds to trial. The plaintiff presents the case first, followed by the defendant(s). Each side presents its expert witnesses, who try to persuade the jury or judge that negligence did or did not occur, and that it was or was not related to the injury. Damage experts will also attempt to quantify the "value" of the case. Eventually, a jury (or judge) will render a verdict of either medical malpractice (plaintiff verdict), or no cause (defendant verdict). If there is a malpractice verdict, monetary damages will be awarded to the plaintiff.

If there is a plaintiff verdict, the defendant may appeal if sufficient legal grounds exist. This may result in a decision from a higher court that upholds or overturns the original verdict, reduces the damages, or orders another trial.

Genesis of Medical Malpractice Lawsuit in England and Wales

Important changes in the way the civil justice system is administered in England and Wales have recently been introduced in the Civil Procedure Rules 1998, which were devised to: improve access to justice and reduce the cost of litigation, reduce the complexity of the rules and modernize terminology, and eliminate outdated practice and procedures.

A claim is initiated when a pre-action letter is sent from the claimant's solicitors to the defendants or their solicitors informing them that a claim is intended. The current ruling under the Pre-action Protocol for the Resolution of Clinical Disputes requires that the claimant's solicitors also send additional information in a Letter of Claim, providing full details of the claim to be made, and enclosing supportive medical evidence, if available. The defendants then have 3 months to investigate the claim in depth before the proceedings are commenced. The claim can be settled at this stage if, on the advice of the defendants' professional experts, it is clearly indefensible.

The Letter of Response that must be sent to the claimant within 3 months outlines the defendants' position, after which the claimant can reconsider the facts before proceeding. This exchange of letters is a valuable process to clarify the position of each party. Many claims are taken no further than this stage and an increasing number are settled. This stage is the equivalent to the Notice of Intent in the United States' system.

The next step is issuance of a writ; in general terms, it must be issued within 3 years of the medical treatment that gave rise to the claim. However, in medical negligence cases in which a child has sustained a disability, the limitation period of 3 years does not start until the child has reached adulthood and is capable of administering his property and affairs. As a result, in some cases, the time limit for issuing a writ is effectively indefinite.

The writ is served with a Statement of Case, and a Defense has to be served on the claimant within the next 28 days. Depending on the financial value of the claim, the Court allocates the case to one of three tracks or timetables, and imposes a time limit for the exchange of relevant documents, witness evidence, experts' reports, and the start of the trial. The Court also ensures that each party adheres to the timetable, which may place pressure on medical expert witnesses who often have heavy clinical responsibilities.

After the exchange of the experts' reports, the Court will usually order the experts for the claimant and defendants to meet and prepare a joint report delineating all the issues that cannot be agreed upon. Often, both sets of experts will find common ground and the case can be settled or withdrawn at this stage. Damages can be revalued on the basis of the terms of the agreement and, even if the case proceeds to trial, it will take less time for the evidence to be heard.

Many medical negligence cases are funded from the public domain by Legal Aid although Conditional Fee agreements are becoming more widespread. The procedural efforts toward greater efficiency should result in reduced costs, but this is also likely to put additional pressure on medical experts. It remains to be seen whether medical experts will find it increasingly difficult to respond to the demands of the Court in the face of intense clinical responsibilities. High level expertise is likely to be derived from active involvement in clinical practice; it would be to the disadvantage of claimants and defendants if, instead, there is increased utilization of the "professional expert" who has limited knowledge of everyday clinical practice.

The use of a single expert appointed by the Court is likely to increase. In a recent case, The Lord Chief Justice opined that non-medical evidence should be given by a single expert unless there were "special circumstances," especially in matters relating to the assessment of damages, where it may be possible to agree to life expectancy and associated costs of nursing care. In low value cases, the Court will order a single expert to examine the claimant and report for both parties. In higher value cases, however, the Court of Appeal has preserved the chance for the parties to instruct their own experts, but those experts have to be identified to the Court and to the other side, and their reports (and all correspondence) must be disclosed to the Court. Parties are no longer able to "buy" a supportive report.

The time for the trial is usually fixed at the second case management conference held with the Court and the parties. Once this date is agreed upon, the witnesses and experts will be expected to appear despite other commitments, and will be held accountable if they do not. Trials should take less time in the new system; joint experts and joint reports lessen the need for lengthy cross-examination. Moreover, the witnesses' statements and some of the experts' reports may be admitted as written evidence, so the evidence they give in court may be confined to a focused cross-examination only. Under the old civil procedure, a trial involving birth injury lasted between 10 and 15 days in court. Now this can be reduced to 1 week.

The judgment can be given at the end of the case, but in complex cases it is usual for the judge to take the time to consider the evidence in depth, and to give his or her judgment at a later date. At that time, he or she also deals with the question of legal costs and the possibility of the successful claimant seeking a structured settlement.

In 1999/2000, the average time to settle a non-cerebral palsy claim was 5.5 years. However, claims involving cerebral palsy claim take much longer. There is a governmental plan to reduce the excessive time period and reform the system of dealing with clinical negligence in the National Health Service.

Role of the Expert Witness

In the United States, expert witnesses must be qualified to give expert testimony by reason of knowledge, skill, training, or education. Qualification may be conferred by the Court if a judge feels that a witness has knowledge that will aid in the understanding of the evidence. In England and Wales, experts must include, in their written reports, details related to their experience and qualifications. Prior to giving evidence in court, this information is presented to the judge. Although there is no formal qualification procedure, the testimony of an expert witness will inherently not have credibility unless he or she is appropriately qualified. Occasionally, barristers will explore the expert's qualifications during cross-examination.

Expert witnesses in the United States may be compensated for their time at reasonable rates. They may not be compensated on a contingency basis, in which fees are paid according to the outcome of the case. In England and Wales, medical experts are not prevented from receiving fees on a contingency basis, but if they choose to do so it inevitably raises doubts about the credibility of their evidence.

Expert witnesses must be unbiased and objective, without any personal interest in the outcome, and must not be an advocate for the party who retains them. The Civil Procedure Rules 1998 in England and Wales demand that expert witnesses conclude their reports with a statement that (a) the expert understands his duty to the Court, and (b) that he or she has complied with that duty. The expert's report must also state the substance of all material oral or written instructions on which the report was based. Experts must be familiar with rulings on the scope of expert testimony and on court procedure, and they should display a highly professional demeanor in the courtroom (Table 1). Their primary role is to help the Court understand the facts of a case, and to offer an opinion on the standard of care and whether the plaintiff's injury was caused by substandard care. Experts may also offer opinions on the condition of the plaintiff, and the prognosis, life expectancy, and nature of the services required.

The arguments that appeal to judges and jurors are simplified, logical, and can be readily understood. It is not helpful for an expert simply to relay complex scientific principles while making little attempt to offer an overall conclusion about what it indicates for the plaintiff "on the balance of probability." Indeed, an expert who focuses on impenetrable research reports, especially on experimental animal models, may be viewed as the "eccentric professor" whose evidence cannot be relied upon (because it cannot be understood by the Court).

Table 1

Guidelines for the Conduct of Expert Witnesses

- Prepare for the case thoroughly.
- Be objective.
- Distinguish between expert and fact testimony.
- Stay within your field of expertise.
- Make sure you understand attorneys'questions before responding.
- Do not confuse "probability" with "possibility."
- Do not baffle the Court with obscure answers to questions.
- If you do not know, do not use conjecture—simply state, "I don't know."
- Do not offer unsolicited information unless you are certain it will help the Court.
- Be assertive and direct. Do not become emotional or demonstrate impatience, frustration, or anger.

The Rules of Evidence

Rules of evidence govern the admission of facts and opinions used in a malpractice case. Courts will usually disallow hearsay, a statement made outside of court by someone other than the testifying witness. However, there are some exceptions, including statements made for the purposes of medical diagnosis or treatment, factual statements in the medical record, and vital statistics. Nonexpert (fact) witnesses can testify only to firsthand knowledge, or to an opinion that is rationally based on firsthand knowledge and which is helpful to a clear understanding of the testimony.

The scope of testimony offered by a qualified expert witness must also conform to the rules of evidence. An important issue is the approach used by the Courts in determining whether the care received by the plaintiff was below a required standard, resulting in negligence. Whether there is a duty of care rests with the law, whereas the appropriate standard of care is a matter of medical judgment. The "standard of care" is that practiced (at the time) by a responsible body of clinicians, even though other physicians may adopt a different practice. Courts are understandably wary about dogmatic and persuasive experts who seek to impose a minority view, which may not truly reflect the opinions of a responsible body of medical opinion. Therefore, opinions must also stand up to logical scrutiny.

The United States Supreme Court ruled in 1993 that there should be standards of acceptance of evidence. The intent of this ruling was to eliminate the use of "junk science" in the courtroom. It stipulates that medical or scientific evidence must have a firm scientific foundation, which extends beyond its publication in peer-reviewed literature. Judges have the discretion to determine, based on their perceptions of the scientific validity, whether an expert's testimony is acceptable. This may seem paradoxical, given the usual lack of scientific and medical training of most judges, and it has unfortunately led to the continued proffering of junk science to juries. Juries are also not scientifically or medically trained to be able to discern "good" from "bad" science. One example of this is the recurrent testimony offered by a pediatric neurologist who has created his own theory of birth injury. He has testified on multiple occasions regarding causation issues in cases of neurologically impaired children. He determines that, although there was insufficient hypoxia to produce any clinical or laboratory findings, and although there was insufficient trauma to produce any clinical signs, the combination of the two acted synergistically to produce the children's deficits. Another expert witness, a pediatric neuroradiologist, has opined on multiple occasions that he can tell the exact time of brain injury solely by interpreting neuroimaging. He analyzed magnetic resonance brain imaging scans performed at several months of age and convincingly told the juries that, from these scans alone, he was able to determine that hypoxic-ischemic injury occurred 30 minutes before the children had been delivered. Unfortunately, this type of evidence is rarely, if ever, subjected to peer review or scientific scrutiny, and in many instances leads to an incorrect jury verdict.

Causation: Beyond the Science

Expert witnesses may be asked to give their opinion as to whether a child's disability was caused by cerebral hypoxia-ischemia, when the insult that caused the injury occurred, and whether alternative management would have avoided the damage. Opinions offered by expert witnesses should be based on epidemiologic and experimental scientific data. However, many of the arguments that arise in litigation cannot be substantiated by reference to scientific publications, because the information does not exist. Instead, the expert witness must resort to presenting a logical, common sense argument based on the scientific information that does exist, currently held views that might be ascertained by reference to textbooks or journals, and personal experience. When these sources of information are insufficient to provide a reasoned opinion, the expert must acknowledge this by saying, "I don't know."

In the following section, the authors present some of the more common difficulties that arise when arguing whether or not a child's disabilities were caused by intrapartum asphyxia and, if so, the timing of the insult. Controversial views that are sometimes put forward by expert witnesses are included. Elucidating these issues may stimulate debate among perinatal neuroscientists and facilitate the direction of further research.

Criteria for the Causal Link Between Intrapartum Asphyxia and Neurologic Disability

Given that asphyxia prior to or around the time of birth is responsible for only a minority of cases of neurodevelopmental disability in childhood, it is essential for the Court to understand when asphyxia might be a consideration as the cause of an individual child's disability. Table 2 provides a broad set of criteria that support an association between intrapartum asphyxia and neurologic disability. The basis for some of these criteria was reviewed in Chapter 2.

These criteria are largely based on epidemiologic and other research data that are population-based, but the Court is interested in the individual claimant who may be in the minority (approximately

Table 2

Criteria Supporting a Causal Association Between Intrapartum Asphyxia and Neurologic Disability*

- Evidence of severe intrapartum hypoxia
    Occurrence of a major injurious event (e.g., prolapsed cord, abruption, uterine rupture, etc.)
    Clinical signs of fetal distress
    Abnormal fetal heart rate tracing
    Fetal scalp pH ≤ 7.0
- Severe depression of vital signs at birth, requiring resuscitation
- Cord blood pH ≤ 7.0
- Neonatal encephalopathy with no cause more likely than cerebral hypoxia-ischemia
- Features of ischemic injury to other organs, e.g., renal impairment
- Dominant disability is spastic cerebral palsy, usually affecting all four limbs

*This table illustrates the broad principles behind causation arguments following birth asphyxia. Controversy remains about the interpretation of many of these individual criteria, and how many need to be present to "prove" causation (see reference 5).

15%) of children with cerebral palsy caused by intrapartum asphyxia. Attempts to impose something more rigorous than broad criteria, and to argue instead that each of a set of requirements must be met in their entirety, are not helpful because they do not allow for individual variation.

The medico-legal analysis of alleged intrapartum asphyxial brain injury is not an exact science, and the Court is interested in probabilities rather than certainties. Some of these criteria are stronger than others. A more detailed discussion is provided in the following sections.

Evidence of Intrapartum Hypoxemia and Injury

If it is argued that cerebral damage occurred as a result of intrapartum hypoxemia, there is an assumption that there should be some marker indicating that fetal hypoxemia might have occurred. Indeed, cases often center around the allegation that the obstetrician failed to heed the evidence of hypoxemia.

During labor, the mother is a "captive patient," and normally the progress of her labor is monitored. A lawyer may erroneously equate proxies for fetal hypoxemia, such as a nonreassuring fetal heart rate tracing and an abnormally low fetal scalp pH level, with evidence of injurious fetal hypoxemia. Courts need to understand that these proxies, along with cardinal clinical events, such as prolapse of the umbilical cord, uterine rupture, and placental abruption should not be equated with hypoxic brain damage, for which additional criteria are needed.

Often, a lawyer may aggressively question an expert witness as to when, during labor, the injury occurred. This is relevant to whether there was a window of opportunity in which an injury could have been avoided by expediting the delivery. Even if it can be shown that a child's disability was caused by intrapartum hypoxia, the issue is not one of knowing when the injury occurred but when the causative or triggering hypoxic insult occurred. There is a variable time lag between the onset of fetal hypoxemia, and the onset of hypoxemia of sufficient severity to trigger the damage (i.e., cerebral hypoxia-ischemia).

Lawyers are generally not interested in the additional facts that cerebral injury itself evolves over a period of time extending into the neonatal period, and that there is a further variable time lag between the onset of the triggering hypoxic insult and the start of irreversible brain damage. In a litigation context, once the insult has been sufficient to trigger damage, "the writing is on the wall." Perhaps if neural rescue therapy ever becomes established, litigation will be directed towards a failure to respond to a window of opportunity to commence neonatal neuroprotective therapy.

A useful starting point when considering the timing of the causative hypoxic insult is to determine whether the hypoxemia was the prolonged, partial, and intermittent type that may become worse with recurrent uterine contractions, or an acute near-total hypoxic insult, as might occur in cord prolapse or uterine rupture. In the former case, an otherwise healthy and well-grown fetus may withstand many hours of hypoxemia before the onset of circulatory insufficiency and cerebral hypoxia-ischemia (see Chapter 11). The point at which this state is reached cannot be determined, but expert witnesses need to present a logical opinion that does not conflict with the main body of research findings. For example, it may be possible to recognize a time period during which the fetal heart rate pattern became worse or fetal pH deteriorated. Other factors to be considered which influence the ability of the fetus to withstand hypoxemia include the nutrition of the fetus at the start of labor, other indices of antepartum health, and the pace of labor, especially if accelerated with oxytocin.

In presumed acute, near-total hypoxemia, as may be suggested by a cardinal clinical event such as cord prolapse or uterine rupture, or a sudden adverse change in the fetal heart rate, the trigger for permanent brain damage may occur within 10 to 30 minutes. In this situation, there may not be a window of opportunity to expedite the delivery and prevent injury. In these examples, there should be additional evidence of acute near-total hypoxemia. This evidence might include severe depression of vital signs at birth and the need for extensive resuscitation, the onset of at least a moderately severe hypoxic-ischemic encephalopathy, brain scan findings of damage to the basal ganglia with relative sparing of the cerebral cortex, and athetoid cerebral palsy.

Antepartum Versus Intrapartum Hypoxemia

Among the population of children with cerebral palsy, or among newborns who have suffered an encephalopathy, the presence of antepartum risk factors is far more common than intrapartum factors; when the latter exist, they often occur in association with antepartum factors. Defense lawyers are usually well aware of this, but if cases are to be successfully defended on the grounds that the injury was incurred before the onset of labor, expert witnesses will need to provide more evidence than simple citation of the epidemiologic research that points to antepartum risk factors.

The argument for causal antepartum hypoxemia is strengthened if the expert witness can point to several indices consistent with antepartum hypoxemia, such as a cardinal clinical event (e.g., severe maternal illness associated with shock or hypoxia), severe fetal growth restriction, reduced fetal movements, recurrent antepartum bleeding, or abnormal tests results of fetal well-being (e.g., Doppler flow studies, amniotic fluid volume, fetal heart rate, fetal breathing).

The problem in making a case for antepartum hypoxemia is that, prior to labor, the mother is not usually a "captive patient" exposed to continuous monitoring; as such, the evidence for antepartum hypoxemia is often weak. However, for those mothers admitted to the maternity unit before the start of active labor, a nonreassuring fetal heart rate at admission provides helpful information, especially if it is combined with other pre-admission features that are consistent with antepartum hypoxemia.

It would appear from epidemiologic studies that depression of vital signs at birth and neonatal encephalopathy may be associated with antepartum hypoxemia. This raises issues that have yet to be resolved by scientific research. It is easy to understand that if hypoxic brain injury has already been established well before birth, then the infant may be born lacking in vigor and have low Apgar scores as a result of the antepartum brain injury. It is more difficult to explain a time lag that might be as much as several days between presumed antepartum hypoxia severe enough to injure the brain, and the onset of neonatal encephalopathy. It may be that the neonatal encephalopathy is simply an extension of a clinically silent fetal encephalopathy, with the neurotoxic biochemical cascade commencing some time before birth. Alternatively, it is possible that severe antepartum hypoxia lowers the threshold for neonatal encephalopathy, which is then triggered during a period of otherwise benign intrapartum hypoxia in those cases in which labor occurs.

These concepts are especially relevant to medical litigation alleging that, although antepartum injury might have occurred, there was also a significant contribution to the child's disabilities from intrapartum hypoxemic injury. In general, expert witnesses should not be tempted to apportion disability in this way because there is no scientific basis for this opinion.

Condition at Birth

A difficult situation arises where there is very strong evidence to suggest that a child's cerebral palsy was caused by intrapartum hypoxemia, yet at birth the infant was only mildly or moderately depressed and responded rapidly to simple resuscitation measures. In these circumstances, the notion that a brain-injuring insult occurred in the last 30 minutes or so before birth is probably unsustainable.

The question remains as to whether it is possible for the infant to suffer intrapartum hypoxemia earlier in labor, severe enough to permanently injure the brain and to generate a neonatal encephalopathy, and yet display only mildly depressed vital signs at birth. This seems improbable because, as labor progresses and contractions become more frequent and stronger, the cardiocirculatory state might be expected to deteriorate progressively following a severe hypoxemic insult that occurred earlier in labor.

The concept of "intrapartum recovery" of the fetal circulation is sometimes controversial. For example, against a background of "placental insufficiency," the overzealous use of oxytocin may lead to uterine hyperstimulation and act as the "final straw that broke the camel's back" in triggering brain injury. The idea here is that cessation of the infusion may lead to recovery of fetal vital signs with the infant born depressed, though not markedly.

Another concept is that an acute and reversible near-total hypoxemic insult occurring early in labor may be sufficient to trigger brain injury, yet relief of the insult may allow the fetus to survive and recover vital signs. Situations that come to mind are maternal circulatory collapse followed by prompt resuscitation, and a self-limiting episode of near complete cord occlusion.

Finally, it is sometimes argued that when an intermittent hypoxemic insult occurs gradually over a prolonged period of time during labor, gross circulatory impairment may not occur because there are intermittent periods of recovery between contractions. The concept here is that the duration of the hypoxemia is sufficient to trigger intracerebral biochemical changes associated with neonatal encephalopathy, but insufficient to cause gross cardiorespiratory failure at birth.

Cord Blood pH Level

Taken in conjunction with the other factors shown in Table 2, an umbilical cord blood pH level of 7.0 or below is supportive evidence of preceding hypoxemia of a degree that is potentially brain-injuring if it is metabolic in origin. When a cord blood pH measurement has been omitted, the pH level in neonatal arterial blood measured soon after birth may be helpful. Lawyers may ask expert witnesses to "work backwards" and indicate what the cord pH level would have been, based on blood samples taken an hour or more after delivery. Indeed, they may ask what the fetal scalp pH level would have been some hours before birth. Expert witnesses, however, should refuse to speculate on these issues because there are so many confounding variables.

Allegations of Failure of Care at Resuscitation

When an infant has depressed vital signs at birth and requires extensive resuscitation, it is often assumed by those without medical expertise that the causative hypoxemic insult has occurred after birth because of the failure of the infant to breathe. Experts must clarify to lawyers that birth actually represents the relief of the hypoxemic insult (escape from the hostile womb); birth provides the opportunity to oxygenate the infant and improve the circulation. If prolonged resuscitation is required, it is sometimes alleged that this is evidence that the pediatrician or medical professional who treated the newborn infant must have done something wrong.

One difficulty is that the details of the resuscitation may not be recorded in sufficient detail to defend allegations of substandard care (see "Risk Management"). It should be routine practice to document that the breath sounds were heard symmetrically in response to positive pressure ventilation, if that was the case. Also, if intubation is difficult, the fact that positive pressure ventilation was given by a face mask between intubation attempts should be recorded.

Neonatal Encephalopathy

An encephalopathy of at least moderate severity is one of the more powerful criteria for arguments that cerebral palsy was caused by intrapartum hypoxemia. A case may center on whether the newborn suffered an encephalopathy and, if so, the severity. Seizures distinguish a moderate or severe encephalopathy (Sarnat stage II or III; see Chapter 12) from a mild one (stage I). There may be considerable difficulty, however, classifying abnormal movements, and differences of opinion may arise during observation at the bedside. Also, the early use of anticonvulsants (given prophylactically) may suppress the occurrence of minor seizures.

Severe encephalopathy implies that the infant is stuporous or comatose. Documentation in the medical records of an infant's level of consciousness may be surprisingly lacking even in the situation of coma (see "Risk Management"). Perhaps the attitude of staff is that it is "understood," that a very ill infant will not move or respond to painful stimuli. Yet, many years after the event, this information may be crucial in a fair assessment of the cause of the child's cerebral palsy.

When there are preceding factors that suggest intrapartum hypoxemia, it is often assumed that a neonatal encephalopathy is hypoxic-ischemic in origin. As a result, expert witnesses may argue about the cause of an encephalopathy many years after the event with no investigations available to guide them. Neonatal units should develop protocols for the investigation of neonatal encephalopathy. There are two questions to be considered: (1) Are there circumstances where the intrapartum history and condition at birth are so compelling that it is reasonable to assume that an encephalopathy commencing within 12 hours of birth is of hypoxic-ischemic origin – and therefore further investigation of the cause is not justified? (2) What are the minimum requirements of an investigative protocol?

Injury to Other Organs

The requirement that organ system impairment outside the brain exists in order to attribute cerebral palsy to intrapartum hypoxemia is not always absolute; the syndrome of acute near-total intrapartum hypoxemia has been reported with no or only minimal signs of injury to other organs. Severe intrapartum hypoxemia in infants with overt cardiac failure usually results in death, rather than survival with cerebral palsy. It is doubtful whether causation is clarified by electrocardiogram (ECG) analysis, and there is always the temptation for some experts to overinterpret the ECG with arguments of the existence of "subtle ischemic myocardial changes."

Impairment of renal function is the most common type of organ dysfunction following severe intrapartum hypoxemia, with the clinical focus normally on the rate of urine production and trends in the plasma creatinine level. Again, in individual cases there is sufficient room for arguments about whether or not there was evidence of renal impairment, especially when urine output has not been properly measured, and only infrequent plasma creatinine levels are available.

Further confusion may exist if fluid restriction was chosen as a therapeutic intervention.

Unresolved Issues of Causation

Many scenarios are argued in court for which there is a paucity of scientific data that can be utilized by expert witnesses. Two common scenarios involve the interface between intrapartum hypoxic-ischemic brain injury, and that attributed to birth trauma or perinatal infection.

Contribution of Birth Trauma to Hypoxic-Ischemic Brain Injury

Severe examples of intracranial birth trauma are uncommon, and the extent to which more subtle forms are implicated in brain injury is unknown. Neonatal encephalopathy may occur when there are risk factors for birth trauma, such as cephalopelvic disproportion, failure to progress in the second stage of labor, failed instrument delivery, or the need to disimpact the fetal head from the pelvis during a cesarean section performed in the second stage.

Clinically, the encephalopathy may be indistinguishable from hypoxic-ischemic encephalopathy, and subsequent magnetic resonance or computed tomographic brain imaging may not indicate subdural hemorrhage. On pathophysiologic grounds, excessive forces acting on the fetal head may be associated with raised intracranial venous pressure and reduced perfusion pressure, resulting in ischemic brain injury, but generally, these forces must be severe. If the risk factors previously described are prominent, if there is no evidence suggestive of hypoxemia in a carefully monitored labor, and if no other cause for the encephalopathy was found, then the notion of reduced perfusion pressure caused by excessive forces is difficult to dismiss. The relevance of this to litigation relates to allegations that "traumatic injury" could have been avoided if a cesarean section delivery had been performed earlier.

It is difficult to accrue clinical and imaging data on this type of injury because intrapartum hypoxemia often acts as a confounding variable. Indeed, if there are risk factors for birth trauma, and it is alleged that brain injury was negligently caused by failure to heed signs of intrapartum hypoxemia, expert witnesses may argue that while there was evidence of intrapartum hypoxemia, it was insufficient to have expedited the delivery, and the cerebral palsy was caused by non-negligent "traumatic injury."

Contribution of Perinatal Bacterial Infection to Hypoxic-Ischemic Brain Injury

The role of fetomaternal infection and inflammatory mediators in generating white matter injury in preterm infants was reviewed in Chapter 4. Understandably, the "cytokine theory" of white matter injury has opened up an area of litigation in relation to the appropriate use and timing of maternal antibiotic therapy. Also, in allegations of negligent neonatal care of the preterm infant, it has provided expert witnesses with an alternative possible cause of injury.

Risk factors for fetomaternal infection have also been identified in term infants with neonatal encephalopathy, and in children with cerebral palsy who were born at term. Problems in proving causation arise when, during labor at term, the mother has a fever or there are other signs of fetomaternal infection. It may be impossible to distinguish electronic fetal monitoring features of hypoxemia *per se* from those secondary to infection, and they may coexist. Similarly, depressed vital signs at birth and neonatal encephalopathy may be the results of intrapartum hypoxemia *per se*, fetomaternal infection (even in the absence of a positive blood culture in the baby), or both. Even if it can be shown that delivery should have been expedited because of abnormalities on the electronic fetal monitor or because of a low fetal scalp pH, some experts will argue that this would not have prevented "cytokine-initiated injury" secondary to infection. The problem is that we do not yet understand the *pace of events* following fetomaternal infection.

Risk Management

A direct effect of the medical malpractice litigation crisis and involvement of insurance companies has been the development of risk management programs within health care organizations. Such programs attempt to minimize the exposure to liability by trying to control the risks of health care that can result in unfavorable outcomes. This should not be thought of merely as "defensive medicine," aimed solely at reducing the risk of litigation because it also enhances clinical practice and therefore benefits patients. Typical risk management programs utilize a process to investigate a potential problem, evaluate the exposure to risk, and plan, organize, and implement an interventional strategy. Risk management also involves quality assurance and quality improvement initiatives to evaluate patient outcomes. Many health care institutions have a risk management department, headed by a full-time risk manager.

Risk management programs are both reactive (retrospective) and proactive (prospective). Reactive measures are taken when an event that may increase exposure to liability has been identified. There are numerous examples of adverse incidents that may arise related to the occurrence of birth asphyxia. An adverse event, such as the lack of immediate availability, or the failure to function, of a component of neonatal resuscitation equipment in the delivery room, is reported to the risk management office. The risk management team then investigates the cause(s) of the problem, and discusses with relevant staff members how such an incident might be avoided in the future. When it is warranted, the results of such an investigation can be incorporated into revised policies and procedures. Some might argue that risk management programs are yet another example of a growing and unnecessary bureaucracy in medical practice. However, by developing and implementing a formal procedure that can be applied to a wide range of adverse incidents, staff are more likely to learn from errors and avoid their recurrence. Furthermore, by assigning responsibility for conducting a formal investigation to a designated department, it is more likely that all the information will be considered and that parents can be appropriately counseled based on the facts. An open and honest approach to parents led by an experienced risk manager will often resolve potential litigation issues before legal representation is sought.

Early reporting of high-risk events enables the risk manager to gather information and recollections about the event when it is fresh in the minds of the relevant health care providers. Actively involved risk managers may attend departmental meetings, grand rounds, follow the quality indicators for departments, and present pertinent risk management topics to clinical staff.

High-Risk Scenarios in Birth Asphyxia

An important key to the successful application of a risk management program for birth asphyxia is the recognition that there are commonly occurring clinical scenarios that form the basis of many, perhaps most, of the claims related to brain injury from birth asphyxia (Table 3). Understanding these clinical concepts should increase our awareness of risks when these scenarios occur. Also, given

Table 3

Some High-Risk Clinical Scenarios Related to Birth Asphyxia

Obstetric Factors
- Failure to take into account past obstetric history
- Failure to predict cephalo-pelvic disproportion
- Failure to act on admission findings that suggested a compromised fetus
- Injudicious use of oxytocin
- Failure to recognize lack of progress during labor
- Failure to correctly diagnose malpresentation or malposition of the head
- Delay or failure to diagnose fetal distress while under observation
- Delay in performing a cesarean section or operative delivery
- Substandard operative delivery technique

Resuscitation at Birth
- Failure to arrange for pediatrician to be present at the birth
- Late arrival of the pediatrician
- Faulty equipment
- Substandard resuscitation technique

Post-Resuscitation Care
- Failure to transfer the baby immediately to neonatal unit
- Failure to be vigilant for seizures
- Failure to recognize hypoglycemia
- Failure to be vigilant for infection

that the management of labor and delivery is frequently scrutinized when the baby is born with depressed vital signs and develops an encephalopathy, there should be an increased awareness of the risk associated with obstetrical nurse (or midwife) shift changeovers – especially during a prolonged or complicated labor, when continuity is so important.

Documentation in the Medical Records

The notion that medical record keeping must be accurate, and the entries timed, legible, and signed has been asserted so many times that the appeal sometimes becomes tedious. Yet, when cases come to court, inadequacies are often apparent for all to see. Reliance is placed on the records because they are assumed to be an accurate representation of events around the time that they occurred. Many years after an incident, it is understandable that a judge or jury is more likely to believe what was written in the records, rather than the recollection of a witness who was present at the time. Furthermore, plaintiff lawyers sometimes use poor record keeping to hint or imply that there was a deliberate attempt to falsify the facts.

Table 3 lists common clinical risk situations related to birth asphyxia, which should forewarn the staff of scenarios in which careful documentation is especially important. It is sometimes unclear whether a timed entry in the records represents the time of the event or the time that the staff member made the entry. This confusion would not arise if staff clearly indicated entries made after the occurrence of the event.

In view of the frequency of allegations of failure to expedite delivery in a situation of fetal distress, it is not surprising that arguments in court focus as much on the timing of onset of electronic fetal heart rate changes, and other allegedly adverse signs, as on whether or not the fetus was truly hypoxic. A problem may arise, for example, when the electronic and handwritten timings on the fetal heart rate rate tracing are different. Moreover, both timings sometimes differ from the timing that was noted in the records.

In terms of risk management, resuscitation at birth is an obvious focus of attention. New staff members may arrive on the scene during a shift changeover and encounter a baby who requires urgent medical attention in the tense, emotional circumstances of childbirth. The accurate recording of events is particularly important because: (1) the condition at birth and response to resuscitation shed light on whether or not a child's disability was caused by intrapartum hypoxia; and (2) it is sometimes alleged that medical negligence during resuscitation caused or contributed to a child's disability. Table 4 lists important risk management concerns related to the documentation of resuscitation.

The occurrence of hypoxic-ischemic encephalopathy is an important factor in deciding whether or not a child's disability was caused by birth asphyxia (see Chapter 12). However, not all neonatal encephalopathies are caused by cerebral hypoxia-ischemia and the need for neonatal units to develop protocols for the investigation of encephalopathy was mentioned earlier in this chapter, together with the importance of accurate documentation of the severity of the encephalopathy.

Risk Management and Communication with Parents

Another aspect of risk management involves the awareness of the potential for litigious behavior by some parents. One of the indicators in the neonatal intensive care unit is repeated expression of dissatisfaction

Table 4

Documentation of Resuscitation at Birth*

- Time of attendance at resuscitation
- Any resuscitation care given by other staff prior to arrival
- Description of vital signs *in addition to* Apgar scores
- Time of onset of any positive pressure ventilation even if only by bag and mask
- Time of intubation, with comment on ease (or difficulty) of intubation
- Movement of chest wall, and auscultation findings in response to positive pressure ventilation
- Timed sequence of changes in heart rate, spontaneous breathing, and color change in response to resuscitation
- If reintubation is needed, state reason

*This list is based on the authors' experience of common issues that arise in clinical negligence cases in relation to birth asphyxia. It is not an exhaustive list and drug administration must also be documented.

with medical care. Disgruntled parents may occasionally become verbally abusive to staff, exhibit unacceptable behavior, and may threaten litigation or other forms of reprisal. Risk management in this situation involves the use of interpersonal communication skills to assuage the parents' attitudes and to establish a better relationship between the parents and the health care team. It may require that the risk management team works directly with hospital staff to foster an understanding that some parents have an exaggerated grief response or limited coping mechanisms, and to assist neonatal staff in developing ways to help the family cope. Indeed, a potentially "inflammatory" situation exists when neonatal staff respond to parental accusations by becoming more and more defensive instead of informative. Parents may then develop the firm belief that they have not been told everything because of a deliberate attempt on the part of the staff to "cover up."

Parents of infants who are seriously ill with presumed hypoxic-ischemic encephalopathy need answers to their questions; when inquiries relate to the obstetric care, the temptation exists for neonatal staff to simply refer the parents to their obstetrician for further information. However, neonatal staff should not give opinions to parents about the standard of obstetric care of their colleagues. Even general observations about the obstetric course must be made carefully because nuances of terminology may lead to a misinterpretation. The risk management team has an important role in coordinating joint discussions between the parents and obstetric and neonatal staffs. As such, the risk management team, rather than the parents, should take an early lead in facilitating these discussions.

The development and implementation of an early notification system based on a trusting professional relationship is the key to any successful risk management program. Trust between the risk manager and the staff is developed over time by his/her involvement in departmental meetings and improvement projects, by face-to-face time spent on informal rounds, and by responses to requests for assistance with difficult situations. Once staff members are involved in the process of effective early conflict resolution and the restoration of good family/health care provider relationships, they are quicker to involve the risk manager in future events. This, in turn, has a direct, positive impact on the risk reduction related to professional liability of individual physicians, nurses, and the hospital or health care system.

Suggested Reading

1. Capstick B: Risk management in obstetrics. In Clements RV (ed): *Safe Practice in Obstetrics and Gynaecology*. Churchill Livingstone, Edinburgh, 1994, pp 405–416.
2. Chiswick ML: Intrapartum asphyxia and cerebral palsy. In Clements RV (ed): *Safe Practice in Obstetrics and Gynaecology*. Churchill Livingstone, Edinburgh, 1994, pp 269–281.
3. Donn SM, Fisher CW (eds): *Risk Management Techniques in Perinatal and Neonatal Practice*. Futura Publishing Company, Armonk, NY, 1996.
4. Donn SM, Faix RG, Roloff DW, Goldman EB: Medico-legal consultation: an expanded role of the tertiary neonatologist. J Perinatol 1987; 7:238–241.
5. MacLennan OA: A template for defining a causal relation between acute intrapartum events and cerebral palsy: international consensus statement. BMJ 1999;319:1054–1059.
6. Volk MD (ed): *Obstetric and Neonatal Malpractice: Legal and Medical Handbook*. 2nd ed. John Wiley & Sons, New York, 1996.

Index